Molecular Biology Biochemistry and Biophysics

16

Sidney Shulman

Tissue Specificity and Autoimmunity

With 32 Figures

Springer-Verlag Berlin · Heidelberg · New York 1974

Professor SIDNEY SHULMAN, Ph. D.

Department of Microbiology
Sperm Antibody Laboratory
New York Medical College
Flower and Fifth Avenue Hospitals
5th Avenue at 106th Street
New York, NY 10029

ISBN-13:978-3-642-80798-5 e-ISBN-13:978-3-642-80796-1
DOI: 10.1007/978-3-642-80796-1

Sidney Shulman

Tissue Specificity and Autoimmunity

With 32 Figures

Chapman & Hall Limited · London
Springer-Verlag Berlin · Heidelberg · New York 1974

Dedicated to the Memory of
Professor Ernest Witebsky

Preface

This book had its origins in some conversations held several years ago. It was felt that a monograph on the subject of tissue specificity might have some merit and interest for a number of scientific workers in the relevant disciplines. Writing was begun slowly, with interruptions; more recently, there has been much more activity, and the relevant literature has been searched and cited up to early 1973. This book was never intended as an exhaustive coverage of all possible topics related to tissue specificity. The tissues and organs covered in six chapters constitute a selected group, representative of areas in which the author has worked and which are thus directly familiar to him, plus several other areas where illustrative and important discoveries have been made. There are other areas of equal importance and interest, but the book would have been much too large if I had tried to cover all of them.

The author had several groups of readers in mind, including students of immunology and the related fields of immunochemistry, biochemistry, and immunopathology. Students of general biology could find it useful. For students of medicine and practicing physicians it may provide a useful review in a field that has many clinical correlations in human disease. The author assumes that the reader has a basic knowledge of immunological concepts and technics, but for some purposes elementary treatments are cited for background reference.

It should be made clear that this book is primarily devoted to *tissue specificity* (or organ specificity), as an expression of biological specificity phenomena. A modest amount of discussion of autoimmunity and autoimmune disease is included, in order to give a more rounded treatment. The use of autoimmune systems provides sharper and more convenient approaches to the study of tissue specificity, in addition to being of interest in its own right.

I must take this opportunity to express appreciation to a number of colleagues who have helped me. First, I must express my debt to the late Professor Ernest Witebsky, who did so much to foster and develop the whole sub-discipline of immunology that has been termed organ (or tissue) specificity. I was with him from 1952 to 1967 as his immunology student, research colleague, and friend. His untimely death in December 1969 was a great loss to many persons throughout the world and to this field of research and teaching. Next, I am grateful to Professor Felix Milgrom, a research colleague for a number of years, with whom I held a number of the early discussions on the preparation of this book. I must also thank several colleagues and assistants for preparation of figures, searching of bibliographic references, and other technical tasks; among these persons are Dr. Mohammad Ghayasuddin, Dr. Eduardo Zappi, Miss Charlotte Pann, Miss Barbara Flouton, and Miss Yanick Boulet. Most of all, I must express my deep and sincere gratitude for the unstinting and devoted assistance of my wife, Joanna, who spent much time in searching for obscure references, proofreading the manuscript, correcting errors, and even typing many of the pages; her careful reading of the entire manuscript contributed to whatever degree of clarity in expression has been achieved, and her immunological knowledge often led to a better detailed exposition. Having made these acknowledgments, I must accept the blame for any errors or important omissions; I hope that they are few.

Much of the work involved in the preparation of this manuscript, as well as much of the research described herein, has been supported by a grant from The John A. Hartford Foundation, Inc.

New York, January 1974 S. SHULMAN

Contents

Chapter 1

Concepts of Specificity

The discovery by BORDET that such innocuous substances as blood or milk were antigenic when injected into a foreign species of animal led to the understanding that species differences were important antigenicity [8, 9]. Next came the realization that immune sera could be used as reagents to distinguish the species origin of various animal substances. In 1900 the American investigator FISCH [19] demonstrated differences in the antigenic properties of bovine, human, and goat's milk; similar observations were made by WASSERMANN and SCHÜTZE [89] in Germany. As a result of these studies, the concept of "species specificity" came into being. A species-specific antigen may be defined as an antigen which is present in all members of a given species and which differs antigenically from the corresponding or analogous substances in other species. Though usually held to indicate the immunological properties of serum, the term can equally well indicate cellular components, as long as they are characteristic for each species. This concept, following upon the more general concept of serological specificity, became well established through the early investigations of BORDET, EHRLICH, and UHLENHUTH.

Most of the early experiments on species specificity used blood serum as the antigen. In the pioneering studies of NUTTALL [65] several hundred blood specimens were studied by means of 30 rabbit antisera made by immunization with serum samples originating in various other species. Nuttall used a simple precipitation method and observed both homologous and heterologous systems. By a "homologous system" (*or* mixture, reaction, etc.) we mean a mixing of antiserum with the material used in the immunization to produce this antiserum. By a "heterologous system" (*or* mixture, reaction, etc.) we mean a mixing of antiserum with some similar or analogous antigen, but not the one used to elicit the antibody. A reaction that occurs in such a mixture is termed a "heterologous reaction" or a "cross-reaction". The strongest reactions are seen in systems of homologous mixtures. In heterologous systems, stronger cross reactions are obtained with (antigen) sera originating from species closely related to the one which provided the immunizing antigens than with (antigen) sera of biologically more distant species. There are practically no cross-reactions between sera originating from different classes of vertebrates. There is in general rather good correlation between reaction strength and taxonomic closeness.

It was soon realized that the species of the immunized animal is also an important factor in determining the properties of an antiserum; this concept has sometimes been called "immunological perspective" [17]. Rabbit antisera can clearly distinguish between antigens from rodents, *i.e.* between rat serum or mouse serum, but hardly at all between antigens from different birds, *e.g.* chicken serum and duck serum. As a result of such observations, LANDSTEINER coined the term "faulty perspective" [36]. Thus, instead of a rabbit, a third species of bird should be used to produce avian antiserum. More subtle antigenic differences between closely related species can be detected by a procedure developed by UHLENHUTH and referred to as "cross immunization" [85]. A chicken immunized with duck serum would produce a good reagent, an antiserum that would react with duck serum but not with chicken serum. The concept of perspective has been enlarged in recent years, members of a species being injected with antigens from other members of the same species; this enables the histocompatibility antigens and the allotypic determinant groups of immunoglobulins to be studied.

The principle of species specificity has been applied for medicolegal investigations in the serological identifications [86, 93] based on antigenic differentiation between analogous components from different animal species. A major forensic application has been the study of blood stains in investigations of homicide. The specificity of antisera for human blood proteins, as distinguished from those of other animals, can be readily utilized, provided cross-reactions are excluded between animal species that are quite close in the taxonomic scheme. In addition to the serum proteins the major blood groups have been much employed, in particular, the ABO system. Generally, rabbit antiserum against human serum has been utilized. There may be some problem of cross-reaction with blood serum from other mammals: antisera that are poorly specific must be found by testing and discarded. Presumably a more specific type of antiserum could be obtained by the immunization of monkeys or apes with human serum. Absorption procedures have been applied to rabbit antisera, although not too helpfully. The adulteration of beef by horse meat has been detected by the use of antiserum. Antigenic analyses of this type have also been applied to the study of semen residues in cases of assault and rape; this example is more properly a question of tissue (not species) specificity, but is mentioned here along with other procedures of forensic science [90].

While the early work on species specificity used whole serum as if it were a single antigenic component, more recent investigations employ individual serum proteins. Measurements of quantitative precipitation have shown about 25% of cross-reaction between bovine and human gamma globulins (BGG and HGG) when each is tested with antisera to both antigens. In other words, BGG precipitates about 25% of anti-HGG and HGG about 25% of anti-BGG. Similarly, a cross-reaction of about 15% was found for bovine and human serum albumins, although values were lower when less intensive immunization was used to obtain the antisera [47, 48].

This degree of cross-reaction indicates that serum proteins of the same kind have common features in various species. This is readily demonstrated in gel diffusion plates (Fig. 1.1) where cross-reaction and spur formation between human and bovine gamma globulin occurs on addition of antiserum to one of them; adding the alternative antiserum to the other gives a symmetrical and inverse picture. We can also demonstrate (Fig. 1.2) the partial, but incomplete, antigenic identity between thyroglobulins from several species. Although analogous serum proteins, such as gamma globulins or thyroglobulins, derived from various species possess some definite antigenic similarity, the different kinds of serum proteins are antigenically distinct within the same species. This is illustrated by the nonidentity reaction between bovine gamma globulin and albumin presented in Fig. 1.3.

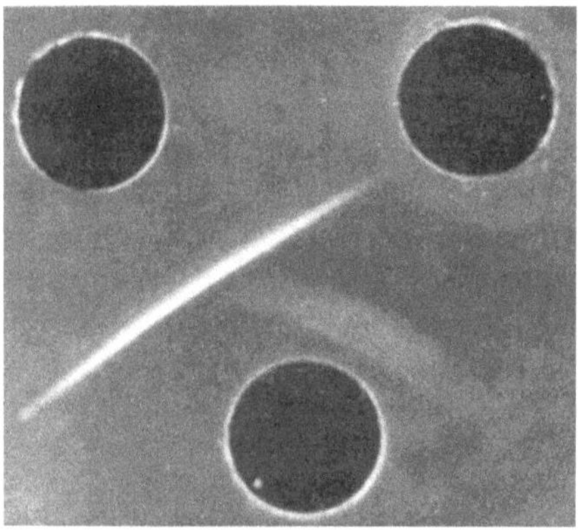

Fig. 1.1. Double-diffusion gel precipitation of antiserum and gamma globulins. Upper left well: gamma globulin fraction of bovine serum. Upper right well: gamma globulin fraction of human serum. Lower well: rabbit antiserum to bovine gamma globulin

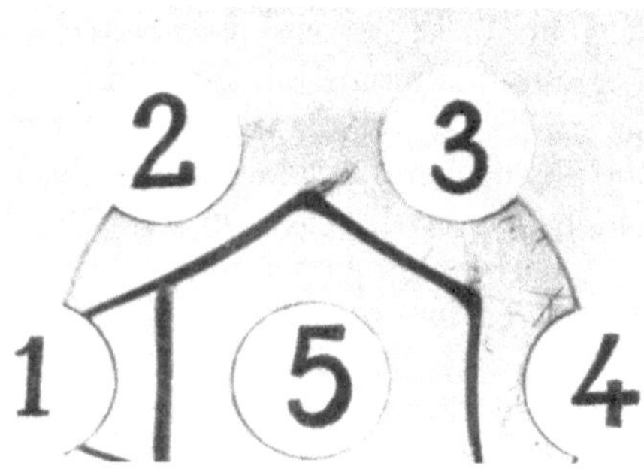

Fig. 1.2. Double-diffusion gel precipitation of antiserum and thyroglobulins. Central well: rabbit antiserum to human thyroglobulin. Peripheral wells: 1. hog thyroglobulin, 2. and 4. human thyroglobulin, 3. monkey thyroglobulin

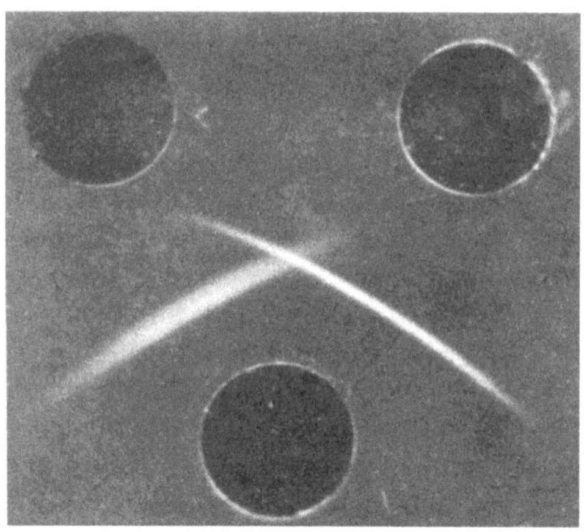

Fig. 1.3. Double-diffusion gel precipitation of antiserum and serum proteins. Upper left well: gamma globulin fraction of bovine serum. Upper right well: albumin fraction of bovine serum. Lower well: rabbit antiserum to bovine serum

A tissue-specific antigen is an antigen characteristic for one particular tissue; we need to be more precise than this. Serum albumin may be considered a tissue-specific antigen of liver cells and gamma globulin a tissue-specific antigen of plasma cells, but both these antigens are shed into the circulation and will thus be present in all tissue extracts. This was why, before any clear-cut identification of individual serum components was made, serum antigens were usually considered to be species-specific, meaning that they could be found in the tissues of any animal of a given species.

The first tissue-specific antigens were described in organs from which extracts could be prepared with relatively little contamination by serum proteins. In 1903, UHLENHUTH [84] described the tissue specificity of the lens of the eye; he produced antisera by injecting rabbits with homogenates of bovine lens. These antisera contained essentially no antibodies to serum proteins and therefore did not react with extracts of bovine tissues other than the lens. Being lens-specific reagents, these antisera also reacted with homogenates of lens from other species, not only mammals but also birds, amphibia, and fish. Later studies revealed several lens-specific antigens which bear witness to evolutionary differences in the phylogenetic development of this organ [28, 43, 44, 45]. The various antigens of lens will be discussed in some detail in Chapter 6.

Many far-ranging studies on antigens characteristic for various tissues were conducted in the early years of immunological research [94—97, 101, 102]. Another historic example is brain tissue specificity: WITEBSKY and STEINFELD [89] used rabbit antisera to bovine brain suspension to demonstrate the existence of a brain-specific antigen. This antigen was believed to be of lipid (generally termed "lipoid" in older literature) nature because both alcoholic and aqueous extracts of the tissue contained the activity, which was present in brain extracts from all vertebrate classes. Another brain-specific antigen—this one of protein nature—had in addition to tissue specificity a considerable degree of species specificity. The antigens of brain will be more fully discussed in Chapter 4.

HEKTOEN and his associates [30, 31] identified thyroglobulin as a tissue-specific antigen that carries both tissue specificity and some species specificity. This question was further explored in the studies of ROSE and WITEBSKY [70]; they showed that an antiserum against human thyroid, when absorbed with bovine or porcine thyroid extract, combined only with thyroid extracts from homologous species. Unabsorbed, the antiserum would show various species interactions. The antigens of thyroid tissue will be further discussed in Chapter 2.

The alternative term *organ specificity* has been used to indicate an antigenic property characteristic of a particular organ, regardless of species (cf. the classic examples of lens and brain). A similarity was seen in the corresponding organ in many different species, and has been called "organ specificity of the second order". Another type of organ-specific antigen is *limited* to a particular species; for example, an antiserum against the red blood cells of the horse reacts with alcoholic extract of horse red blood cells but with no other tissue extract of horse and with no red cell preparation from any other species [37]. Termed by some early workers "organ specificity of the first order" or "tissue specificity", this indicated the presence of an antigen characteristic of a particular organ within a single species [20—22, 37]. The early workers maintained some strict distinction in the use of the terms "organ specificity" and "tissue specificity", but over the years the terms have come to be used interchangeably and the original distinction has been lost. The author prefers the term "tissue specificity" as offering more precision and better clarity of definition, since organs generally contain two or more tissues. For example, there will be antigens that are characteristic of the adrenal gland: this is a single organ but it is a pair of tissues, and detailed study will generally reveal that an adrenal-specific antigen is either medulla-specific or cortex-specific and hence better so characterized.

To illustrate the contrast between tissue specificity *not* restricted to species and species-specific tissue specificity, we can consider the report of WITEBSKY and MILGROM [98] on the characteristic autoantigen of adrenal tissue. In their study a large number of guinea pigs were immunized with pooled guinea pig adrenal gland homogenate combined with complete Freund's adjuvant; similarly, a large number of rabbits were immunized with pooled rabbit adrenal homogenate combined with complete Freund's adjuvant. Studies were made on the tissue specificity and species specificity of the response in each group of animals. A large proportion of animals in both groups responded with the production of antibody which was in fact specific for adrenal tissue. This antibody reacted in a number of test cases with the adrenal tissue of the immunized animal's own body and was thus an autoantibody. A striking contrast was observed between the behaviour of the rabbit and the guinea pig antisera: the rabbit antisera reacted not only with rabbit adrenal extract but also with adrenal extracts from other mammalian species, including guinea pig, man, and rat, but not dogfish. Conversely, guinea pig failed utterly to react with adrenal tissue from any of several other species tested, reacting only with guinea pig adrenal. No complete explanation was available for this difference in specificity, but the rabbit adrenal extract had more antigenic groups than a cross-reacting preparation, for example, bovine adrenal extract. Thus it seems that a group of adrenal antigens occurs in the corresponding tissue of different species, but that the activity of the total extract varies for different species; however, the precise details are not yet understood. Additional discussion of adrenal antigens will be found in Chapter 3.

Much earlier, in the 1920s, FLEISHER and his collaborators, working with antisera to guinea pig liver, kidney, muscle, spleen, testis, and brain, had found that several antisera reacted best with the homologous organs but showed strong cross-reactions with other guinea pig organ extracts [20—22]. Using elaborate absorption procedures, they identified three types of antigen: 1. species-specific antigens present in all organs of the animal, 2. tissue-specific antigens characteristic of each organ, and 3. antigens possessed in common by several different organs. The existence of the first two types of antigen is now commonly recognized; the third category is less frequently considered.

Years ago, identification of tissue-specific antigens by serologic procedures was usually possible only when the particular tissue extract contained strong tissue-specific antigens and was relatively little contaminated with serum protein. Today's serologic and immunochemical procedures will reveal even the minor tissue-specific antigens in tissue extracts, as illustrated by studies on adrenal specificity [60]. Rabbits immunized with suspensions of bovine adrenal gland developed antisera containing antibodies that combined with extracts of *all* bovine tissues. Complement fixation and tanned-cell hemagglutination tests failed to reveal adrenal specificity. However, the use of double-diffusion gel precipitation gave an indication of the presence of adrenal-specific antibodies. Further studies based on several chemical treatments of the antigenic preparation enabled the adrenal-specific antigen, a thermostable, alcohol-insoluble material, to be more precisely characterized. It proved to be a mucoprotein or glycoprotein substance which withstands *boiling* and precipitation by 70% *ethanol* and was thus termed BE antigen by the original authors [60].

Other tissue-specific antigens of the BE type are obtained from brain, liver, testis, pituitary, polymorphonuclear leucocytes, intima of large vessels, and kidney. All these antigens show distinctive tissue specificity along with various degrees of species specificity. A full discussion of this class of antigens is beyond the scope of this book; the original publications may be consulted [12, 32, 54, 57—59, 68, 77].

The function, or physiologic role, of most tissue-specific antigens is unknown. Recently, much attention has been devoted to the antigenic properties of certain hormones; these are proteins having well-defined physiologic activities [103]. An antigenic hormone is secreted into the circulation but can still be considered a tissue antigen, characteristic for the gland that produces it; *e.g.* insulin may be considered pancreas-specific. Studies on insulin have been particularly interesting, since it is a comparatively small protein molecule and it should not be too hard to find the chemical basis for its antigenic specificity. The details of the chemical structure of insulin have been reviewed by us [79]; other structural details and comparisons are now available for this protein [15] and for a recently discovered precursor, "proinsulin" [11]. The chemical basis for the species specificity of insulin has been elucidated in terms of molecular structure, but the tissue-specific characteristics need further study. Many of its antigenic properties have been reviewed by POPE [67]. We return below to insulin and other pancreatic antigens.

Antigens characteristic for certain organs (lens, brain, thyroid, etc.) are capable of stimulating the formation of antibodies that can react with the corresponding antigens derived from the same tissue of all other animals of the species and of the antibody-forming animal. The formation of autoantibodies against tissue antigens has been discussed in a number of reviews [14, 23, 51, 52, 61]. Immunization with tissue extracts obtained from the same species, frequently termed "iso-immunization", has turned out to be a convenient procedure for producing tissue-specific antisera. The advantage of immunizing in this way is that many antigens, especially the serum proteins, do not usually express themselves, and the immune sera obtained are very frequently pure tissue-specific reagents, a goal seldom reached upon immunization with tissue antigens from a foreign species.

In addition to the soluble antigens there are some, apparently derived from cell membranes or other particulate structures, that are generally water-insoluble and cannot be extracted in the usual way by homogenization in saline solution. With cells that can be obtained in a stable suspension, like erythrocytes or leukocytes, cell-membrane antigens can be demonstrated by agglutination tests. Otherwise, they can be conveniently studied by means of mixed agglutination procedures; these methods were pioneered by COOMBS [13] and by FAGRAEUS and ESPMARK [18]. A modification which involves use of cell culture monolayers was developed and used by MILGROM *et al.* [55]: antibodies bound to the cell cultures are detected by an indicator system, consisting of erythrocytes sensitized by antibodies and agglutinated by an anti-gamma globulin serum. A major insoluble antigen of living mammalian cells turned out to be a component characteristic for the species under investigation [55]. Table 1.1 summarizes

Table 1.1. *Mixed agglutination with cell cultures of bovine adrenal medulla*

Antiserum dilution	Antiserum against bovine: Adrenal suspension	Brain suspension	Liver suspension	Liver extract	Serum
1:10	4+	4+	4+	±	2+
1:100	4+	4+	4+	±	1+
1:1000	4+	4+	3+	–	–
1:10000	4+	3+	3+	–	–
1:100000	2+	2+	1+	–	–
1:1000000	–	±	–	–	–

the results of an experiment reviewed by MILGROM [53], in which cell cultures of bovine adrenal medulla gave strong reactions with antisera to suspensions of bovine adrenal, brain, and liver; the reaction was very weak or negative when the antisera used were obtained by immunization with extracts from bovine tissues or with bovine serum. The brain antiserum, which in this experiment reacted with cell cultures up to a dilution of 1:100000, was also examined against various extracts of bovine tissues. This antiserum by a number of methods (complement fixation, gel precipitation, and tanned cell hemagglutination tests) gave strong reactions with brain extracts from various species, but it failed almost completely to react with extracts of bovine tissues other than brain. If it were not for studies by the method of mixed agglutination, this antiserum might have been thought to contain only antibodies to tissue-specific antigens and none that recognizes species specificity. This would have been a wrong conclusion, for in fact the cell membrane antigens under discussion showed only a slight degree of interspecies cross-reaction. These cross-reactions could be removed completely by suitable procedures of absorption. These antigens of the cell surface might even be taken as outstanding examples of species-specific antigens, since they are present on most if not all cells of a given species, independently of the cellular differentiation.

The following chapters will provide extensive and detailed discussions of specific antigens and autoantigens of certain tissues. A few additional examples are added at this point. Let us take skeletal muscle: antigenic studies of muscle acquired special interest and incentive when it became clear that sera from many patients with myasthenia gravis contain antibodies to antigen(s) found in muscle tissue [7, 63, 78, 80, 87, 91]. Using especially the technique of immunofluorescence, researchers demonstrated that this is a specific reaction and that these antibodies are autoantibodies, since they react with muscle tissue from the same patient [7]. Myasthenic sera can also react with muscle taken from other animals, and the rhesus monkey in particular has proved a useful source

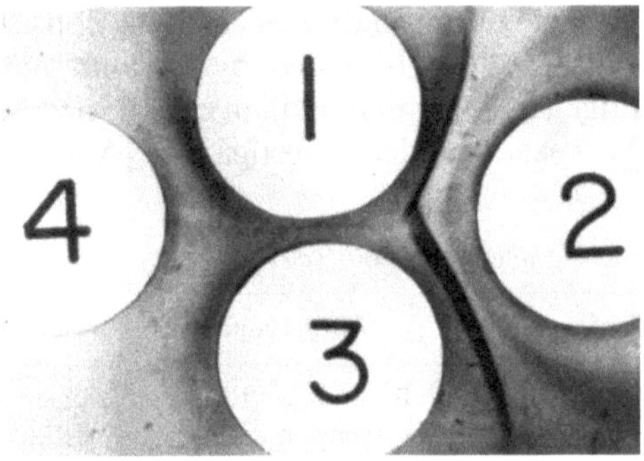

Fig. 1.4. Double-diffusion gel precipitation of sera and muscle extracts. Wells were filled as follows: 1. sucrose extract of monkey muscle, 3. water extract of monkey muscle, 2. myasthenic serum, and 4. normal human serum

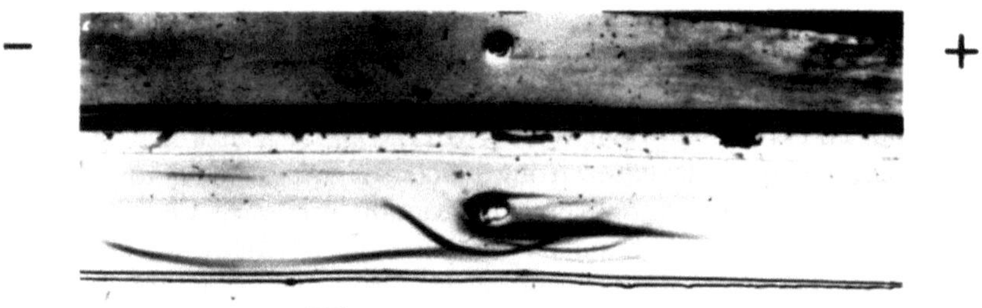

Fig. 1.5. Immunoelectrophoresis of normal human serum and myasthenic human serum. The upper well contained normal serum; the lower well contained myasthenic serum. The upper trough was filled with a sucrose extract of monkey muscle. The lower trough was filled with a goat antiserum to human serum

of antigenic material for studies of this type which need no longer be restricted to human tissue [7]. Specific precipitation tests for interactions between muscle extracts and myasthenic serum have been developed, both fluid procedures utilizing thin capillary tubes, and gel diffusion procedures utilizing both Ouchterlony and immunoelectrophoretic methods [38, 39, 74]. The gel diffusion precipitation pattern in Fig. 1.4 reveals that there are two precipitating components rather than one. Fig. 1.5 illustrates a typical immunoelectrophoretic study: two major arcs of precipitation are observed and there is the suggestion of a third antigen-antibody system. Such studies should permit further purification and characterization of these antigen-antibody systems [16, 29, 62, 81].

One of the major frustrations in the study of muscle-specific autoantigens and their significance in the autoimmune disease, myasthenia gravis, had been the lack of a model system in experimental animals. However, it was more recently reported [24—27, 34, 66] that guinea pigs or rats, when injected with extracts of thymus or skeletal muscle with complete Freund's adjuvant, developed thymitis, antibodies to thymus and muscle, and a neuromuscular block resembling myasthenia gravis. Such experimental models may be expected to advance the study of these autoantigens and the autoimmune response.

A second tissue of some interest is the pancreas. The tissue-specific antigens associated with the pancreas have been studied by isoimmunization of experimental animals with saline extracts of pancreas emulsified in Freund's complete adjuvant, as described at some length by WITEBSKY and his collaborators [49, 50, 69, 99, 100]. The demonstration of pancreas-specific antibodies is more readily achieved with some animal species than with others. Some pancreatic antigens can be described precisely in terms of chemical structure; in particular, the tissue-specific antigen and hormone insulin, supplies an exquisitely detailed model for correlating the chemical structure of this molecule and its antigenic specificity.

The insulin molecule [15, 79] consists of two polypeptide chains linked by two disulfide bridges. Chain A contains 21 amino acids and chain B 30 amino acids, giving a total molecular weight of 5700. Although there is considerable cross-reactivity between an antiserum to the homologous insulin species and other insulin species, there can also be fine differences involved, and these should be related to the differences in amino-acid composition or sequence within the insulin molecule. We can assume that an animal injected with insulin produces several antibody types, each specifically related to one antigenic determinant group. Variations in the amino acid sequence could presumably affect the immune response to that particular portion of the antigenic molecule. Where species comparisons have been made, there are usually only two or three sites where the amino acids are different, and these sites must represent the points of major antigenic distinctiveness. Antibodies directed against portions of the molecule that are constant in insulin structures from different species have, however, to be eliminated, before the distinctive interactions can stand out clearly.

Efforts have been made to distinguish between the antigenic properties of the two polypeptide chains [67]. If the chemical structure of insulin is examined in relation to its activity and antigenicity, it can be concluded that neither chain separately will inhibit the binding of insulin by its antibody. The terminal portion of the B chain, from amino acid positions 23 to 30, does not seem to take part in the combination with antibody.

Antibody variations have been studied in rabbits and guinea pigs in efforts to evaluate the different antigenic determinant sites on the insulin molecule. ARQUILLA and FINN [4, 5] found that antibodies from rabbits will bind to certain portions of the insulin molecule, and that antibodies from other rabbits or from guinea pigs cannot bind to these same portions, the individual variations being caused by antibodies directed to different determinant groups. This would suggest that the insulin molecule has more than one antigenic determinant site. Inbred strains of guinea pigs showed genetic differences: strain 2 guinea pigs produced antibodies to certain portions of the insulin molecule and strain 13 guinea pigs did not, but no such contrasts were observed among guinea pigs *within* either strain. Even such a relatively simple molecule as insulin resisted attempts to give precise chemical definition to each antigenic determinant group. The effect of minimal iodination as a modification was also studied [6]. More recent studies of the binding sites of the insulin molecule have emphasized the importance of the B chain. Antibodies to insulin reacted to a significant degree with B-chain derivatives, but not with A-chain derivatives, as shown for several species by YAGI *et al.* [104], VARANDANI [88], and KERP *et al.* [35]. SURMACZYNSKA *et al.* [82, 83] have shown that derivatives with several amino-acid residues removed from the molecule show different reactivities with different varieties of antibody. Recent reports have suggested some relationship between autoimmunity and insulin-dependent diabetes [15, 33, 92].

Another attempt to pinpoint the relation of definite antigenic determinants of specificity to the detailed molecular structure of the antigen concerns the immunological properties of cytochrome *c* [46, 64]. Cross-reactions were observed with this protein as obtained from 25 different species. Where an identical amino-acid sequence exists, no immunological distinction could be made, but where the primary structure of the various forms of cytochrome *c* differs, a distinction could be made by means of a suitable antiserum. Sometimes a single amino-acid substitution could change the activity.

Let us take one more brief example to illustrate how far distant taxonomically we can search for tissue specificity. This example derives from studies on the venom sac of the bee and other hymenoptera. The venom sac is a distinctive organ; its antigenic components and contents have been extensively explored in studies dealing with human allergic reactions to insects. Many of the investigations in this field have been reviewed by us elsewhere [71, 72]. Some of the major points can be summarized here. The antigens, the allergens, and the discernable protein fractions were described in extracts of bees, wasps, and yellow jackets [40, 75]. Antigens were found that were specific for the venom sac extracts of each of these three insects, in contrast to the components of the bodies without the sacs [41]. The bodies (but not the venom sacs) contained antigens that were common to various pairs of these insects [3]. The major components were fractionated of the whole body and of the venom sac of bee [76], wasp [42], and yellow jacket [2].

From the honey bee, pure venom could be readily obtained and was found to be a purer antigenic fraction that the venom sac extract, so that a venom-specific antigen did in fact exist [73]. The proof is strikingly shown in Fig. 1.6, where double-diffusion gel precipitation (with anti-venom serum) has revealed the presence of a strong specific antigen in bee venom. This antigen also appears in venom-sac extract, accompanied by a second component which is also seen in body extracts. We have written about this in more detail elsewhere [72].

In conclusion, we may note that *the distribution in nature of the biochemical substances that are the antigens is really at the root of the phenomena* that we describe as *species specificity* and *tissue* (or organ) *specificity*. We shall not deal here with other areas of immunologic specificity. For example, Forssman (*or* heterophile) specificity will not be considered for, while interesting, it is more relevant to the discussion of *species* than of *tissue specificity*. Adequate introductions to the Forssman (and related) antigens can be found in the standard texts [1, 10] and there is a very extensive review by SPRINGER [79a]. A useful listing of the biological distribution of the Forssman antigen is given by BOYD [10]. We also omit the antigens of transplantation and histocompatibility since these alloantigens constitute a basis for distinctions between individuals of (non-inbred) species rather than between tissues of an individual or between species themselves.

The point of major interest here is that *each tissue* of the, let us say, vertebrate body may have *one or more specific antigens*, characteristic of and localized in (or at least produced by) this tissue. These antigens might also be polymorphic,

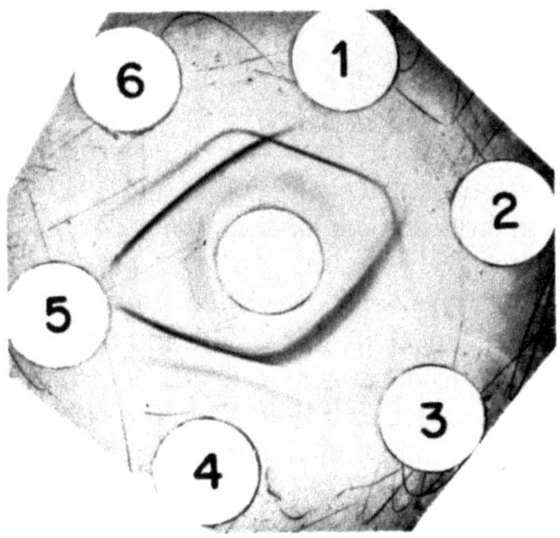

Fig. 1.6. Double-diffusion gel precipitation of rabbit antiserum to bee venom and various bee body tissues. Central well: rabbit antivenom serum. Peripheral wells: 1. whole body extract, 2. sacless body extract, 3. venom, 4. and 6. venom sac extract, 5. normal rabbit serum

although much remains to be clarified in this regard. Each such antigen may or may not be restricted to the species in question. As to the significance of tissue specificity, we could speculate on the role such antigenic constituents may play in embryonic differentiation, in the mechanisms of tumor growth, in the phenomena of cancer growth (with formation perhaps of new antigens) and occasional cancer regression, among other possibilities. We do know that many of the tissue-specific antigens can also be autoantigens, and the study of autoimmunity has already contributed much to our understanding of a number of human diseases.

Chapter 2

The Thyroid Gland

One of the first antigenic systems to reveal the property of tissue specificity was that found in aqueous extracts of the thyroid gland; this system further indicated a protein rather than a lipid material basis for this specificity. The thyroid is the most extensively studied of the organ-specific (or tissue-specific) systems; it has yielded some very interesting correlations between antigenic properties and the biochemical nature of the molecules that are responsible for this specificity. The thyroid antigens can therefore be considered the model for our knowledge of tissue specificity. For additional discussion of these antigens, and especially the forms of autoimmunity to them, see the review recently presented by us elsewhere [128].

1. Early Findings of Tissue Specificity and of the Protein Composition of Extracts

The earliest immunological studies of the thyroid were made by Hektoen and his colleagues. In 1923, HEKTOEN and SHULHOF [42] studied thyroid extracts and even partially purified the major component, thyroglobulin. They prepared thyroglobulin from a variety of mammals, including bear, anteater, kangaroo, sloth, tapir, deer, fox, baboon, and zebra, in addition to the usual laboratory animals. They also prepared antisera and discovered that antisera which precipitated thyroglobulin did not precipitate similarly prepared globulins from other organs of the body. On this basis the thyroid protein was supposed to be a tissue-specific antigen [41]. The antisera to various mammalian thyroids gave cross-reactions with thyroglobulins isolated from a number of other mammals, but failed to react with chicken thyroglobulin. The pattern of cross-reactions seemed not to be determined solely by the criterion of taxonomic closeness but to occur rather randomly within the class of mammals.

The work of HEKTOEN and his colleagues was confirmed, at least in principle, by WITEBSKY [184] and by ADANT and SPEHL [1]. These workers emphasized that the reactions obtained with heterologous preparations were very weak compared to the reactions with homologous preparations, as obtained by both precipitation and complement fixation methods. Somewhat later, quantitative precipitation methods were applied by STOKINGER and HEIDELBERGER [149] who sought to measure in a precise manner the degree of cross-reaction that could occur among thyroglobulins from various mammals. WITEBSKY *et al.* [188] used a different approach to evaluate the serological specificity of crude extracts of thyroid gland and to compare the observed cross-reactions. We shall return to these studies after a brief discussion of the biochemical properties of the thyroid proteins.

Investigations of the constituents of the thyroid gland were begun around the end of the last century. The earliest study on the proteins of the thyroid gland worthy of mention is that of GOURLAY [38], who in 1894 described a "nucleo-albumin" which he extracted from the thyroid gland of ox. In 1896 HUTCHINSON [45] suggested that the colloid of the thyroid gland—a well-known histological structure—was made up largely of a globulin, claiming that "nuclein"-type substances were present as minor components. He also recognized that iodine was present in extracts prepared from sheep thyroid. The most memorable work of this period was that of OSWALD [81], who in 1899 isolated the major protein substance from the thyroid and demonstrated its globulin properties. Globulins and albumins had recently been defined as proteins, insoluble and soluble, respectively, in 50% saturated solutions of ammonium sulfate. OSWALD christened this protein thyroglobulin (in German: Thyreoglobulin), now often shortened to Tg. Using the then popular method of ammonium sulfate precipitation, OSWALD found that protein precipitation began when the tissue extract was 26% saturated with ammonium sulfate and was essentially complete at 44% of saturation; some additional protein could be brought down by adding saturated salt to the supernatant fluid. Essentially all the iodine was contained in the first product, so OSWALD considered the second precipitation to be unimportant. Because this iodinated protein was so easily extracted in high yield, he presumed that it came from the colloid of the gland. This was the type of preparation Hektoen and his colleagues [41] used for the serological studies mentioned above.

HEIDELBERGER and PALMER [39], using hog thyroids, introduced a preliminary step of adjusting the pH to 5.0 in the cold; this gave a precipitate that had the properties of a nucleoprotein (like GOURLAY'S). After removal of this product, the solution was neutralized and sodium sulfate at half-saturation and at 35 °C was used to precipitate the fraction of interest. This material was considered to be purified thyroglobulin, although only a rather limited analytical comparison was made between the product and the original crude extract. The physicochemical properties of this hog thyroglobulin were studied by HEIDELBERGER and PEDERSEN [40], who found the sedimentation coefficient to be 19.2 S. Using a partial specific volume of 0.72 ml/g, and a diffusion coefficient of 2.39×10^{-7} cm^2sec^{-1}, they obtained a molecular weight of 700000; with equilibrium ultracentrifugation, they obtained a molecular weight of 675000. They also made studies of the electrophoretic properties and determined that native hog thyroglobulin had an isoelectric point of pH 4.6 and that a preparation denatured by exposure to acetic acid had an altered isoelectric point, namely, 5.0.

Twenty years later, the isolation and biochemical properties of the major thyroid proteins were studied again by SHULMAN *et al.* [132]. They prepared saline extracts of hog thyroid glands and used them for immunization of animals, for serological and immunochemical testing, and for various physical and chemical measurements. The theories and methods for a number of the physicochemical procedures have been described by us elsewhere [140]. Examination in the analytical ultracentrifuge showed *five* sedimenting components to be present in crude hog thyroid extract [132], and the characteristic patterns are shown in Fig. 2.1. From measurements made at various concentrations of total protein, the sedimentation coefficients of the five components were extrapolated to infinite

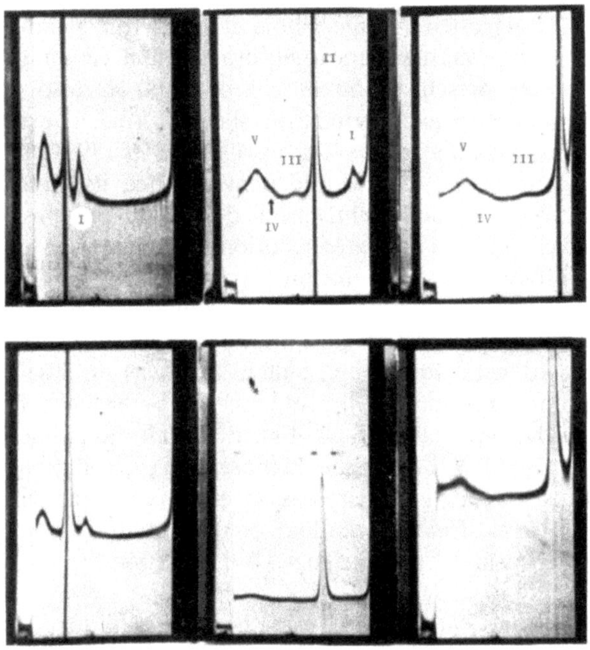

Fig. 2.1. Ultracentrifugal patterns of a hog thyroid crude extract. Upper line: protein concentration, 2.0 per cent; photographs at 8, 26, and 44 minutes after rotor reached speed of 58200 r.p.m. Lower line: protein concentration, 0.8 per cent; photographs at 8, 26, and 34 minutes after rotor reached speed of 59700 r.p.m. Direction of sedimentation is to the right

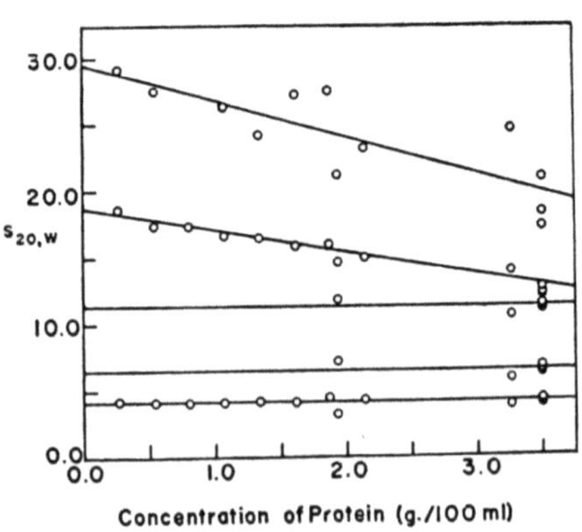

Fig. 2.2. Sedimentation coefficient plotted against protein concentration for 13 runs from three preparations of hog thyroid crude extract

dilution and the following values were obtained: I, 29.5 S; II, 18.7 S; III, 11.3 S; IV, 6.5 S; V, 4.2 S. A composite graph of these sedimentation rates is shown in Fig. 2.2; there is considerable concentration dependence for components I and II. The 18.7 S component was thought to be the classical thyroglobulin, partly because of its predominance in the total pattern and partly because HEIDELBERGER and PEDERSEN [40] had selected a 19 S component as the

Table 2.1. *Relative proportions of the sedimenting components of hog thyroid crude extract*

	Concentration of extract (g/dl)				
	4.46	2.23	0.89	0.45	0.00
	Proportions (%)				
Tg	84.0	81.9	81.2	79.7	(79.8)[a]
F	2.1	4.3	5.6	6.6	(6.7)
S (IV + V)	13.6	13.6	13.6	13.6	(13.6)
Total	99.7	99.8	100.4	99.9	
IV	2.2	—	—	—	
V	11.4	—	—	—	
V/IV	5.2	—	—	—	

[a] Values in parentheses are obtained by extrapolation.

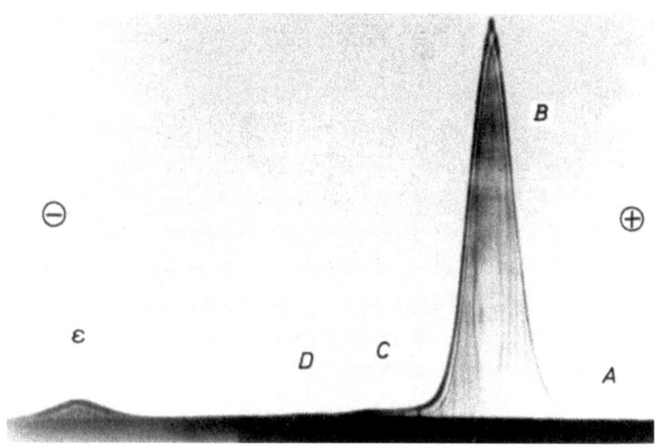

Fig. 2.3. Electrophoretic pattern (descending) of a hog thyroid crude extract. Protein concentration, 0.65 per cent; barbital buffer, pH 8.60; ionic strength, 0.10; electric field strength, 6.8 volts/cm; time, 180 minutes

thyroglobulin. We found that the 18.7 S component comprised approximately 80% of the total protein in the mixture. Clearly, direct estimates of this composition could be misleading if only a single total protein concentrate was examined, because of optical anomalies in the ultracentrifuge. Our figure of 80% was obtained by extrapolating the measurements to zero concentration, which gave the proportion of component I (or F, for fast peak) as 5 to 10% of the total, and components IV plus V (or S, for slow peak) as 10 to 15%. Where peak III could be seen at all, its contribution was only 1 or 2% of the total. Resolution of S into peaks IV and V was generally poor, but repeated measurements showed the ratio of peak V to peak IV to be generally about 5. Table 2.1 shows the proportions in a typical set of hog thyroid extracts. It was suspected that peaks IV and V contain, respectively, serum globulin and albumin, representing contamination of the tissue with blood. We were able to show definitely [132] that serum proteins do not make up the total composition of these two ultracentrifugal components and that proteins of thyroidal origin were present. Each of the slower sedimentation peaks corresponds, in fact, to a mixture of proteins, and evidence on this polydispersity will be presented below.

When the total hog thyroid extract was subjected to filter-paper electrophoresis, only one component could be seen and this traveled at pH 8.6 like a

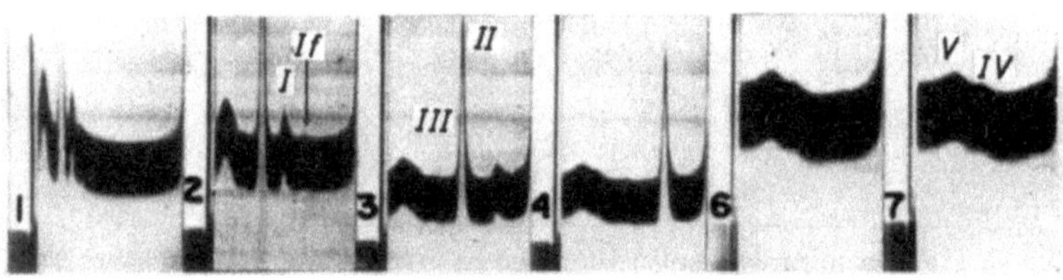

Fig. 2.4. Ultracentrifugal patterns of an extract of normal human thyroid. Protein concentration: 1.6 per cent. Photographs at 0, 8, 16, 24, 40, and 48 minutes after attaining speed of 59700 r.p.m. Direction of sedimentation is to the right

Table 2.2. *Ultracentrifugal analysis of normal human thyroid extract*

	Peak					
	If	I	II	III	IV	V
$S_{20,w}$ (S)	~70	29.3	19.5	10.8	6.4	4.1
Per cent	7.5	10.9	58.3	1.8	4.4	17.1

serum α-globulin. In a later study [136], moving-boundary electrophoresis was used, and a typical pattern is shown in Fig. 2.3: peak B accounted for 92% of the total, and in barbital buffer, at pH 8.5, ionic strength 0.10, it was estimated to have a mobility of -4.8 × 10^{-5} $cm^2 volt^{-1} sec^{-1}$. This component apparently represents the thyroglobulin, along with additional minor components that are not resolved in electrophoresis; there were also three very small peaks: A, C, and D.

WITEBSKY *et al.* [189] reported in 1956 that ultracentrifugal examination of extracts of normal human thyroid tissue gave patterns very similar to those obtained for hog thyroid. The five major peaks, with approximately the same distribution, were augmented by a sixth (faster) component; these are labeled If, I, II, III, IV, and V in Fig. 2.4. The sedimentation coefficients and percentages are indicated in Table 2.2. The main peak, II, again had the sedimentation characteristics of thyroglobulin. An extract from human cancer of the thyroid gave a completely different pattern, indicative of drastic changes in the proportions of the components, the thyroglobulin component, in particular, being reduced by a factor of at least 10. The data are listed in Table 2.3. We return below to this phenomenon of abnormal proportions.

Table 2.3. *Ultracentrifugal analysis of malignant human thyroid extract*

		Peak					
		cI	cII″	cII′	cII	cIII	cIV
Primary	$s^0_{20,w}$	78.0			17.4	6.0	3.8
	Per cent	2.8			4.9	18.3	74.0
Metastasis	$s^0_{20,w}$	68.0	~44	~31	18.5	6.1	4.3
	Per cent	6.0	3.2	2.6	4.3	9.4	74.5

The electrophoretic pattern of normal human thyroid extract revealed the presence of four components, one of which constituted 62% of the total and should therefore be thyroglobulin; the cancer extract, on the other hand, gave a different pattern of nine, poorly resolved components [189]. Ultracentrifugal patterns have been described for human thyroid extract of normal [16, 18, 64, 162] and cancerous [146, 147, 171] glands, and also from goiters [16, 18].

Investigations have been carried out on the ultracentrifugal components of thyroid extracts from several other species. Rat thyroid tissue has a pattern similar to that found for hog thyroid: ROBBINS *et al.* [100, 192] found 27 S, 18–20 S, 10 S, and 6 S or 7 S components. Working with a transplantable thyroid tumor of the rat, they found that the proportions of the components resembled those of the human cancer extract, described above. There was a conspicuous 4 S iodinated component which they termed "thyroid S-1 iodoprotein", similar in its properties to hog thyralbumin to be described below. The proteins in sheep thyroid tissue were found to be similar to those in human thyroid [17, 101], and similar patterns and sedimentation coefficients have been reported for thyroid proteins from cattle [23, 99].

Studies on the components in extracts from human carcinomas or other tumors of the thyroid gland generally indicate a very high proportion of a 4 S component and a relatively low proportion of the 18–20 S component, and efforts have been made to evaluate the extent to which they are identical or similar to those components of normal thyroid tissue which have the same sedimentation coefficients. STANLEY [146] studied salting-out curves of various preparations and found good correlation between the 19 S components and a fraction that salted out between 35 and 45% saturation of ammonium sulfate, as described below. The lesson of these data is that in various pathological states the thyroid gland cannot synthesize thyroglobulin as it does in the normal state. Similar descriptions have been reported by VALENTA *et al.* [171]. These reports confirm the importance of measuring the proportions of 19 S and 4 S components, as originally indicated by WITEBSKY *et al.* [189].

2. Purification of Thyroglobulin and other Thyroid Proteins: Problems of Heterogeneity and Instability

a) Early Studies

DERRIEN *et al.* [19, 20] worked on the purification of hog Tg and studied its physical and chemical properties. They used, as a stock solution, phosphate salts at a total concentration of 3.5 *M*, and constructed solubility curves in considerable detail over a wide range of salt concentrations. A group of three major and three minor components could be seen; the three major components had similar salting-out properties and were considered to be three fractions of thyroglobulin because their iodine content was identical. It seemed reasonable to suppose that the heterogeneity of the thyroglobulin material in these three forms indicated diverse states of aggregation of a single protein, since the preparations were homogeneous by ultracentrifugal and electrophoretic criteria. DERRIEN *et al.* proposed that thyroglobulin is a protein of essentially constant amino-acid structure and composition, but that the degree of iodination may vary under different physiological and nutritional conditions. The hog thyroglobulin had an extrapolated sedimentation coefficient of 19.4 S, a diffusion coefficient of $2.6 \times 10^{-7} cm^2 sec^{-1}$, and a partial specific volume of 0.72. From these three values, a sedimentation-diffusion molecular weight of 650000 was determined. Thyroglobulins from hogs, cattle and dogs were compared and showed only small differences in amino-acid composition. The thyroid protein of each species contained variable amounts of iodine, but the content of tyrosine and other amino acids was constant. We have described the molecular dimensions and three-dimensional structures of these iodinated amino acids in detail elsewhere [124].

b) Fractionation by Chromatography—Early Approaches

Methods of purifying these proteins gradually improved and INGBAR *et al.* [46] studied sheep thyroid proteins by gradient-elution chromatography on the anion exchanger, diethylaminoethyl (DEAE)-cellulose. They observed what was essentially a single peak with an asymmetrical trailing region; the two components were pooled and examined for homogeneity in the ultracentrifuge. Each showed a 19 S component; the trailing material showed an additional faster component. No slower components were seen. However, as the studies were carried out on rather dilute solutions, it was difficult to make a critical analysis of homogeneity of the product. INGBAR *et al.* also found non-uniform labeling of the protein material with radioactive iodine; they therefore concluded that thyroglobulin is heterogeneous, even when obtained from a single animal.

ROCHE *et al.* [102] examined the heterogeneity of hog Tg; they also employed DEAE-cellulose. The distribution of protein and of radioactively-labeled iodine in the eluate led them to conclude that thyroglobulin itself was heterogeneous, in addition to the observed multiplicity of proteins in the total extract, as determined by SHULMAN *et al.* [132].

SHULMAN and STANLEY [134, 136] obtained from hog thyroid extract two major protein peaks on DEAE-cellulose. On re-chromatographing the products, they found some indication that resolution had occurred during chromatography on DEAE-cellulose. The best final product contained 96% of the 19 S component. The content was studied of iodinated amino acids in the first peak and at three positions of the broader second peak and analyses were made for the iodotyrosines, monoiodotyrosine (MIT) and diiodotyrosine (DIT), and for the iodothyronines, triiodothyronine (T3) and thyroxine (T4). There was a steady increase in the iodothyronines in the four samples, ranging from 1.9 in the earliest eluted material up to 8.8 in the latest eluted material. There must therefore be a series of molecules, presumably all or mostly in the thyroglobulin group of proteins, which differ to some slight degree in the amount and nature of iodine content. This confirms the findings of INGBAR *et al.* [46].

c) Fractionation by Ammonium Sulfate Precipitation: Thyralbumin and Thyroglobulin

Fractional precipitation with ammonium sulfate as used in the early studies [123, 133, 136, 137] led to the isolation of the major globulin and albumin fractions of thyroid extract; 1.60 to 1.70 *M* ammonium sulfate was required for preparation of thyroglobulin and 2.50 to 3.00 *M* for the preparation of a new fraction, thyralbumin (Ta). The thyroglobulin was about 97% homogeneous and the thyralbumin was 100% homogeneous in ultracentrifugal analysis, the latter being the 4 S component or peak V of crude extract. The yield of thyralbumin was approximately 1% and that of thyroglobulin approximately 10 to 15% of the original total protein. This method had the advantage of not requiring any special equipment so that it could be used to handle large quantities of extract.

Studies by moving-boundary electrophoresis of thyralbumin prepared in this way showed the material to be heterogeneous. Seven or eight migrating components could be detected; one component constituted about one-third of the total material, and had the same electrophoretic mobility as serum albumin. For comparison, a sample of hog serum was fractionated in a similar way to the thyralbumin and was found on electrophoretic examination to reveal the albumin peak plus two slower migrating components. These three components could therefore be matched up with the pattern of thyralbumin, leaving four or five constituents which seemed thus to be truly of thyroidal origin [127]. The iodine content in this type of preparation was approximately 0.10% iodine [127], which would correspond well to the iodoproteins of 4 S class, isolated from thyroid tissue by indirect means by other investigators [6, 7, 94, 100, 109, 160, 192]. This will be discussed below.

Ui *et al.* [168, 169] showed that thyroglobulin purified by an ammonium sulfate procedure (1.55 to 1.75 M salt at low temperature, or 1.50 to 1.70 M at 20°C) still contained a 28 S component in addition to the 91% of 19 S component. After chromatography on DEAE-cellulose, using stepwise elution with buffers of increasing ionic strength and a constant pH of 6.5, the 19 S material showed a high degree of homogeneity in the ultracentrifuge: the fraction that was eluted at an ionic strength of 0.22, following a level of 0.15, had the highest purity and was essentially homogeneous in the ultracentrifuge. Despite the satisfactory ultracentrifugal picture, the protein concentration examined was only about 0.6%, and more rigorous conditions might be preferable. Some of the fractions showed a considerable enrichment of the 28 S component (which Ui *et al.* called the F-component), accompanied by a still faster one. From the iodine analysis of the various mixtures, the 28 S component was expected to be an iodoprotein. The chemical analysis of the various chromatographic fractions showed an increasing ratio of iodine to nitrogen in the sequential fractions eluted from the column. This gave further support to the concept that there are a large number of iodoproteins, differing in degree of iodination but apparently very similar in sedimentation properties, belonging to either the 19 S or 28 S families.

d) Fractionation by Centrifugation; Dissociation of Thyroglobulin

A new method of purification was introduced by Edelhoch in 1960 [23], using preparative ultracentrifugation. The thyroglobulin of calf thyroid saline extract was first precipitated by salting out, and this preparation was centrifuged for 260 minutes at 40000 r.p.m. at room temperature in the Spinco Model L ultracentrifuge. The top portion, approximately 70% of the centrifuged solution, was pipetted off and the bottom portion was decanted as the product, leaving the packed pellet behind. This process was repeated several times, and a product was obtained which showed a high degree of ultracentrifugal homogeneity. In an alternative preparation, the differential centrifugation technique was applied directly to the saline extract of the thyroid tissue.

The sedimentation coefficient of the purified protein was found to be 19.4 S. This was in close agreement with the value that had been reported by O'Donnell *et al.* [80] for hog Tg. A diffusion coefficient of 2.49×10^{-7} was reported, slightly smaller than the value of 2.60×10^{-7} reported by O'Donnell *et al.* [80] and by Derrien *et al.* [19] for hog Tg. Using a partial specific volume of 0.713, a molecular weight of 669000 was then calculated from the Svedberg equation [140]. This value for bovine thyroglobulin was in close approximation to the values already reported for hog Tg of 665000 (Derrien *et al.* [19]) and 660000 (O'Donnell *et al.* [80]). The molecular weight was also determined by light scattering, and a result close to 690000 was obtained; this, however, is a weight-average molecular weight and can be strongly influenced by small amounts of higher molecular weight material.

A series of reversible changes of shape was observed in the thyroglobulin molecule, depending upon the pH and ionic strength of the solution [23]. With increasing pH from 6.0 to 12.7 there are several changes, and at least four new molecular species are formed in a sequence of progressive disorganization of this molecule. While the relative proportion of 19 S material falls, there is at first an increasing quantity of a 12 S boundary; at higher pH levels 15 S, 8 S, and 3 S components appear. The 12 S component involves the formation of a particle with sedimentation properties similar to the α-protein of LUNDGREN and WILLIAMS [65]. This product was thought to result from the dissociation of thyroglobulin into two subunits. At pH above 9.5, 15 S components come into existence, and at the highest pH levels only the 8 S and 3 S material are found. The changes produced up to pH 11 are at least partially reversible but after that are largely irreversible, depending upon the duration of exposure to the elevated pH value.

e) Fractionation by Chromatography—Later Approaches; the Thyroid Family of Proteins

Purification of hog thyroid proteins was studied by use of DEAE-cellulose chromatography, in a stepwise elution technique [129]. The extract was separated into five major fractions or elution peaks. Thyroglobulin was found in its most homogeneous form in peak 3 of the effluent pattern, illustrated in Fig. 2.5, and this protein could be obtained in an ultracentrifugal homogeneity of 99 to 100%, with a yield of 7 to 8% of the original protein. Another 7 to 8% was recovered with a purity of 98–99%, and a total of 35–40% of the material could be obtained with homogeneity above 95%. Immunochemical homogeneity of this thyroglobulin preparation was also demonstrated. By means of an anti-serum to hog serum, the essentially complete removal of the serum contaminants

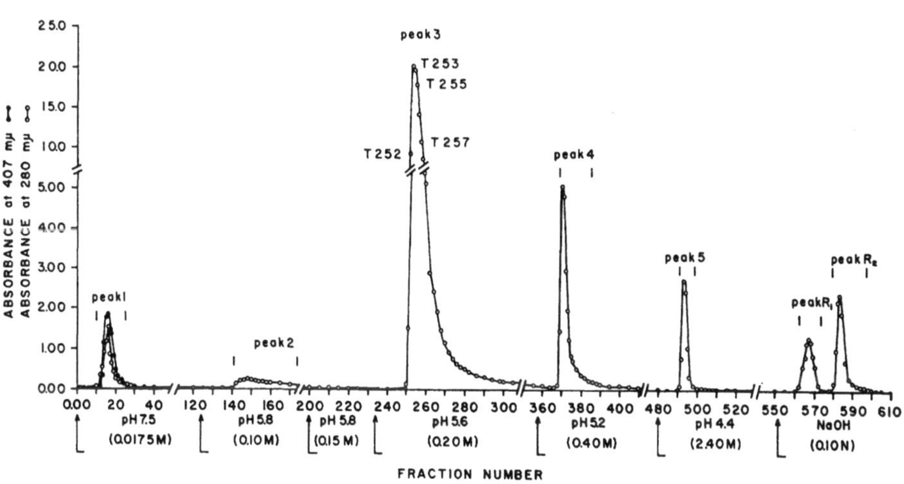

Fig. 2.5. Elution pattern from DEAE-cellulose chromatography of a hog thyroid crude extract. Column size was 2.2 × 25 cm (12 g). The sample was applied as 1.38 g in 0.0175 *M* sodium phosphate buffer, pH 7.5, to a column of 2.2 × 25 cm, and a stepwise gradient was employed, introducing the successive buffers, as indicated. An additional elution was performed with 0.10 *N* NaOH. The short vertical lines indicate the tubes which were pooled to form the numbered peaks

from the initial crude extract was demonstrated, to some 1/10000 of their initial level.

Other investigations on fractionation of thyroid proteins in more recent years have been based on filtration with either dextran gel (commonly obtained as Sephadex) or granulated agar (or agarose). For example, in human thyroid extracts three major elution fractions were eluted by gel filtration on Sephadex G-200 [131]. Only moderately pure thyroglobulin and 27 S component could be obtained (in one of the eluted fractions). However, the 7 S and 4 S components could each be subdivided into two approximately equal fractions by means of zone electrophoresis on paper curtain. In addition, there was evidence for the existence of 12 S, 19 S, 27 S, and 34 S components [121]. Thus, the initial thyroid extract yielded a total of 8 distinctive protein fractions, in 6 sedimentation classes. Components that are 33 S and 38 S have also been mentioned by SALVATORE *et al.* [122]. Recent measurements on highly purified preparations gave extrapolated sedimentation coefficients of 27.7 S and 32.3 S for two of the components [139].

PERELMUTTER and colleagues [86, 87] applied a very similar procedure to bovine thyroid extract and obtained similar elution patterns; here the later-eluted materials were not examined, since the aim was the isolation of thyroglobulin, which was obtained in a state that was described as 100% pure. Procedures of this sort were also applied in other preparations of pure thyroglobulin [12, 74, 173].

SALVATORE *et al.* [121] applied similar procedures to rat, guinea pig, cattle, and sheep materials, obtaining similar results, although they gave few experimental details. They introduced an improved procedure, agar gel filtration, for the isolation of the 19 S and 27 S materials, utilizing a resin with a much higher exclusion value than Sephadex. Additional studies on the 27 S protein by SALVATORE *et al.* [122] and VECCHIO *et al.* [175] have definitely characterized it as an iodinated component, although the exact relationship between this molecule and the 19 S molecule is not yet clear. The 27 S protein usually containes more iodine than the thyroglobulin obtained from the same thyroid tissue: in one pair of human preparations, for example, iodine levels were 1.0% and 0.7%, respectively. The heavier iodoprotein, with an extrapolated sedimentation coefficient of 27.0 S, and a diffusion coefficient of 1.91×10^{-7} cm^2 sec^{-1}, had a calculated molecular weight of 1200000. TARUTANI *et al.* [126] explored the disruption of human 27 S protein by means of sodium dodecyl sulfate and concluded that there were probably two forms of thyroglobulin differing in stability. They suggested that 27 S protein was a mixture of combinations of dissociable and non-dissociable thyroglobulin molecules, paired with like or unlike subunits.

The iodoproteins in a variety of vertebrates have been examined and compared by ROCHE *et al.* [103]. Interesting extremes were found concerning subunits (half-molecules) and their degrees of stability, as shown in the lamprey by ALOJ *et al.* [2] and in the guinea pig by SALVATORE *et al.* [120].

The three major thyroid protein groups that contain iodoproteins are the 27 S, 19 S and 4 S components. The two major subfractions of the 4 S proteins found in human material can be compared to the electrophoretically polydisperse hog thyralbumin and to the analogous rat protein, the S-1 iodoprotein, isolated by ROBBINS and colleagues [100, 192]. A 4 S thyroid protein was isolated from normal rat thyroid extracts by ROITT *et al.* [109] using sucrose density-gradient ultracentrifugation. A 4 S iodinated protein, similar to serum albumin in some properties, has been reported in the serum of patients with a variety of thyroid diseases [94, 160]. One report claimed it was immunologically identical to human serum albumin [94], another that it was unreactive with antiserum to serum albumin [160]. Perhaps these authors were studying different members of the 4 S family of proteins. Patients who have 4 S iodoprotein in their serum generally have an unusually large proportion of 4 S iodoprotein in their thyroid tissue. As already mentioned, electrophoretic studies of a human thyroid cancer extract revealed 3 to 5 poorly resolved components, all associated with a 4 S ultracentrifugal component [189]. BECKERS *et al.* [6, 7] found non-iodinated proteins in certain human thyroid extracts of the 4 S class and called them pre-thyroglobulin because of their electrophoretic mobility. LISSITZKY and his colleagues have also described certain iodoproteins that were not thyroglobulin: they obtained an iodoprealbumin from both the thyroid tissue and blood serum of a patient with a eumetabolic goiter [61]. They also found an iodoalbumin in the tissue of congenital goiters and concluded that this protein was carried by the serum to the thyroid tissue where it was iodinated [59, 60].

The relationship of these components to the thyralbumin of hog or the two major 4 S fractions of human thyroid tissues has yet to be clarified. JONCKHEER and his colleagues [52, 82], having isolated from normal human thyroid tissue what they termed a well-purified preparation of thyroid albumin for further study of its physical and chemical properties [50, 51], concluded that it was an iodinated protein synthesized within the thyroid gland, and different from serum albumin. Various other preparations of thyroid iodoalbumins and other abnormal iodoproteins have been described [22, 30, 32, 54, 163, 164, 174].

f) Biochemical and Immunochemical Heterogeneity of Thyroglobulin

Chemical heterogeneity among the molecules presumed to be thyroglobulin has been confirmed in a number of reports, many of which have already been mentioned. It is important to agree on fundamental criteria for defining the thyroglobulin molecule or group of molecules. The criteria that are currently rather widely accepted [98] are as follows:

1. thyroglobulin contains iodine,
2. thyroglobulin has a sedimentation coefficient of 19 S,
3. thyroglobulin has an electrophoretic mobility at pH 8.6 which resembles that of a serum α-globulin,
4. thyroglobulin is salted out at approximately 40% ammonium sulfate saturation.

Heterogeneity within this type of *apparently* homogeneous material has been related most frequently to characteristics of the iodine metabolism, that is, that subfractions of otherwise identical protein materials have varying contents of different iodinated amino acids which affect their chemical activity [10, 90].

Earlier studies had also generated the concept of micro-heterogeneity of thyroglobulin, based on salting-out differences, or, solubility differences at high salt levels [20]. More recently, ASSEM *et al.* [4] applied starch-gel electrophoresis as well as various chromatographic separations to reasonably well purified human thyroglobulin prepared by salting-out procedures, and their results indicated that several components were present. All three components seen in the starch-gel electrophoresis were identified as thyroglobulin by all other criteria, except ultracentrifuging, but the iodine contents were low and poorly reproducible. The iodine/nitrogen ratio and also the content of sialic acid (one of the carbohydrate units of Tg) differed in the different components. These results were thus analogous to those of INGBAR *et al.* [46] who were the first to use DEAE-cellulose to show a difference in iodine/nitrogen ratios among the different fractions. Similar reports had been made by UI *et al.* [169], SHULMAN and STANLEY [134], and ROBBINS [96, 97].

The heterogeneity of thyroglobulin can also be indicated in terms of antigenic determinant groups of several kinds, and this type of analysis is most important with regard to the immunochemistry of this molecule. These studies will be discussed at a later point.

There are also types of thyroglobulin which are really quite abnormal, for example, in their very low level of iodination. Essentially noniodinated thyroglobulin is obtained from certain carcinomas and adenomas of the human thyroid gland, and similar products are isolated from experimental animals after treatment with anti-thyroid drugs. These preparations generally do contain a very low level of iodine, if it is not completely absent; perhaps they should be termed hypoiodinated. STANLEY [147], who studied human thyroid glands containing discrete malignant nodules, found that the iodine content of thyroglobulin from the malignant portions was less than that from the normal portions, and in one case was negligible. Other more extensive findings, reported quite recently [172], showed thyroid carcinomas and adenomas to contain iodine only 0.1 to 0.001 % of that in thyroglobulin obtained from normal thyroid tissue, suggesting a block in the iodination of thyroglobulin. There are strong indications that these varying levels of iodination cause conformational changes in the thyroglobulin molecule, it is not yet known whether they influence the antigenic groups that cover the surface of this molecule, but we may anticipate that such influences should exist. Studies should therefore be conducted on the antigenic properties as a function of iodination of this molecule.

3. Subunit Structure of the Thyroglobulin Molecule

Let us consider now in some detail the various physical and chemical properties of the thyroglobulin molecule and its composition. The sedimentation and diffusion coefficients and the estimated molecular weight have been reported by a number of workers and require little further discussion. Detailed reviews have been presented by EDELHOCH and RALL [28] and EDELHOCH [24]. The shape of the molecule has been studied by a number of methods, including sedimentation, viscosity, light scattering, optical rotation, and relaxation time measurements [27, 29, 148]. These studies revealed many properties of this complex molecule, including the conclusion that it behaves as a compact and rigid particle. It was also observed, according to optical rotatory dispersion and fluorescence polarization measurements under various conditions, that the molecule can undergo several forms of dissociation into smaller units, but does not appreciably change in its content of helical, that is, secondary, structure, even when subjected to any of a number of denaturing agents. Direct observations have also been made by electron microscopy [9, 49]. In particular, BLOTH and BERGQUIST [9] showed that it has the shape of a flexible helix with two turns, a total length of 220 Å, and a maximal diameter of 110 Å. Thus the molecule actually has a much smaller axial ratio than had been indicated by hydrodynamic measurements, and is much less compact.

We now consider the chemical structure of thyroglobulin, beginning with its carbohydrate content: it is a glycoprotein, containing in the carbohydrate portion, galactose, mannose, fucose, glucosamine, and sialic acid [96, 141, 144, 145, 170, 193]. The carbohydrate content varies slightly, ranging from 8.0% to 10.0% for human, ovine, bovine, and porcine types of thyroglobulin [71]. Studies by SPIRO *et al.* [141, 144] and CHEFTEL *et al.* [11] indicated the existence of two types of carbyhydrate residue, each a mixture of glycopeptides, which could be separated by dialysis. The glycopeptides can be released from thyroglobulin by the proteolytic enzyme, pronase, obtained from *Streptomyces griseus*.

CHEFTEL *et al.* [11] described both non-dialyzable and dialyzable glycopeptide fractions of sheep thyroglobulin. These fractions were estimated by ultracentrifugal examination to have molecular weights of approximately 3500 and 1700, respectively. NARASIMHA MURTHY *et al.* [76, 77] isolated and purified a major glycopeptide from sheep thyroglobulin by utilizing a succession of ethanol fractionation, gel filtration, and Dowex-50 chromatography. This peptide contained at least 12 amino acids, plus sialic acid, glucosamine, galactose, mannose, and fucose. Since the yield of this peptide was approximately 5 to 6%, it was thought to represent at least 60% of the carbohydrate of thyroglobulin; it contained little or no iodine. The molecular weight of 2400 was measured in the ultracentrifuge by the Archibald procedure and the sedimentation equilibrium method. When molecular weight was estimated by means of chemical analysis for aspartic acid in the form of the DNP residue, basing this calculation on the extinction coefficient of DNP-aspartic acid and assuming a single residue per peptide, the result was 2600. The carbohydrate analysis showed the presence of glucosamine, hexose, fucose, and sialic acid. If the Tg carbohydrate were a single entity, the molecular weight of the glycopeptide would be approximately 50000; since this major glycopeptide has a molecular weight of 2600, there would be some 20 units of this type distributed throughout the molecule, assuming all the carbohydrate units were identical. There was no evidence at that time as to whether these entities would be in fact identical, or whether there would be a variety of different glycopeptides or polysaccharide units.

The carbohydrate composition of calf, sheep, pig, and human thyroglobulins was determined by SPIRO and SPIRO [145]. In every case, the monosaccharides were galactose, mannose, N-acetylglucosamine, fucose, and sialic acid. The sialic acid was in the N-acetyl form, except in pig thyroglobulin, where 10% was in the N-glycolyl form. Using a molecular weight of 670000, they calculated that there were approximately 290 monosaccharide residues in the calf, sheep, and pig proteins, and 350 residues in the human protein, per molecule of the glycoprotein. The higher percentage (10%) of carbohydrate in the human thyroglobulin corresponds to its greater content of mannose and glucosamine.

SPIRO [142] described two distinctive types of carbohydrate unit in bovine Tg which were quite different in size and composition. One unit had a molecular weight of 1050 and was composed of five residues of mannose and one residue of glucosamine; the other had a molecular weight of 3200 and consisted of sialic acid, fucose, galactose, mannose, and glucosamine, with respectively, 2, 1, 4, 3, and 5 residues. Each molecule of bovine thyroglobulin was thought to consist of approximately nine of the smaller units and fourteen of the larger units, attached at 23 linkage points in the polypeptide chain. Many of these 23 amino acid residues were judged to be aspartic acid.

TARUTANI *et al.* [151, 152], using neuraminidase, removed some 80–87% of the total sialic acid from human thyroglobulin; they concluded that the remainder was buried inside the molecule and therefore inaccessible. Desialization of thyroglobulin did not involve any appreciable conformational change in the molecular structure. Chromatographic separation of the native protein molecule produced a series of fractions with variable amounts of sialic acid, in parallel with the variation in iodine content. Thus, the heterogeneity in purified thyroglobulin seems to be related not only to the iodine content, but also to the sialic acid content [153]. The sialic acid content was different in thyroglobulins prepared from normal thyroid and from several goitrous thyroids [154]. Removal of galactose from the desialized preparations was also explored [155].

Relatively little work has been done on the amino acid composition and the arrangement of amino acid and carbohydrate units in the polypeptide chains of this large and complex molecule. Several reports have appeared on the total amino acid composition of thyroglobulin preparations [111, 143]; some of the most recent data are tabulated in Table 2.4. The first attempt to explore the physicochemical nature of the Tg molecular subunits seems to have been the 1965 study by PIERCE *et al.* [88]. They prepared highly purified human thyroglobulin from normal thyroid glands and from those of subjects with non-toxic colloid goiters and performed amino-acid analyses on both, as well as on preparations of hog and sheep thyroglobulin. They found some 180 half-cystine residues per molecular weight of 660000, in disulfide linkage. Hence, there are approximately 90 disulfide linkages holding the molecule in its configuration and presumably connecting whatever polypeptide chains there may be. Chemical reduction and alkylation of Tg gave a resultant product that showed slow sedimenting components in the ultracentrifuge, especially a component with a sedimentation coefficient of 3.2 to 3.4 S. The molecular weight of this dissociated species was estimated to be approximately 110000 to 125000; this suggested that there may be 5 or 6 subunits or polypeptide chains in the original thyroglobulin molecule.

Other investigators have concurred in finding essentially all the cysteine units in disulfide form but the actual number has been widely accepted as about 11 or 12% higher. The half-disulfide content has been given as 202 [14, 15, 91] and as 200 [62], and even as high as 208 [111]. PITT-RIVERS and SCHWARTZ [91], mentioning the 202 half-cystine residues per molecule,

Table 2.4. *Amino acid composition of thyroglobulin from different species, expressed as residues per mole*

Amino acid	Human				Bovine	Porcine
	Sample 1	Sample 2	Sample 3	Mean		
Asp	397	387	390	391	373	361
Thr	284	274	267	275	250	271
Ser	468	464	490	474	509	485
Glu	719	704	747	723	671	675
Pro	317	325	336	326	361	388
Gly	409	416	406	410	442	446
Ala	404	408	378	396	469	493
Val	312	323	308	314	306	314
$^1/_2$-Cys	205	210	210	208	218	224
Met	74	72	79	75	59	55
Ileu	149	161	155	155	131	121
Leu	476	473	493	480	498	518
Tyr	120	123	111	118	129	111
Phe	258	262	256	258	272	243
Lys	166	166	168	166	137	123
His	77	79	79	68	63	69
Arg	281	296	271	282	322	331
MIT		4	4			7
DIT		4	2			10
T_4		2	2			3
$^1/_2$ I_2(%)		0.33	0.29			0.79

The number of residues per mole was calculated for a molecular weight of 650000, of which 65000 represents the carbohydrate fraction, 7000 represents the iodinated amino acids, and 578000 is the protein portion. The average amount of tryptophan is estimated as 2.2% by weight.

described a careful study on the very small number of free sulfhydryl groups; they concluded that there were 5 such groups, only 2 of which are accessible without some denaturation.

Other laboratories have also explored the subunit structure of the thyroglobulin molecule, including EDELHOCH and colleagues [14, 15, 26, 78] and LISSITZKY and colleagues [62, 63]. A subunit molecular weight of about 165000 was found by the former group [15]. The product of complete reduction of bovine Tg was obtained by splitting all these disulfide bonds; the molecular weight was estimated by a combination of sedimentation and viscosity data. The molecular properties of the reduced molecule were studied by a number of physical technics, and a rigid, two-chain, highly permeable, sponge-like structure was proposed [26]. Reversibility of the reduction process was explored, and considerable success was achieved [14]. Two sedimenting units may be formed by mild reduction; these have been separated and further analyzed, although no new light was shed on the controversial question of the minimal subunit molecular weight [78].

LISSITZKY *et al.* have made a detailed analysis of this problem [63]. They achieved full reduction and alkylation of the disulfide bonds of purified sheep

Tg. Applying a variety of methods for molecular weight determination they obtained under some conditions values of 80–85000, and under other conditions, 114000 or 160000. They concluded that 80000 was the most likely result. They suggested there were two different kinds of polypeptide chain of 80000 molecular weight to be assembled, in suitable numbers, in the thyroglobulin molecule [62, 63].

Another type of approach for the separation of chain units by non-enzymatic methods is treatment with succinic anhydride [112]. Very recently, SMITH and SHULMAN [138, 139] reported that several slower-sedimenting species varied in proportion for different molar ratios of reagent to protein, and also differed for normal and goitrous human Tg. The two slowest species, a major 11 S peak and a minor 9 S peak, were seen in addition to a minor 16 S peak at low concentrations of reagent. Their changing proportions at higher levels of succinylation suggested that there are two stages in the molecular disruption. The abnormal Tg protein was more completely broken down into the 9 S type of component, indicating again the importance of the iodination for strengthening the subunit interactions.

The dissociation of the thyroglobulin molecule into subunit forms has also been studied by means of sodium dodecyl sulfate, and it appears that the degree of dissociation is related to the degree of iodination of the molecule. From this TARUTANI *et al.* [157–159] concluded that non-iodinated thyroglobulin is structurally different from the iodinated form. NUNEZ *et al.* [79] have described some data that indicate, from sedimentation analyses, a relationship of molecular conformation to iodination, and EDELHOCH *et al.* [25] have discussed this relationship again recently. These differences must affect the antigenic properties, especially with regard to autoantigenic or heteroantigenic forms. Many exciting new leads can be expected to arise from explorations of the detailed architecture of the various antigenic units as chemically defined structural groups.

4. Detailed Studies of Thyroid Specificity

Let us return to the matter of the tissue specificity of the thyroid gland. In the initial work, in 1955 [188], saline extracts of macerated thyroid glands from hogs, as well as other hog organs, were prepared as gently as possible, with the specific aim of avoiding denaturation of the proteins. Rabbits were given several courses of either intravenous injection or intradermal injection with complete Freund's adjuvant—the latter being then a new route for experimental immunization. The intradermal-adjuvant procedure was found to be superior, because of the very small amount of extract needed for successful immunization and also because of the absence of the danger of anaphylactic reactions which sometimes occur with intravenous injections.

Thyroid-specific antibodies appeared as early as two weeks after the beginning of intradermal-adjuvant injections of thyroid extract. Antibodies against hog serum were also elicited, but were of considerably lower titer than the thyroid antibodies. Various tests for specificity were performed with extracts from other tissues, but cross-reactions were much weaker than homologous reactions. The existence of thyroid specificity could also be confirmed in another way, as illustrated in Table 2.5. The reactions of antisera produced against another organ, *e.g.* kidney, when tested with dilutions of kidney and of thyroid extracts, contrasted with the behavior of a thyroid antiserum, tested with kidney and thyroid extracts at various dilutions. In the first case, both dilution titrations were small and

Table 2.5. *Reactions of hog thyroid and hog kidney extracts with their corresponding antisera, in complement fixation tests*

	Antigen:	
	Thyroid extract	Kidney extract
Rabbit antiserum to:		
Hog thyroid	400000	25
Hog kidney	125	625

Figures indicate the greatest dilution of antigen which gave complete inhibition of hemolysis.

of similar magnitude; with thyroid antiserum, the kidney titer was small but the thyroid titer was of a much higher magnitude. Tissue-specific antibodies were also demonstrated by absorption studies. Antisera that were absorbed with hog serum showed a subsequent lack of species-specific antibodies, but they continued to demonstrate potent levels of thyroid-specific antibodies.

a) The Species Distribution of Thyroid Antigens

The cross-reactions of anti-thyroid antisera were studied in order to determine the extent to which thyroid proteins were shared by the thyroid glands of various animals [117]. Cross-reactions between various species were irregular and unpredictable, in agreement with the results of HEKTOEN *et al.* [41], using isolated thyroglobulins. Absorption of a rabbit antiserum to human thyroid by human serum eliminated the human species-specific antibody but did not reduce the level of thyroid-specific antibodies. When this same antiserum was absorbed with human thyroid extract, on the other hand, the entire antibody content of the serum was removed. Thirdly, the absorption of such an antiserum with hog thyroid extract eliminated the cross-reaction with hog thyroid and cattle thyroid extract, but it did not detectably reduce the strong reaction with the homologous human thyroid extract. Thus, the cross-reactions between anti-thyroid antisera and thyroid extracts of various species were found to be thyroid-specific; in other words, no reactions were detected with other organs of the various animal species.

Several of the preliminary comparisons are shown in Table 2.6, taken from the work of ROSE and WITEBSKY [117]. Rabbit antisera were prepared against thyroid extracts of hog, cattle, man, and dog. These were then tested with saline extracts of thyroid glands from a large number of animals. It can be observed that reciprocal cross-reactions occurred between hog and cattle, hog and dog, cattle and dog, and dog and man. In addition, the antisera to cattle and dog gave cross-reactions with sheep and horse, and the antiserum to hog cross-reacted with horse. These various cross-reactions seemed to occur in a surprisingly unpredictable manner. At this time, no reaction with *rabbit* thyroid

Table 2.6. *Reactions of anti-thyroid antisera with crude thyroid extracts from various species*

	Crude saline extracts of thyroid glands from:								
	Hog	Cattle	Man	Dog	Sheep	Horse	Cat	Guinea Pig	Rabbit
Rabbit antisera to thyroid extracts of:									
Hog	+	+	−	+	−	+	−	−	−
Cattle	+	+	−	+	+	+	−	−	−
Man	±	±	+	±	±	−	−	−	−
Dog	+	+	+	+	+	+	−	−	−

+ = definite reaction in complement-fixation and precipitation tests.
− = no definite reaction by complement-fixation or precipitation tests.
± = disparity between different techniques, or among different antisera.

was shown by any of these rabbit antisera. However, this observation was to be reversed in later studies on autoantibody formation.

Another principle of great importance must be emphasized, and that is the individuality of the antibody response in different animals within a group. Antisera that are prepared in different individual experimental animals can vary considerably in the degree of cross-reaction they exhibit. Therefore, any conclusion on

Table 2.7. *Cross-reactions of three different rabbit antisera to human thyroid, in complement fixation tests*

	Crude saline extracts of thyroid glands from:					Human Serum
	Man	Cattle	Dog	Hog	Sheep	
Rabbit antisera to human thyroid:						
R 46 b	16000	625	25	0	5	2000000
R 47 b	80000	80000	80000	16000	625	2000000
R 51 a	16000	125	5	0	5	0

Figures indicate the greatest dilution of antigen which gave complete inhibition of hemolysis.
Since a single pipette was used for preparing serial dilutions of each antigen, the figures may be regarded as having relative, but not absolute, significance.

the nature of organ specificity and tissue specificity may well be in error if this feature is not adequately explored. Let us consider, as an example of this important parameter, data for three individual rabbits, each immunized with human thyroid extract, shown in Table 2.7. All three of the antisera reacted strongly with the homologous human thyroid extract. Two of them reacted strongly with human serum as a contaminating antigen, but the third did not react with this material at all. With regard to thyroid extracts from other species, two of the antisera exhibited very weak cross-reactions, but in contrast the third reacted very strongly with the other thyroid extracts. Thus, if one had studied only rabbit 47b one would have concluded that there was no organ specificity in thyroid. The third rabbit, 51a, illustrates a very important factor in such studies, namely, that an occasional animal is found whose antiserum is already highly specific for the tissue extract being studied. Bleedings from such animals are extremely useful, as they can be used directly as reagents. In general, however, one must improve on the tissue specificity of the bleedings that are obtained, and this can be done by selective absorption.

In conclusion, it can be stated that antisera produced in rabbits by injection of crude extracts of thyroid glands will give cross-reactions with thyroid extracts of various other species in an unpredictable and irregular manner. Antisera produced by similar immunization of dogs contain thyroid-specific antibodies, but the cross-reactions with thyroid extracts of other species are considerably less prominent than is the case with rabbit antisera. There is considerable variation in the extent of cross-reaction, depending upon the individual animal used for immunization. An antiserum to human thyroid contains antibodies against human serum as well as against thyroid extracts of different species. Absorption of this antiserum with human serum eliminates the antibody to serum components without removing the thyroid-specific antibodies. The cross-reactions of thyroid antisera with thyroid extracts of other species are thyroid-specific [117]. This fulfills the definition of tissue specificity.

Rabbit antisera to various mammalian thyroid extracts contain several kinds of specific thyroid antibodies [113]. Two varieties could be easily distinguished: those that reacted only with the homologous thyroid extract as used for immunization, and those that cross-reacted with thyroid extracts of other species. This was readily evaluated by means of double-diffusion techniques of agar precipitation. For example, one of the two lines produced by the reaction of a hog thyroid antiserum with hog thyroid extract gave a reaction of partial identity with a single precipitation band produced by the same antiserum with the thyroid extracts of certain other species. The two types of thyroid-specific antibodies may well be directed againly different antigenic sites on the thyroglobulin molecule. One of these groupings would be present on thyroglobulin from many different species and the other only on the homologous thyroglobulin molecule.

b) The Substance Responsible for Thyroid Specificity

Thyroglobulin was identified as the component of the thyroid extract responsible for tissue specificity [114, 137]. Salting-out procedures with ammonium sulfate were utilized to obtain Tg and Ta preparations for serological testing. Most of the organ-specific thyroid antigen was indeed precipitated in the thyroglobulin fraction, and very little species-specific antigen. The thyralbumin fraction, on the other hand, was found to contain little or no detectable thyroid-specific activity, but did react with antiserum to hog serum. It is not yet clear whether this indicates a lack of thyroid antigens or, as is more likely, that the corresponding antibodies were not expressed in the antisera that were used.

5. The Formation of Autoantibodies

a) Isoimmunization and Thyroiditis

A useful development in the study of thyroid specificity, as reflected in its antigenic properties, was the discovery that autoantibodies can be produced against one or more components of thyroid material. It had been thought that antibodies of this type could not be experimentally stimulated, but the effort to produce them was successful, largely, it would seem, because of the use of complete Freund's adjuvant in the intradermal immunization procedure [136, 187]. The antibody activity was manifested by complement fixation, precipitation, and passive hemagglutination procedures. These antibodies were tissue-specific, showing a remarkably high degree of thyroid specificity. They were in fact autoantibodies, as judged from the positive reactions seen with thyroid material from any rabbit tested, including the antibody-producing rabbit. Animals could even be thyroidectomized or partially thyroidectomized and, when immunized with preparations of their own thyroid glands, produced antibodies which would react with their own thyroid extracts and also with the thyroid extracts of all other rabbits tested. In subsequent studies, it was shown that many of these rabbits developed severe histological changes in the thyroid glands, corresponding to partial replacement of the thyroid tissue by infiltrating mononuclear cells. This experimental autoimmune response has been the subject of many subsequent studies, and has been discussed in a number of reviews [57, 73, 118, 119, 128, 185]. These lesions were eventually found to be closely comparable to those observed in humans suffering from chronic thyroiditis, also called Hashimoto's thyroiditis, or struma lymphomatosa. It was subsequently discovered by the London group [107] and also by the Buffalo group [191] that many patients with chronic thyroiditis did in fact have circulating autoantibodies against human thyroglobulin, or at least human thyroid extract, when tested for this possibility. A number of reports and reviews have appeared concerning the autoantibodies in thyroid disease [47, 48, 55, 70, 83–85, 89, 92, 95, 128].

A few additional points may be mentioned concerning the experimental situation in the rabbit [136]. The development of hemagglutinating activity in successive bleedings after the initial injection of rabbit thyroid extract can be seen for six rabbits (Table 2.8). Five were shown to have a precipitating serum and, of these, one animal clearly showed a tendency to demonstrate two lines of precipitation (Fig. 2.6). This double precipitation, surprising in a situation of such high specificity of antigen-antibody interaction, was checked in several alternative gel-diffusion arrangements (Fig. 2.7); it could not be readily attributed to an extreme imbalance of antigen and antibody proportions. This is further discussed below.

Table 2.8. *Passive hemagglutination tests: Titers of all bleedings from rabbits immunized with rabbit thyroid extract*

Trial bleeding	Week	Rabbit 876	Rabbit 877	Rabbit 878	Rabbit 879	Rabbit 880	Rabbit 881
First test:							
a	0	0	0	0	0	0	0
b	1	27	243	81	81 p	243	27
c	2	81	81 p[a]	243 p	243	243	81 p
d	3	243	243	810	729	729	243
e	4	243	243	2430	729	2187 p	2187
f	6	2187	2187	21870	6561	6561	19683
g	8	2187	6561	21870	6561	6561	19683
h	11	729	6561	21870	6561	6561	19683
Second test:							
h	11	7290	65610	65610	65610	65610	65610
i	15	–	65610	65610	65610	65610	65610
j (final)	21	–	65610	196830	196830	–	196830

[a] p = First bleeding to show demonstrable precipitation in gel diffusion plate.

Several additional points are of importance with regard to the study of human autoantibodies against thyroid components. Thyroid material was obtained from a patient who also had autoantibodies in her serum [190]; it was thus possible to prove definitely that the thyroid antibody reacted with extract from her own thyroid gland as well as with extracts of thyroid glands of other people, thus proving that humans have autoantibody. The serum was further tested with ammonium sulfate-fractionated products from the extract, and it was shown that the thyroglobulin fraction reacted quantitatively much like the saline extract itself. This was a strong indication that the antigen that

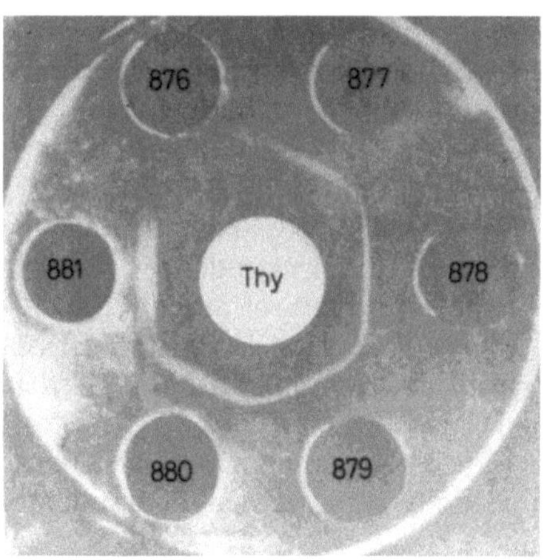

Fig. 2.6. Double-diffusion gel precipitation between rabbit thyroid extract (central well) and sera of bleeding g from six immunized rabbits (peripheral wells)

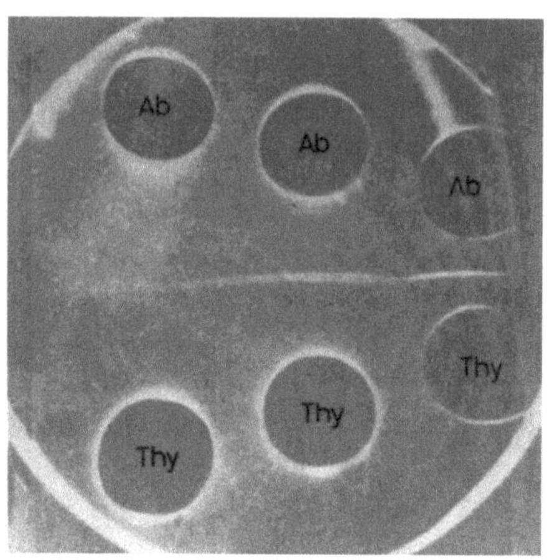

Fig. 2.7. Double-diffusion gel precipitation between rabbit thyroid extract (lower wells) and antiserum 881 g (upper wells), with edge-to-edge separations of 1.0, 2.0, and 3.0 cm

stimulated autoantibody formation, in other words, the autoantigen, was in fact thyroglobulin.

Unlike the antisera obtained by experimental stimulation, human sera which show antibody activity by means of tanned-cell hemagglutination do not indicate any activity when tested by means of the complement fixation test. In fact it used to be said that human autoantibodies do not fix complement with human thyroid extract or human thyroglobulin, whereas rabbit autoantibodies do so with rabbit antigen. It was later found that human serum could fix complement if the antigenic preparation was obtained from a thyrotoxic goiter rather than from normal thyroid material or from simple non-toxic goiters [167, 183]. It was then discovered [44, 105, 106] that these reactions of complement fixation were due to a second antigen, associated with the microsomal fraction of the thyroid homogenate rather than with the thyroglobulin. Immunofluorescent techniques were applied in experiments reported by BEUTNER and WITEBSKY in 1962 [8]: three different types of antibody could be seen in the fluorescent antibody staining of human thyroid slices by means of human sera from thyroiditis patients. The antigens were characterized by staining of a) the colloid of the thyroid, b) the cytoplasm of the cells of the thyroid epithelium, and c) the nuclei of the thyroid. The reaction with nuclei does not really concern us, since this type of reaction is non-tissue-specific and is found in all organs of the body. The other two reactions, however, indicated that antibodies against thyroglobulin were localized in the colloid, and antibodies against the microsomal[1] antigen in the cellular cytoplasm. The serum of various patients may contain one or another antibody or various proportions of them. These antigens can also be studied in organ culture preparations [31].

ROITT and his group [5, 108] reported finding a third autoantigen, also revealed by immunofluorescent studies and involving staining of the colloid, but in a pattern distinct from that obtained with antibodies to thyroglobulin. This antigen has been designated the CA-2 antigen. It was also studied by HJORT [43].

Studies of the molecular nature of the thyroglobulin antigen have been discussed above. A number of detailed explorations on the various autoantigens and the induced antibody activities, have been made by Rose and his colleagues [3, 21, 53, 115, 161], using the monkey as an experimental model [56]. KITE and WITEBSKY and associates [13, 186] based their experimental model on a strain of chickens. The original rabbit model has been extended by WEIGLE and colleagues [75, 176–182] to cover many parameters of autoantigenicity, tolerance, and related factors. These and other animal models and the various mechanisms thought to be involved in thyroid autoimmunity are discussed in some detail in a recent review of this topic [128].

On the complementary question of the nature of the immunoglobulin response in thyroiditis there has been a considerable body of somewhat contradictory

---

[1] It had been reported in a number of studies that the autoimmune response to the thyroid microsomal antigen did not occur in experimental animals, except for monkeys. It was generally concluded that this autoantigen is active only in primates. A very recent report, however, claims that this microsomal autoimmunity can be achieved in rabbits [65a].

literature, reporting variously that human thyroiditis patients have their autoantibody in the form of a 19 S molecule and a 7 S molecule. (PRESSMAN *et al.* [93]; KORNGOLD *et al.* [58]; TORRIGIANI *et al.* [165, 166]). Undoubtedly, the disagreements reflect genetic differences and probably also the different stages of the disease process. To discover whether the stimulation of autoantibody might follow the schedule now well accepted for ordinary antibody responses, that is, the production of early 19 S antibody followed by later production of 7 S antibody, studies were made with experimental animals, where the time sequence could be controlled. GHAYASUDDIN *et al.* [34, 130] showed that the early response in rabbits stimulated to produce autoantibodies to their thyroglobulin consisted primarily of 19 S antibody, although in very weak titer and difficult to measure precisely. The later bleedings contained overwhelming quantities of 7 S antibody.

b) Autoantigenic Determinant Groups

ROITT *et al.* [104] and SHULMAN *et al.* [135], using somewhat different techniques, worked on quantitative precipitin curves for human autoantibody reacting with human thyroglobulin and found two kinds of curve, one resembling the typical rabbit precipitin curve, and the other resembling the classical horse-type flocculation curve with strong inhibition by excess antibody. In contrast to the earlier studies of STOKINGER and HEIDELBERGER [149], who found that precipitates formed by a heteroantibody (*e.g.* rabbit antibody with human thyroglobulin) the molecular ratio of antibody/antigen ranged from 40:1 to 60:1, it was now observed that with autoantibodies (human antibody with human thyroglobulin) these ratios ranged from 2:1 to 6:1 [104, 133]. These very much smaller values suggested that the autoantibodies are directed to a more restricted portion of the thyroglobulin molecule than are the heteroantibodies. The inference was drawn that the recently developed concept that thyroglobulin can be an autoantigen must be revised. The new hypothesis states only that *certain portions* (or *determinants*) of the thyroglobulin molecule can be autoantigenic [109]. It was reasoned that, of the approximately 50 antigenic determinant groups which might exist on each thyroglobulin molecule, only about 6 would be immunogenic in the stimulation of autoantibody [125, 126, 135], so it should be possible to isolate from the thyroglobulin molecule peptide portions which would interact only with heteroantibodies, and other portions which would react either with autoantibodies alone or with both autoantibodies and heteroantibodies. This will be further discussed below.

It has been pointed out that gel diffusion precipitation between thyroglobulin and its corresponding autoantibody can occur as a split line [136]. This phenomenon was further studied by GOODMAN *et al.* [37] to see whether it might be due to the contribution of antibody in different molecular forms. They concluded, however, that this could not be the explanation. They showed that occasionally as many as three "parallel" lines could be formed. The pattern is always rather peculiar in that the ends of the precipitation arcs are fused, with the middle portions showing a separation; this is just the opposite of the split lines that have been described with regard to extreme excess of antigen or antibody. GOODMAN *et al.* thought some kind of molecular heterogeneity of the antigen must be responsible for the phenomenon.

The hypothesis that only a small fraction of the antigenic determinant groups on the thyroglobulin molecule are actually autoantigenic determinant groups, inspired several further studies[2]. In immunodiffusion experiments, MATES *et al.* [66] showed that the reaction of heteroantibody (rabbit) with a human thyroglobulin sample produced a spur of precipitate over the reaction of autoantibody with the same antigen; this spur formation would seem to be quite consonant with the above hypothesis. Further, rabbit anti-human thyroid antisera gave precipitation with various trypsin-induced molecular fragments of human Tg, whereas a human thyroiditis antiserum, thus containing autoantibodies, did not. MATES *et al.* [67] later showed by means of the passive hemagglutination method that some of the fragments formed from human thyroglobulin after extensive trypsin hydrolysis are in fact able to give some reaction with the human autoantibody, though the same fragments were unable to affect the precipitation reactions.

Artificial mixtures of 19 S thyroglobulin with different quantities of either 27 S component or 12 S component failed to produce precipitation in the split line form; it was therefore concluded that some heterogeneity of the 19 S molecule itself must be responsible for the split line [68]. The antigenic groups on the 4 S and 7 S tissue-specific thyroid proteins were also studied, as they resemble those on the 19 S thyroglobulin molecules [69].

Molecular splitting of human thyroglobulin was carried out by ROSE and STYLOS [116, 150], using material purified by methods previously described [129, 137]. The product was only little characterized physicochemically, but

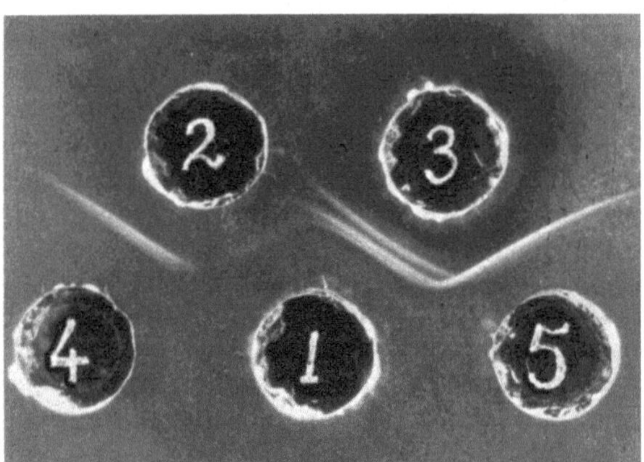

Fig. 2.8. Double-diffusion gel precipitation between (1) a pool 1 sample from a 10-hour tryptic digest of rabbit thyroid extract, (2) an autoantibody serum of rabbit, and (3) a heteroantibody serum of goat, with comparisons of (4) and (5) rabbit thyroglobulin

[2] Recent studies of thyroglobulin by SALABÈ and his colleagues [119a, 119b] have added further support to the concept of distinctive antigenic determinant activities, and have extended the modes of differentiation between autoantigenic and heteroantigenic types of reactivity.

it did show a loss of precipitating reaction with autoantibody and not with heteroantibody. Pepsin fragments behaved quite similarly to trypsin products. Papain fragments precipitated with both kinds of antibody, and chymotrypsin fragments precipitated with neither. No extensive biochemical characterization of the mixtures of peptides was performed, however, and it is not yet feasible to associate these antigenic activities with definite molecular units.

A group of similar studies has been made with rabbit Tg, rabbit autoantibodies and goat heteroantibodies being used for evaluation. Again tryptic digestion was employed, patterned in part after the earlier report of METZGER *et al.* [72]. An interrupted tryptic digest, containing 91 % of a 1.2 S component, showed different patterns of reaction with the two types of antibody. GHAYASUDDIN *et al.* [33, 35, 36] separated these peptide fragments by gel filtration, obtaining eight pools; only pools 1 and 2 precipitated with heteroantibody and only pool 1 precipitated with autoantibody. The pool 1 fraction, that is, the earliest eluted fraction, showed 4 lines of precipitation in gel diffusion with heteroantibody, and 2 lines with autoantibody. This curious pattern is shown in Fig. 2.8, where the merging of lines is also apparent. The fact that some of the peptides failed to precipitate with the autoantibody was taken to confirm that they carried none, or at most one, of the autoantigenic determinant groups. At any rate, these fragments carried more heteroantigenic determinant groups than autoantigenic groups [36]. Further observations of this sort, along with the related problem of precipitating and nonprecipitating forms of the autoantibody, are beyond the scope of this treatment; they have been recently discussed elsewhere [128].

Chapter 3

The Adrenal Gland

We come next to the adrenal gland, which also gives us the opportunity to introduce a special class of tissue-specific antigens that are highly thermostable in character. It is important first to distinguish between the adrenal medulla and the adrenal cortex, which are really two tissues in one organ. Many studies have in fact indicated that a particular antigen of interest is localized in either the medulla or the cortex; other studies have not.

1. Thermostable Antigens of Adrenal

A bovine medulla-specific antigen has been described as thermostable, resisting exposure to boiling water for one hour, and even autoclaving at 120 °C [49]. After this treatment, the material of interest remained soluble and could be precipitated with an appropriate antiserum. A second step in preparing and concentrating this antigen was its precipitation by 71 % ethanol at room temperature. The resulting precipitate could be dried and redissolved in saline. These preparations were termed BE, meaning non-precipitable by *boiling* and insoluble in *ethanol;* this nomenclature was established before there was any knowledge of the glycoprotein nature of this antigen. Indeed, the authors at first quite reasonably supposed the material to be a polysaccharide. Thermostable antigens of the above type had to be differentiated at the outset from the alcohol-*soluble* thermostable antigens that were the subject of much earlier and more classical studies, responsible for the large body of immunological literature which refers to lipid antigens or lipid haptens. The BE antigens resemble them in being thermostable, but are quite different in being *in*soluble in ethanol. A second thermostable antigen was observed, which was *not* specific for the adrenal [49].

Witebsky and Klinke [72] had much earlier described the existence of a thermostable adrenal antigen. Suspensions of bovine adrenal medulla, after being boiled for 30 minutes could still react with an anti-adrenal serum. The modification that was now introduced consisted of heating the adrenal extracts for one hour at 100°, followed by precipitation in 71% ethanol [49]. The substance was both organ-specific and species-specific and was characterized in immunoelectrophoretic analysis as a rapidly moving component that migrates toward the anode.

Milgrom *et al.* [48] later reported the presence of similar thermostable antigens in bovine, porcine, equine, and human adrenal glands. Two components were demonstrated, one species-restricted and the other detected in all the species tested. These antigens were tentatively described as organ-specific haptens because complete Freund's adjuvant had to be used to elicit antibody formation [47]. The adjuvant was thought to act as a carrier for the specific substance.

The chemical properties of the thermostable, adrenal-specific antigen of bovine origin were studied by SHULMAN *et al.* [60]. Ultracentrifugal and electrophoretic examination revealed these preparations to be quite heterogeneous. Direct analysis in the ultracentrifuge showed three sedimenting boundaries, with sedimentation coefficients of 5.7 S, 2.7 S, and 1.9 S. The corresponding molecular weights were estimated to be well below 50000. Moving-boundary electrophoresis revealed even greater heterogeneity; there were 4 to 7 components in different preparations with mobilities from -12.3 to -1.2×10^{-5} cm^2 volt^{-1} sec^{-1}. The total macromolecular material contained 8% of hexose and 2.8% of hexosamine. Studies on the absorption of light by these preparations suggested that nucleic acid contributed 1/10 to 1/2 as much solute mass as did the protein.

Because of the high degree of heterogeneity in BE preparations, the approach involved using various inactivating agents to destroy the antigenic activity rather than attempting direct characterization of chemical properties. Exposure to sodium periodate failed to destroy the antigenic activity, whereas in control experiments blood-group-A substance was easily destroyed. On the other hand, the specific antigenic property was readily destroyed by chymotrypsin at an enzyme-substrate ratio of 1 to 50. This observation suggested that the antigenic component is most likely of protein nature. Because of this property and the heat stability, along with the high carbohydrate content, it was tentatively concluded that the antigen itself is a mucoprotein [60], but further characterization must await better purification of the antigen.

RIFÉ [56] showed that among the cellular particulates that were separated from a tissue homogenate, the BE antigen of bovine adrenal medulla was predominantly associated with the microsomes. Ribosomes were inactive and this suggested that the antigen may be associated with the endoplasmic reticulum. There is no clear relationship between this localization of the antigen and its chemical nature as a mucoprotein or glycoprotein, but this aspect merits further study. Although not related to the thermostable group, other tissue antigens, notably of liver and kidney, have also been associated with microsomes [19, 53, 55, 65], and a certain human adrenal antigen (further discussed below) has also been associated with the microsomes [21].

2. Thermolabile Antigens of Adrenal

A totally different type of adrenal-specific antigen has been described [73], which is highly thermolabile and found largely in the adrenal cortex. This antigen could also elicit autoantibodies. In the initial study, guinea pigs and rabbits were immunized with the same preparations in adjuvant of adrenal homogenates obtained from a number of species of animal. This procedure yielded excellent examples of the two types of tissue specificity. The rabbit antisera reacted not only with saline extracts of rabbit adrenals, but also with adrenal extracts from guinea pig, man, ox, and rat. In contrast, the guinea pig antiserum reacted exclusively with adrenal extract from guinea pig; the antigen was not present in any other tissues of the guinea pig nor in adrenals of any other species. The antigenic activity was thermolabile and was destroyed by ethanol. It could be fully precipitated by 1.35 *M* ammonium sulfate and it thus corresponded to an adrenal globulin.

Subsequent studies were carried out on the physical and chemical nature of the resulting rabbit adrenal-specific autoantigen [13, 59]. The ultracentrifuge revealed a group of components with a predominant 3.9 S peak and additional components with faster sedimentation coefficients, such as 6.6, 10.0, 11.8, and 18.1 S. There was some evidence that the antigen was associated with the 6.6 S component. Salting out with ammonium sulfate revealed that the antigenic material was precipitated in the range between 0.00 and 1.50 *M* of this salt. Digestion with chymotrypsin readily destroyed antigenic activity, indicating that the antigen is very likely a protein.

CENTENO *et al.* [15] later found a *group* of adrenal antigens of this type. The rabbit antisera prepared by immunization with rabbit adrenal homogenates plus Freund's adjuvant were concentrated and proved to be mixtures of three or four distinct antibodies to adrenal extract. The methods used were extensive removal of water from the antiserum by osmotic concentration with sucrose, or the precipitation of γ-globulin by 1.40 *M* ammonium sulfate, the precipitate then being redissolved in a small volume of saline. The addition to this saline of 25% human serum albumin seemed to reduce the incidence of nonspecific precipitation around the edge of the well in the gel diffusion plate. The pattern shown in Fig. 3.1 illustrates this multiplicity of components. At least three

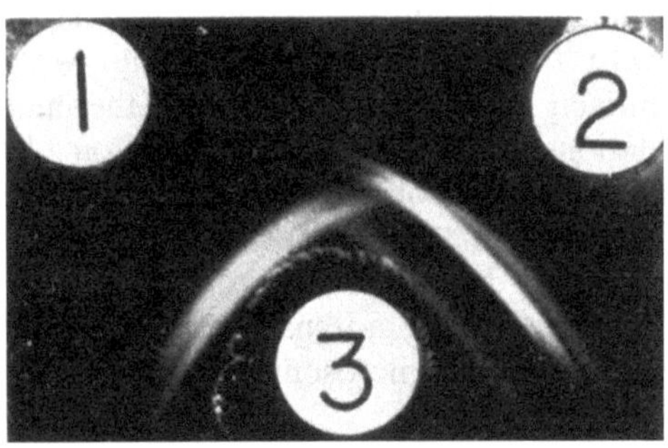

Fig. 3.1. Double-diffusion gel precipitation of (1) bovine adrenal medulla extract and (2) rabbit adrenal extract against (3) γ-globulin preparation from a rabbit antiserum to rabbit adrenal

of the antibodies were proved to be autoantibodies by direct testing with the antibody-producer's adrenal tissue; it was shown that the adrenal medulla contained two of the antigens and the cortex one of the others. However, there are great difficulties in the unequivocal separation of cortex and medulla in the rabbit, so that the evidence is still somewhat incomplete. As there is known to be some antigenic cross-reaction between bovine and rabbit adrenal, the separated medulla and cortex of bovine adrenal were also used, as seen in Fig. 3.1.

HELLE [24, 25] has studied the soluble protein fractions of adrenal chromaffin granules from several species. Gel diffusion tests with a rabbit antiserum to bovine material indicated that ovine and bovine preparations contain common determinants whereas equine and porcine soluble proteins are antigenically different from bovine proteins. It is not yet clear what relationship these antigens might have to the other (labile) antigens of the adrenal described above. Further chemical studies were made by WINKLER *et al.* [71].

3. Experimental Adrenalitis

There have been efforts to induce the formation of adrenal lesions and damage by immunization. The procedures usually employed preparations of whole adrenal glands with Freund's complete adjuvant, and therefore the lesions were localized in both cortex and medulla. In the earliest work COLOVER and GLYNN [17] used material from non-inbred guinea pigs and termed the resulting condition isoimmune adrenalitis. MILCOU *et al.* [46] observed histologically lesions in the adrenal cortical tissue of rabbits immunized with rabbit adrenal glands. They also detected autoantibodies by complement fixation and precipitation methods. STEINER *et al.* [63] found that autoimmunization in guinea pigs produced lesions in medulla and cortex, whereas control animals that received adjuvant alone, or suspensions of other organs with adjuvant, did not show any adrenal damage. They did not examine the sera of these animals for antibody responses. The adrenal lesions consisted largely of focal infiltrations of lymphocytes, plasma cells, and histiocytes, located between the parenchymal cells and the sinusoidal endothelium. KRACHT *et al.* [36] saw circulating antibodies and histologic changes in adrenals of guinea pigs immunized with either homologous or autologous material.

Later work by BARNETT *et al.* [4], indicated that damage was more severe when the adrenal material used came from a different species. These authors failed to produce adrenal lesions in rabbits when rabbit material was injected, whereas with injection of guinea pig material rabbits showed adrenal damage. They also warned that the adrenal antigens found in complement fixation tests might be different from those revealed by immunofluorescence in the cortical cells. This could explain the general observation that in adrenal immunization studies it is difficult to correlate the incidence and degree of lesion development with antibody formation. This same work also indicated some interesting cross-reactions between adrenal antigens and those of testis and ovary; the tissue staining results were especially interesting. When reacted with sera from rabbits immunized with rabbit or guinea pig adrenal, the interstitial cells of rabbit ovary specifically took up fluorescent stain. Cytoplasmic staining in the adrenal involved all three layers of the cortex, but only the cortex. In addition, Leydig cells and spermatids were stained, as were also mature epididymal sperm, after exposure to serum from rabbits immunized with homologous adrenal; in contrast, with sera from rabbits that had been immunized with guinea pig adrenal, only the Leydig cells were stained. This was thought to suggest that there is an antigen common to sperm and adrenal cortex of rabbit that is not present in guinea pig adrenal. On the other hand, other antigens present in rabbit adrenal cortex, ovarian interstitial cells, and Leydig cells are also present in guinea pig adrenal. It would seem from this work that there are at least two antigens in sperm, only one of which is present in adrenal cortex of the same species. Sperm antigens are further analyzed and discussed in Chapter 5.

TERPLAN *et al.* [64] sounded a cautionary note after inoculating guinea pigs and rabbits with homologous or autologous adrenal suspensions in the usual adjuvant preparations. Many of the animals displayed histologic changes, and the sera contained specific adrenal antibodies. However, the appearance and severity of the lesions could not be correlated in any regular way with the serologic data. Further, some of the control animals injected with various other tissue preparations showed very similar histologic changes in their adrenals. The authors concluded that one should not interpret the observed adrenalitis only in terms of an immune response to adrenal antigens.

In a series of more recent studies, LEVINE and his colleagues introduced the rat as an experimental animal for adrenalitis. They showed that inbred (Lewis) rats could develop adrenalitis after a single injection into the foot pad [43] or even directly into cervical lymph nodes [41] of isologous or homologous adrenal homogenate with adjuvants. In some experiments, pertussis vaccine was added to the adrenal-Freund's adjuvant mixture injected into the foot pad, and this produced striking histologic lesions [43]. Lesions also appeared in the absence of pertussis vaccine when isologous tissue was used, but antigen alone in Freund's complete adjuvant gave reactions of lesser severity. With homologous tissue, in contrast, no lesions occurred without the pertussis adjuvant. No serologic studies were reported. Nonetheless, there was adequate control of specificity, since there was complete absence of adrenalitis after injection of the double adjuvant without tissue, or with incorporation of isologous spinal cord, testis, or pituitary tissue. Adrenalitis was also induced by passive transfer from actively immunized donors to normal recipients through the use of living lymph node cells [43]. Transfer could also be achieved by use of whole blood [40], although this required the use of recipient animals which had received a prior thermal injury to the adrenal tissue. Adrenalitis was also established in transplanted adrenals, grafted into immunized animals [42].

Further studies were made of lesion induction and the significance of the blood-tissue barrier. There were clear distinctions between adrenal and neural antigens in the induction of tissue lesions [39]. LEVINE [38] also investigated the role of steroids and showed that they were not involved in the formation or prevention of experimental adrenalitis, since neonatal adrenal is at least as good as adult adrenal in provoking adrenalitis (although neonatal tissue does contain low levels of steroids). This is an indication that the antigen is present immediately after birth and confirms serological findings in the rabbit system by other authors [4]. With regard to the rat, it was found that several heterologous species provided adrenal tissue that could stimulate rat adrenalitis. These species included cow, guinea pig, gerbil, and (better) dog and rabbit, but such lesions were invariably mild and were produced only when the adjuvant included the pertussis vaccine [38]. We may contrast the situation in guinea pig and rabbit where heterologous tissue is quite effective, as was noted above. The different strains of inbred rats were compared as regards isologous systems: the BN strain was as active as the Lewis strain, but the Fischer 344 and Wistar-Furth strains had lower susceptibility. A final point concerning the site of the lesions is that the medulla is probably much less involved than the cortex. In some experiments the medullary tissue was enucleated and the remaining organ was quite effective as either antigenic stimulus or target tissue for adrenalitis [38]. These indications that the cortex contains the principal antigen(s) of interest are in harmony with earlier serological work, which showed the cortex to contain certain autoantigen(s) [4].

Additional studies have been carried out on rats: functional disturbances of the adrenal tissues have been provoked in preliminary form [28], following immunization with a preparation in complete Freund's adjuvant containing either cortical and medullary tissue. The report indicated both morphologic and functional disturbances of the adrenal tissues in the injected animals, apparently correlated with immune responses. Although the studies were rather limited, they are of considerable interest in the light of suggestions that autoimmunization may be a factor in idiopathic Addison's disease, especially where there is atrophy of the cortical tissue in this human disease, as further discussed below. IRINO and GROLLMAN [29] also studied the ultrastructural details in rats that developed immune adrenalitis, as did HOENIG *et al.* [26] in a different approach. The former group emphasized the deterioration of the secretory cells and the development of cortical insufficiency, whereas the latter group showed more interest in the inflammation and emphasized the role of the lymphocyte. Further detailed studies have been made by WERDELIN and colleagues [68, 69] of the mechanisms which might be independent or related phenomena in experimental adrenalitis in rats: cellular proliferation in the draining lymph node, or the circulating lymphocytes, and the adrenal inflammation. They used a method of radio-labeling the popliteal lymph node cells and then tracing their migrations.

In a study by ANDRADA *et al.* [3] Lewis rats of both sexes were immunized with rat adrenal extract in complete Freund's adjuvant, and histologic evidence of adrenalitis was obtained in 37 of 55 females (70%) and 4 of 15 males (27%). Not only was the frequency of adrenal lesions higher in the females, it was also noted that the lesions were generally milder in the male rats. That Freund's adjuvant was necessary to elicit adrenal lesions was shown by giving 10 female rats intradermal injection of adrenal extract alone; only one of these controls showed a very slight histological abnormality, and the other nine had completely normal adrenals. The lesions consisted of mononuclear cell infiltrations, localized in the fasciculata and reticularis zones of the cortex; by contrast, the lesions described in rabbits and guinea pigs were located mainly at the junction of the reticularis zone and the medulla. Rats which received only one injection showed the first adrenal abnormalities 9 days afterwards, the majority of the definite lesions being observed at 11 to 19 days. Later the lesions regressed and subsequent injections did not seem to increase either the frequency or severity of the lesions.

Of serum samples from 76 immunized rats, 12 gave positive results in immunofluorescence tests with rat adrenal sections, but not with sections of other rat organs. The bright fluorescence was usually seen on all three zones of the cortex but never in the medulla. The antiserum titers were rather low. The reactions were thus strictly tissue-specific, inasmuch as these anti-adrenal sera showed no reactions with sections of thyroid, liver, kidney, testis, and ovary. The histological results showed similar specificity: rats immunized with adrenal extract as described above rarely had lesions in other tissues, such as liver, kidney, thyroid, and gonads. Two or three animals showed slight changes in kidney or testis structure; however, this may be evidence of a minor activity of some importance, for in a group of rats injected with testicular extract 2 of 15 animals developed mild adrenal lesions. No such lesions appeared in the 50 rats injected with various other tissue extracts, *e.g.*, thyroid, liver, kidney, pancreas, ovary, or with Freund's adjuvant alone. In complement fixation tests with rat adrenal extract, 69 sera gave unequivocally negative results and the remaining 7 gave weak positive results, which could not be interpreted in any meaningful way.

It has also been claimed that rhesus monkeys injected with homologous adrenal extract in Freund's adjuvant developed mild but significant histological changes in the adrenal cortex, and that there was some evidence of formation of adrenal-specific antibodies; however, no details were presented [3]. Studies have also been carried out on BSVS mice immunized with either bovine or murine adrenal homogenates [67]. The results emphasized and described the tissue- and species-specific adrenal antigens of bovine origin, but left unanswered the question of adrenal-specific antigens in the mouse.

4. Human Adrenalitis

There have been a number of studies to test the possibility that Addison's disease is due to an autoimmune mechanism. STEINER *et al.* [63] and TERPLAN *et al.* [64] had stated that the histologic changes seen in experimental adrenalitis do not constitute a model for the cytotoxic atrophy of the human adrenal that is present in Addison's disease. Nonetheless, antibodies against adrenal have been sought in the serum of patients with Addison's disease. Before any experimental animal studies had been made, ANDERSON *et al.* [2] found complement-fixing antibodies directed against adrenal tissue in two out of ten patients with Addison's disease, whereas tests with other organ extracts were negative, except for thyroid, which gave positive results with the same two sera. BLIZZARD *et al.* [10] used the immunofluorescence method and showed the presence of antibodies in 16 out of 30 patients with Addison's disease. The localization of these autoantigens was in the cytoplasm of the cortical cells; in 14 of the 16 cases, staining was seen in all layers of the cortex, two others showing staining only in the fasciculate zone. In contrast, they obtained completely negative results with sera from 15 cases of Cushing's syndrome or of virilizing hyperplasia. Both groups of investigators found that a significant fraction of their positive sera also reacted with thyroid material; conversely, many sera from patients with thyroiditis were positive only with thyroid and completely negative to adrenal. It was concluded that these two antigen-antibody systems were quite distinct, but that there must be frequent concurrent activity of the two systems. This concept of concurrent activity is not unexpected, since WELLS [66] in 1930 showed that patients with idiopathic Addison's disease had lymphocytic infiltration of the thyroid, whereas patients with tuberculous Addison's disease seldom showed any such infiltration. Similar findings were reported by SLOPER [61]. This association between adrenal and thyroid diseases has also been recorded by others [2, 8, 11, 12, 16, 27, 45]. From histologic and serological findings it was suggested that patients with one type of autoimmune endocrine disease are liable to have another [10]. Despite these definite cross-reactions, the organ specificity of the antigens present in human adrenal disease has been amply demonstrated. Which specific adrenal antigens are involved? The cellular particulates were studied and the activity was apparently found in both the microsomal and mitochondrial fractions of adrenal homogenates [9], but it was not clear how well separated these fractions were. GOUDIE *et al.* [21] produced evidence that all the activity is in the microsomes. All the above studies dealt with circulating anti-adrenal antibodies but recent activity has extended to a search for cellular hypersensitivity in cases of Addison's disease [50–52, 50a]. The cellular antigen, however, has been found in the mitochondrial fraction only. On this basis, and also because they found no correlation between the occurrence of humoral and cellular immunity although both were frequently found, NERUP and BENDIXEN [52] argued that the antigens in the different particulates are quite different.

It has become clear that for immunological purposes one should distinguish two categories of Addison's disease: one caused by tuberculous infection, and the other idiopathic in origin. It seems that the idiopathic form is the one where there is a significant degree of correlation with antibodies against adrenal components whereas such antibodies are hardly ever found in the tuberculous form. The idiopathic form is often associated with hypoparathyroidism and steatorrhea [6, 9, 22, 23, 30–32, 37, 44, 62, 70]. In a recent summation [22] of several studies, involving a total of 178 patients who had been diagnosed as having idiopathic Addison's disease [20, 35], adrenal antibodies were demonstrated by immunofluorescent observation in the serum of approximately 40 to 60 per cent of the patients, whereas incidence was less than 1 per cent in 650 miscellaneous patients who had neither Addison's disease nor hypoparathyroidism. Further, BLIZZARD *et al.* [7] demonstrated adrenal antibodies in 6 of 56 patients with idiopathic hypoparathyroidism, but who did not have overt Addison's disease; this was attributed to the presence of subclinical adrenalitis. The possibility of symptomless chronic adrenalitis has been indicated [57]. GOUDIE *et al.* [22], found that serum from a patient with presumed Addison's disease gave immunofluorescent staining with sections of testis, ovary, and placenta, as well as with adrenal tissue (cf. similar results in studies on experimental adrenalitis). This activity was not absorbed or removed by any of the steroid hormones with which the patient had been treated [21] although it would be quite possible for such steroids to act as haptens in inducing antibody formation [5]. Similar findings of cross-reaction with testis and/or ovary by sera from some cases of Addison's disease have been reported by others [1, 6, 33, 34].

Chapter 4

The Brain

1. The Several Brain-Specific Antigens

In 1926, BRANDT, GUTH, and MÜLLER showed that when rabbits were injected with an alcoholic extract of bovine brain tissue mixed with hog serum as a carrier, the antibodies formed were specific to brain components [22]. This work was extended in 1928 by WITEBSKY and STEINFELD [264] who immunized rabbits by intravenous injection of aqueous suspensions of brain tissue from other species and found that tissue-specific anti-brain antibodies formed. Using the method of complement fixation testing, they observed high titers in reactions between brain antisera and brain suspensions, but much lower titers with other organ suspensions. In some cases slight cross-reaction was seen with kidney suspensions but was destroyed by heating for 2 minutes at 100 °C. Two types of antisera were recognized: some reacted only with brain preparations from the species providing the immunizing material, but others reacted with brain suspensions of other animal species, including rabbit. One type of antiserum had antibodies against a protein that was both organ- and species-specific. The other type of antiserum reacted with a lipid hapten and contained antibodies that were organ-specific but reacted with brain suspensions of all species tested. WITEBSKY and STEINFELD also found that antisera against a heated aqueous homogenate of bovine brain reacted equally well with alcoholic extracts of bovine, rabbit and guinea pig brain, so allowing further clarification of the distinction between two types of brain antisera. One type contained antibodies elicited by the heat-stable, organ-specific brain lipid. The antibodies in the other antiserum were directed against a thermolabile, organ-specific, species-restricted protein component of bovine brain present in the aqueous homogenate along with the lipid. The antibodies against the lipid were found to react with rabbit brain also, and they were designated as autoantibodies. There is a third type of brain-specific antigen, a thermostable protein, which will be discussed below, and yet other protein antigens which will be dealt with in several additional categories. Some similar antigenic classes have been examined in avian brain tissue [77], but the present discussion will be restricted to mammalian systems.

2. The Lipid Haptens

a) Glycolipids as Normal Organ-Specific Haptens

Satisfactory progress has been made with regard to the chemical structure of the original lipid hapten of brain, as described by WITEBSKY [264]. In 1963 JOFFE, RAPPORT, and GRAF [96] identified this hapten as a (galacto)cerebroside and further details were given by RAPPORT *et al.* [212]. This substance is of a type found in the brain tissue of many species; it belongs to the larger group of substances that are termed glycolipids. Glycolipids are compounds which contain one or more carbohydrate residues in addition to one or more residues of lipid nature, such as fatty acids. The history of immunological studies on antigens of various tissues is replete with references to alcohol-soluble antigens. This specific hapten of brain was one of the first to be identified and is a classic example of an alcohol-soluble hapten. Other important milestones in the immunological literature are the Forssman hapten (*or* antigen) and the group-specific substances of erythrocytes. For half a century these alcohol-soluble antigens were assumed to be chemically identified as lipids, but it is now becoming increasingly clear that in all probability they are actually glycolipids. While the lipid residue may be of greater importance for determining extractability into an alcohol phase, it may well be that the sugar residue is more important in determining the antigenic specificity of the substance. There are many types of glycolipids, but the particular sub-group of interest here is that of the cerebrosides. The members of this group do not contain phosphorus, and on hydrolysis they yield a lipid portion and a hexose sugar. In most cases the hexose is galactose and for this reason the members of the group are sometimes termed galactolipids. It is possible, however, to have glucose as a replacement. A typical galactocerebroside molecule is shown in Fig. 4.1. On complete hydrolysis each galactocerebroside molecule yields one molecule each of sphingosine, galactose, and a fatty acid. Since there can be several types of fatty acid, there is a corresponding variety of galactocerebrosides.

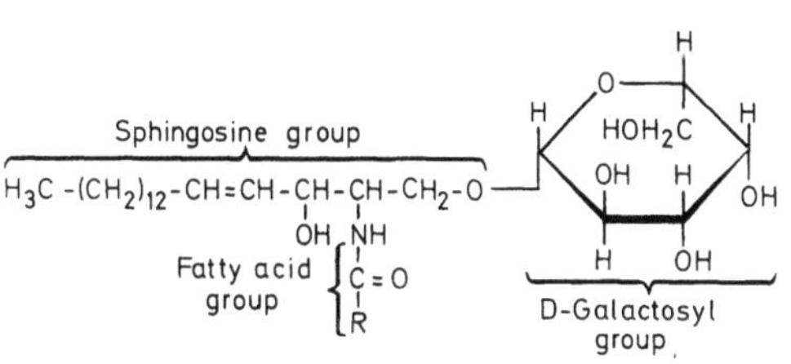

Fig. 4.1. Structural formula for a galactocerebroside

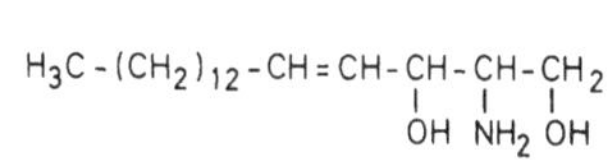

Fig. 4.2. Structural formula for sphingosine

First, let us look at sphingosine, a base that is present in small amounts in many tissues but predominantly in nervous tissue; it is also considered to be a component of all cell membranes. This base occurs most characteristically in the substance termed sphingomyelin. Our interest here is in sphingosine itself. As can be seen from Fig. 4.2, this compound is a primary alcohol, a secondary alcohol, and a primary amine simultaneously. The primary alcohol and primary amine groups connect this residue to the two other residues in the cerebroside molecule. The fatty-acid component of the cerebroside is generally of the 24-carbon variety, although 18-carbon molecules have also been reported. Two important galacterocerebrosides are cerasin (cerasine), which contains lignoceric acid as its fatty acid, and phrenosin (phrenosine), which contains 2-hydroxylignoceric acid. Other examples are nervon and oxynervon, and various compounds in which the double bond of the sphingosine is in reduced form, giving dihydrosphingosine. Rapport and colleagues [96, 212], using the method of complement fixation, found that brain-specific antiserum reacts with galactocerebrosides. The hapten was partially isolated by extraction with chloroform and methanol followed by absorption chromatography on alumina. The fraction that displayed activity was further purified by chromatography on silicic acid, with methanol in chloroform as the eluting agent. The pure active component was a galactocerebroside, either cerasin or phrenosin or both (Fig. 4.3).

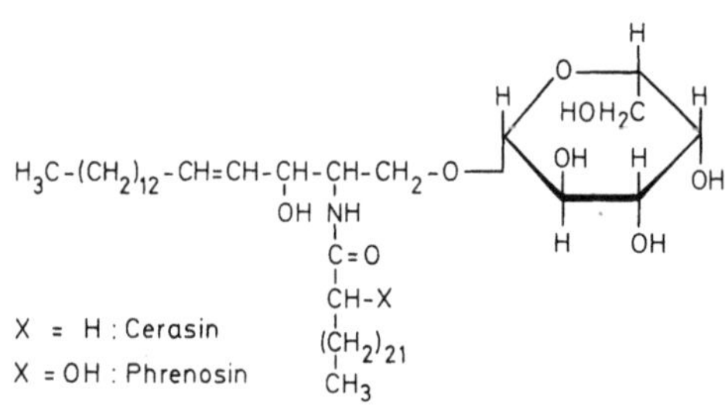

Fig. 4.3. Structural formula for cerasin or phrenosin

RAPPORT *et al.* [96] tested their specific antisera with galactocerebrosides and glucocerebrosides of several kinds. All the preparations of galactocerebroside showed activity but the glucocerebrosides were uniformly unreactive. Obviously the precise structure of the sugar residue determines the antibody specificity in this type of glycolipid; the same will probably be true of other glycolipids. The authors emphasized that these galactocerebrosides are common to the brain tissue of many species but virtually absent from other organs; thus they correspond very well to the brain-specific properties of the lipid hapten described many years earlier. We have thus seen the end of the trail leading to the definition of the classic lipid antigen specific for brain. We can expect related trails of inquiry to be pursued in future studies, such as the antigenic properties of the gangliosides, as discussed in the next section.

b) Gangliosides as Antigenic Markers of Disease

An interesting extension of the earlier studies is the finding that (rabbit) antibodies can be used to distinguish between certain chemical fractions isolated from normal human brain and from brain tissue of infants suffering from Tay-

Sachs disease [193, 194, 268]. The fractions were preparations of the ganglioside groups of glycosphingolipids, differing from the cerebrosides, which are also glycosphingolipids, in containing the additional residues of N-acetylgalactosamine and N-acetylneuraminic acid (sialic acid) along with the moieties shown in both of these subgroups, *i.e.*, glucose, galactose, and ceramide, the latter being sphingosine (or a related base) combined with a fatty acid. This ability to make an immunochemical distinction of brain tissues is based on the complexity of gangliosides that can be present. SVENNERHOLM [241], using thin-layer chromatography, showed that normal brain tissue contains at least ten different gangliosides, although four of them constitute 90% of the total; in contrast,

Table 4.1. *Reactions of isolated gangliosides with antisera to normal human gangliosides (NHG) and Tay-Sachs gangliosides (TSG)*

Ganglioside	Structure[a]	Immunodiffusion reaction with[b]: anti-NHG	anti-TSG
G_1	Cer ← 1 Glu 4 $\xleftarrow{\beta}$ 1 Gal 4 $\xleftarrow{\beta}$ 1 GalNA 3 $\xleftarrow{\beta}$ 1 Gal 3 $\xleftarrow{\beta}$ 2 NANA (Gal) 3 ↑ 2 NANA 8 ← 2 NANA	Negative	—
G_2	Cer ← 1 Glu 4 $\xleftarrow{\beta}$ 1 Gal 4 $\xleftarrow{\beta}$ 1 GalNA 3 $\xleftarrow{\beta}$ 1 Gal 3 (Gal) 3 ↑ 2 NANA 8 ← 2 NANA	Positive	—
G_3	Cer ← 1 Glu 4 $\xleftarrow{\beta}$ 1 Gal 4 $\xleftarrow{\beta}$ 1 GalNA 3 $\xleftarrow{\beta}$ 1 Gal 3 ← 2 NANA (Gal) 3 ↑ 2 NANA	Negative	Negative
G_4	Cer ← 1 Glu 4 $\xleftarrow{\beta}$ 1 Gal 4 $\xleftarrow{\beta}$ 1 GalNA 3 $\xleftarrow{\beta}$ 1 Gal (Gal) 3 ↑ 2 NANA	Positive	Negative
G_5	Cer ← 1 Glu 4 $\xleftarrow{\beta}$ 1 Gal 4 $\xleftarrow{\beta}$ GalNA (Gal) 3 ↑ 2 NANA	Negative	Positive

Table adapted from PASCAL and SAIFER [110].

[a] Cer = ceramide; Glu = glucose; Gal = galactose; GalNA = N-acetylgalactosamine; NANA = N-acetylneuraminic (sialic) acid.

[b] NHG = ganglioside purified from normal human brain; TSG = ganglioside purified from Tay-Sachs brain.

one of the minor gangliosides accounts for 90% of the total in patients with Tay-Sachs disease. Each compound can be distinguished chemically by the content of sialic acid [221]. Enzyme deficiency may be a factor in the disease mechanism [188]. The four major gangliosides in the normal brain were first reported by KUHN *et al.* [124]. Further studies revealed the subtleties in these structures with regard to the points of attachment of the sialic acid residues [121, 125, 126]. SAIFER and colleagues [192] have used quantitative and double diffusion precipitation techniques to reveal a number of details by which the antiserum specificity for several pure gangliosides can be correlated with the structural details of the arrangement and number of saccharide units. Table 4.1 summarizes some of these immunochemical distinctions and also shows the structures of five gangliosides [192].

3. The Basic Proteins; Allergic Encephalomyelitis (AE)

In 1934 SCHWENTKER and RIVERS [223] reported that brain tissue could even be made to be autoantigenic if it were given with vaccinia virus or allowed to autolyze under sterile conditions and then given in repeated injections. They also found that a significant number of animals injected with brain tissue developed paralysis of the hind legs and most of these died within a few days. Histological examination of the brain tissue showed perivascular infiltration and necrosis. This was the beginning of the work on allergic encephalomyelitis (AE), and there have since been numerous studies on this type of severe tissue damage which can be experimentally elicited by an immunization precedure and involves the formation of specific autoantibodies. In 1947, KABAT *et al.* [97] and MORGAN [180] injected brain suspensions in Freund's adjuvant into monkeys. Allergic encephalomyelitis developed after a single injection. FREUND *et al.* [76] made similar studies in guinea pigs. The presence of killed mycobacteria in the emulsion was essential, but the injection of other organ homogenates in this way failed to produce the characteristic paralysis. A very large number of studies, has appeared in recent years concerning the chemical nature of the tissue-specific antigen responsible for this autoimmune response, and much controversy has arisen. STONE *et al.* [239] emphasized the difference between acute and chronic forms of the disease as seen in different strains of guinea pig. A number of review articles have given detailed descriptions of the initiation of this experimental disease, and also of the effective antigenic tissues, the variations in different animal species, the means of transferring the disease to normal animals, the various activities of the autoantibodies formed, the genetic factors in susceptibility to the disease, and the general chemical nature of the autoantigen [4–6, 109, 138, 197, 198, 257].

a) Induction, Transfer, and Suppression of AE

We should first consider a few of the main factors in this experimental autoimmune disease. THOMAS *et al.* [249] showed that injection of dog brain extract in complete Freund's adjuvant to dogs was followed by paralysis in one to two weeks. Histological study revealed extensive demyelination. Complement-fixing antibodies appeared, but there was no correlation between titer and the severity of the disease. A number of other studies published at about the same time described the pathology and histopathology in this disease [2, 20, 41, 91, 94, 114, 122, 166, 182, 186, 231, 237, 240]. It is now well established that it can be produced in most mammals and birds by means of suitable immunization with preparations from brain or from spinal cord. It is a model for the autoimmune diseases and also for the demyelinating diseases of neurological interest. Examination of the nature of the tissue-specific agent and the reasons why some animal species have agents more antigenic than those of other species has proved rewarding. Exploration of the parameters of sensitization in production of the disease and recovery from it has also been important. WAKSMAN *et al.* reported a delayed hypersensitivity response in rabbits immunized in a similar way. The AE developed at the same time as the maximum response to cutaneous testing. Many subsequent studies have yielded added evidence for the involvement of a hypersensitivity mechanism in this disease response [4, 5, 11, 14, 21, 71, 129, 195, 230, 236]. The skin reactivity to a purified encephalitogenic substance, which will be described below, correlates closely with the development of AE [230]. In addition, AE can be transferred to normal animals by transfer of sensitized lymph node cells [70, 72, 73, 131, 195, 215, 216, 236, 238]. Complement-dependent mechanisms do not seem to be involved in the development of lesions [140]. Furthermore, the experimental manipulations that interfere with lymphocytes and delayed hypersensitivity also interfere with AE [21]. Recently, cellular migration and its inhibition has been used in evaluation of the state of hypersensitivity in such studies, as has lymphocyte transformation [47].

In PATERSON'S demonstration [195] that in rats this disease could be transferred in cells, the cells were deposited in recipient rats which had been made tolerant to antigens of the donor rat to allow adequate survival of the cells. The recipient animals did develop characteristic lesions of the nervous system. Later studies in various laboratories emphasized the advantage of using inbred strains to assure cell survival; these have been reviewed in detail [197]. The severity of the lesions decreased if repeated transfers of such cells were made [144, 242]. In a different approach, LEVINE and colleagues studied the effects of radiation [145] and of steroids [151] on the enhancement or suppression of passive transfer results. They also showed that the incubation period after passive transfer can be substantially shortened if large doses of cells are used and the recipients are adrenalectomized [155].

PATERSON and HARWIN [206] and PATERSON *et al.* [200] showed that the complement-fixing antibodies in fact suppressed AE in rats following injection of spinal cord material when an intravenous injection of rat serum containing these antibodies was given at the same time. The antibodies may combine with the antigenic site and so block the action of a cytotoxic antibody or of sensitized cells, or the passively transferred antibody may cause general suppression of active immune responses. PATERSON [196] suggested that AE is a disease of delayed hypersensitivity involving the lymphoid cells and the brain tissue and in which a cytotoxic antibody against myelin is found.

Other methods of inhibition have been studied [9], *e.g.*, injection of encephalitogenic material in *incomplete* adjuvant, as described by ALVORD *et al.* [10], or intravenous injection of the antigen after skin reactivity of AE has developed, as reported by LEVINE *et al.* [142, 143]. A durable inhibiting effect of cyclophosphamide has also been reported [205], and a number of recent reports deal with the action of this immunosuppressive agent [199, 201, 203, 204]. Another immunosuppressive drug, L-asparaginase, has recently been shown to suppress AE [100]. Other aspects of the role of adjuvant, and especially the mycobacteria, have been discussed, along with other parameters in suppression [55, 72, 108, 117, 156, 162, 181, 222, 226–229, 232, 255]. More recent studies have described inhibition or suppression of AE, and even the correction of existing AE, by the use of purified basic proteins, *i.e.*, the encephalitogens, as will be discussed in detail below (EINSTEIN *et al.* [55], LEVINE *et al.* [149], and EYLAR *et al.* [65]).

Levine and colleagues have emphasized the study of AE in the rat. They showed that the Freund's adjuvant could be totally dispensed with, first in a study in CD-F rats [153], although in these animals, guinea pig cord homogenate had to be used in place of rat tissue, and the animals had to be pretreated with pertussis vaccine. AE was induced more easily in the Lewis rat [154], where inoculation with spinal cord material sufficed, and neither Freund's adjuvant nor pertussis vaccine was needed; the active antigen came from Lewis rats. The amount of antigen required in these studies was 200 to 400 times the amount needed in the presence of adjuvant [159]. Correlations between hyperacute and milder forms of AE have been described [146, 156], as well as the genetic factors and histocompatibility barriers among rat strains [150, 158]. The hyperacute form is characterized by an infiltration with polymorphonuclear leukocytes as the predominant form (rather than mononuclear cells), along with edema and fibrin. In some conditions the administration of cyclophosphamide also favors invasion with polymorphonuclear cells [141, 148]. LEVINE and coworkers also described the extent to which brain or cord tissue from heterologous sources was effective in producing AE in the rat; they found that antigen from mammalian (rat, guinea pig, human), avian (chicken), reptilian (turtle), and amphibian (frog) sources was active, but that antigen taken from fish (carp) was ineffective [152].

PATERSON *et al.* [202] have also described a number of factors involved in the induction of AE in rat, and have reported studies on cerebrospinal fluid in rabbits with AE [207]. Metabolic changes in the brain have been described in AE in rabbits [262].

b) Chemical Nature of the Encephalitogenic Factor

The causative antigen(s) of the inflammatory and demyelinating disease, AE, were originally termed the encephalitogenic factor(s) and are now considered to be certain basic proteins of myelin, although several other kinds of substance were earlier proposed as the encephalitogenic factor. The fact that myelin is the antigen-containing component has been well established for some years. There are a number of reasons for this conclusion: lesions are more frequent in white matter than in gray [257, p. 4]; immunofluorescence studies with AE serum show localization on myelin [19]; central nervous system tissue from immature animals, where myelination is absent, is nonencephalitogenic [98, 256]; the activity of fractionated products of neural tissue is in proportion to their content of myelin [127]; white matter is more strongly encephalitogenic than is gray matter [180], and spinal cord, which has a higher content of white matter, is more active than brain [119]; siccacell preparations are sometimes active [157]. Some of the additional evidence has been well summarized by LEVINE and WENK [152] in their studies on AE in rats. They found that the encephalitogenicity of various tissues, including spinal cord, brain, white matter, gray matter, glioma, pineal gland, and peripheral nerve, was proportional to the content of myelin in each.

Some of the most important aspects of the chemical identity of the encephalitogen(s) are discussed below. Additional details of properties and comparative data on various kinds of preparations can be found elsewhere [3, 6].

α) Proteolipids and Collagen-Like Proteins

The first type of antigen proposed as the encephalitogenic factor was the group of proteolipids. These substances have been under examination since 1951, soon after the report of HOTTLE *et al.* [91] that the encephalitogenic factor is dialyzable; it had not then been definitely established that the dialyzable material was a protein. Proteolipids had been discovered only a few years earlier; these compounds, which occur only in nerve tissue, proved to be soluble in certain lipid solvents and insoluble in aqueous solvents. Several specific members of the group were described in the initial biochemical studies by FOLCH *et al.* [74, 75, 134]. In 1951 and later, WAKSMAN and his co-workers found that preparations of this type were encephalitogenic in rabbits [258, 259]. Other workers reported similar activity in mice and guinea pigs [79, 189]. Although these fractions did induce allergic encephalomyelitis and also elicited complement-fixing antibodies to brain (the tissue residues were inactive), problems of interpretation soon developed. The proteolipids, as tested in rabbits, actually had less antigenic activity than did the fresh bovine white matter used as the starting material, when compared on a dry weight basis [259]. Further, the dose-response curve was different from that for whole nervous tissue. It was pointed out that alterations and degradations of proteolipid might occur during extraction, but that several antigens might be involved in the total encephalitogenic activity of whole nervous tissue, and if this were so there was no assurance that all of them were readily extracted with chloroform-methanol mixtures [197]. A number of subsequent studies provided evidence for this latter supposition, except in the case of mouse, in which reactivity to proteolipid is better than that to whole white matter and there is no sensitivity to basic protein preparations [6, 107]. The major significance of the discovery of proteolipid activity was that this fraction was generally used as a starting material for the preparation of more active fractions.

Secondly, we can consider a collagen-like protein. In 1958 ROBOZ *et al.* [113, 219] extracted a protein from bovine spinal cord, and reported encephalitogenic activity of a protein fraction for the first time. It had a nitrogen content of 17.6%, and it appeared homogeneous when examined by ultracentrifugation and electrophoresis. The nitrogen content suggested that the material was primarily a protein rather than a proteolipid, and the amino-acid composition of the protein resembled that of collagen, including large amounts of hydroxyproline and hydroxylysine. This preparation was shown to produce severe allergic encephalomyelitis in guinea pigs. It was the first water-soluble factor to be studied for AE induction, and all standard immunochemical techniques could be applied to its study. However, its activity on the basis of dry weight was not high enough to permit it to be considered the major encephalitogenic antigen. Again, the studies on this material were primarily of value as a starting point for further developments.

Before discussing the proteins and polypeptides of major interest, we should mention several other attempts to isolate various constituents from myelin. These have included a phospholipid-protein complex [116, 250, 252], a protein-lipid complex [95], and complement [1].

β) Basic Proteins

Certain basic proteins have excited most interest in the area of AE antigens in recent years. A number of laboratories have contributed to the now accepted concept that the encephalitogen is a basic protein or group of such proteins [31, 90, 102, 106, 110, 171, 218, 242]. ROBOZ and HENDERSON [218] and KIES and ALVORD [110] were the first to report the extraction of different encephalitogenic fractions from those mentioned above from bovine spinal cord and guinea pig brain in 1959. These fractions differed from the collagen-like protein in that they were obtained by acidic extraction technics. The high isoelectric point of this type of guinea pig encephalitogen emphasized the remarkable basic properties of this protein material. Although it resembled a histone in its properties, the protein found in the tissue was bound to lipid in the myelin sheath rather than to nucleic acids [127, 251]. Encephalitogenic activity of basic protein fractions of defatted CNS tissue was then reported in guinea pig, rabbit, and rat. Active proteins have been isolated from guinea pig brain [118], bovine cord [220], rat brain [106], rabbit cord [101], human white matter [33], bovine brain [190], and porcine cord and peripheral nerve [254]. An acid-soluble protein similar to the basic protein fractions described by these various laboratories has also been isolated directly from two proteolipid sources—petroleum-ether extracts of whole CNS tissue [119] and chloroform-methanol extracts of acidified lyophilized CNS tissue [266]. The similar chemical characteristics of the basic proteins prepared from the various species suggests the presence of a common constituent in these different sources [106].

ROBOZ-EINSTEIN *et al.* [220] isolated this protein from bovine spinal cord by means of several chromatographic procedures and extraction and manipulation at pH levels down to 2. They then found their product induced typical AE in guinea pigs in a dose as low as 8 μg in adjuvant. Similar results were reported by KIES and ALVORD and their colleagues [110, 115, 119], who had used similar methods of preparation. Their final product showed activity with even 1–2 μg of this basic protein.

WOLFGRAM [1956] emphasized the importance of the pH of extraction [266]. He found that the type of proteolipid extracted from homogenates of nervous tissue with a chloroform-methanol solvent depended greatly on the pH level. If the extract was obtained at pH 2, the proteolipid was 70% protein and was digestible by trypsin. If, however, the proteolipid was obtained at higher pH levels, it was resistant to trypsin and the amino-acid composition of the protein portion was different. The final product after extraction at low pH followed by other steps was nondialyzable and freely soluble in water, and it consisted entirely of protein with nitrogen content of 15.9 – 16.4% and electrophoretic migration to the cathode. Tests with acrylamide gel electrophoresis revealed only one component. As little as 5 μg of this protein produced encephalomyelitis. It was concluded that it was similar or identical to the other basic proteins reported.

General properties of the basic protein noted by 1965 include its remarkable stability; its activity withstands exposure to 95 °C, and also extraction with 0.1 N hydrochloric acid, extraction from aqueous solutions with phenol, precipitation from phenol solutions with acetone, and precipitation by picric acid. It was presumed that it was associated with the proteolipid material in complex formation within the nervous tissue, and that the lipid portion was of no consequence for biological activity but of great importance in extraction and purification [197].

At about the same time, indications began to appear that several molecular-weight classes of the basic protein material might be encephalitogenic, or at least that there might be smaller-molecular weight proteins, in contrast to the larger ones discussed in the earlier reports. ROBERTSON, BLIGHT, and LUMSDEN [217] were the first to claim that a dialyzable polypeptide diffusible through cellophane was encephalitogenic. NAKAO and ROBOZ-EINSTEIN [106] prepared an active preparation from the diffused portion of a basic protein preparation and found it was related to the nondialyzable encephalitogen isolated earlier [220]. These reports indicated that small molecular types were important as well as large molecular types, as will be discussed below.

A highly purified and active protein with many properties in common with the basic proteins described by other workers was described in 1964 by KIBLER *et al.* [102]. They examined their final product by ultracentrifugation, and measured a sedimentation coefficient of 0.42 S, which they felt suggested a molecular weight of less than 10000.

KIES and her group [112] then described highly purified preparations of two basic proteins from bovine white matter. It was proposed that these two preparations, termed "major S-7 component" and "component IV", were essentially identical and were higher molecular weight encephalitogens. Their molecular weights were estimated by gel filtration at about 40000. A number of such "large" encephalitogens had been reported by then, as had a number of "small" encephalitogens with molecular weights of about 10000, as emphasized by KIES *et al.* [112]. These observations, like those on dialysis, were another harbinger of the later more precise delineation of large and small encephalitogenic molecules described below. The molecular weights quoted at this stage were later corrected, but the relative weights were confirmed.

In 1967 CARNEGIE, BENCINA, and LAMOUREUX [30] described the purification of a basic protein and a polypeptide fragment which was also encephalitogenic, from both bovine spinal cord and guinea pig brain, starting with an acetone extraction. The molecular weight of the protein was indirectly estimated at 16 500, and that of the polypeptide at 3 500. Amino-acid analyses for both preparations were given, and the protein proved to contain 149 amino acids. Ultracentrifugal examination of the basic protein showed a single peak with a sedimentation coefficient of 0.7 S, a surprisingly low value in view of the molecular weight indicated.

For some years there had been considerable confusion about the true molecular size of the encephalitogenic substance in preparations from nerve tissue. This can be readily appreciated in view of the large number of reports summarized. As mentioned above, it became fashionable to speak of the high-molecular weight, or large, encephalitogen and the low-molecular weight, or small, encephalitogen. CARNEGIE *et al.* [30], and other authors at about the same time [112], attempted to explain these confusing findings by pointing out that the results might depend on whether the initial extraction was performed with chloroform-methanol. The properties of the protein obtained are influenced by the level of activity of an acid proteinase in the nervous tissue, which is high if dehydration and defatting are performed by means of acetone-petroleum ether extraction but considerably lower if defatting is performed with chloroform-methanol. If the proteinase is permitted to have any appreciable activity, it hydrolyzes the basic protein during acid extraction and produces polypeptide fragments. Further studies by this group have explored the encephalitogenic portions of the large (170-residue) protein and especially the relationships to delayed hypersensitivity [29, 32, 137, 173].

c) Chemical Structures of the Encephalitogens

The studies of KIBLER *et al.* [102] on purified preparations from bovine spinal cord were based on extraction of material soluble in 0.1 M sodium citrate, pH 4.3. The material obtained in this step was then fractionated by chromatography on CM cellulose, with a linear gradient of increasing ionic strength and a constant pH of 8.6. One of the peaks eluted in this way appeared homogeneous when examined by ultracentrifugation and electrophoresis, and was encephalitogenic in rabbits in quantities of 200 μg (as against 250 mg of the initial whole-cord homogenate) [101]. When examined in a synthetic boundary cell in the ultracentrifuge, this preparation showed a sedimentation coefficient of 0.42 S. It was judged that the molecular weight "may be less than ten thousand". Actually, a considerably lower molecular weight could have been predicted.

Several years later these workers progressed [104] to a more detailed study of this component, which they prepared from several animal species. In this later study chromatography was followed by gel filtration on Sephadex G-50, and one of the several peaks from this separation was found to be highly active and highly homogeneous. This product, peak 4, was examined in a number of ways. Calculation of the minimum molecular weight from amino-acid analysis gave an average figure of 4100. The N-terminal amino acid was shown to be phenylalanine and there was probably one N-terminal residue per molecule, suggesting a molecular structure made up of a single polypeptide chain. The results of elution in gel filtration and centrifugation in a sucrose density gradient were compared with those obtained with other proteins. A molecular weight considerably lower than that of ribonuclease was suggested, and it was concluded from all these observations that the molecular weight was between 4000 and 8000, probably nearer the smaller figure.

Several other reports have made similar contributions to our knowledge of the molecular structure. The work of PALMER and DAWSON in 1969 [191] was based on a preparation of encephalitogenic protein taken from bovine spinal cord by the method of MARTENSON and LEBARON [170]. Ultracentrifugal examination showed a single symmetrical peak with an extrapolated sedimentation coefficient of 1.33 S, a diffusion coefficient of 7.80×10^{-7} cm^2/sec and a partial specific volume of 0.72 ml/g; a molecular weight of 15100 was calculated from these data. Amino-acid analysis was performed on this preparation, and 137 amino-acid residues per molecule were found. Treatment with cyanogen bromide caused splitting into at least two fragments. The smaller type of fragment contained 13 amino acids and had no encephalitogenic activity. The larger fragment was believed to contain all the remaining residues of the original molecule and it did have encephalitogenic activity. It was obvious from these results that the methionine residues liable to attack by cyanogen bromide are near the end (or ends) of the molecule and that the antigenicity is not very much affected by cleavage at these positions, so that cyanogen bromide would not be very useful in location of the antigenic site. Further studies on the several molecular forms of encephalitogen have also been published by KIES and colleagues [51, 171] and EINSTEIN and co-workers [37–39, 54, 56, 213]. Three-dimensional structures have quite recently been proposed for this protein [234].

A fairly recent report from the laboratory of KIBLER *et al.* [105] provided a complete amino-acid analysis of one of the encephalitogens. In addition, the comparative data on a number of preparations from other laboratories were discussed. The molecular weight of bovine and rabbit encephalitogenic protein was found to be 4700. KIBLER *et al.* confirmed that phenylalanine was the N-terminal amino acid and stated that histidine was the C terminal amino acid. The protein they had purified was found to be a single polypeptide chain of 45 amino-acid residues and the complete sequence of residues was determined through preparation and analysis of tryptic and chymotryptic peptides; the sequence is shown in Fig. 4.4, which also indicates the peptides cleaved from this preparation in the initial step in the sequence analysis. A total of seven tryptic peptides was ultimately prepared although initially there were five peptides, two of which were then each split into two peptides.

The relationships between this protein and the higher-molecular weight encephalitogens isolated and described by other workers were also explored and discussed [105]. The high-molecular weight preparation of KIES *et al.* from bovine spinal cord [120] was isolated and analyzed. In all 144 amino acids were found in this unit. About 20 tryptic peptides were obtained, 3 of which were identical to 3 of the 7 obtained from the small encephalitogen. Other

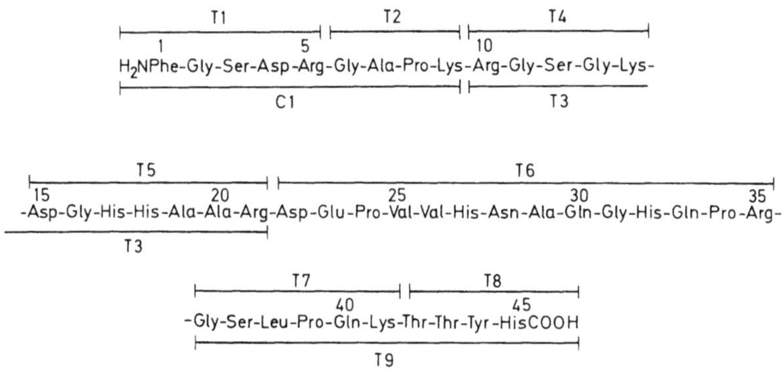

Fig. 4.4. Amino-acid sequence in the 45-residue encephalitogen molecule, according to KIBLER *et al.* [56]. Peptides obtained by trypsin (T) and chymotrypsin (C) digestion are indicated

Table 4.2. *Amino-acid composition of several preparations of encephalitogenic protein and fragments (number of residues per molecule)*

Amino acid residue	Basic Protein					Peptide Fragments		
	1 Bovine	2 Porcine	3 Bovine	4 Human	5 Bovine	6 Bovine	7 Bovine	8 Bovine
Lys	12	11	10	12	13	6	2	3
His	8	8	8	10	9	4	0	5
Arg	14	14	14	15	16	6	3	4
Asp	10	9	9	10	9	4	1	4
Thr	6	6	6	7	6	3	0	2
Ser	13	12	13	13	13	6	4	3
Glu	10	9	9	8	9	5	2	4
Pro	11	11	10	10	9	6	1	4
Gly	21	21	20	20	20	12	7	7
Ala	12	13	11	10	11	5	2	4
Val	3	3	2	3	4	1	0	2
Met	2	2	2	2	2	0	0	0
Ile	3	3	2	3	3	1	0	0
Leu	8	8	8	7	8	3	0	1
Tyr	3	4	3	3	3	2	1	1
Phe	7	7	7	7	6	3	2	1
Try	1	1	1	1	1	1	1	0
Total	144	140	135	141	142	68	26	45

Table adapted from KIBLER *et al.* [56].

Column 1: KIES *et al.* [69]. Analysis from [56].
„ 2: TOMASI and KORNGUTH [144].
„ 3: CHAO and EINSTEIN [18].
„ 4: ENG *et al.* [25].
„ 5: EYLAR and HASHIM [26].
„ 6: CHAO and EINSTEIN [18].
„ 7: EYLAR and HASHIM [26].
„ 8: KIBLER *et al.* [56].

peptides showed similarities to the remaining units of the small protein. The data indicated that the small protein of KIBLER and SHAPIRA [104] was in fact a portion of the large basic protein of KIES *et al.* [120]. Table 4.2 shows these comparisons and the analyses of several other preparations of high-molecular weight encephalitogen.

TOMASI and KORNGUTH [253] were not really interested in the encephalitogen as such, but in the basic proteins of animal tissues. They isolated and purified a basic protein from porcine brain and studied a number of its physical and chemical properties. They started with a chloroform-methanol extract, and after several steps they obtained a product extracted at pH 2.4–2.6. This was further purified by ammonium sulfate precipitation, gel filtration on Sephadex G-100, and chromatography on Amberlite IRC-50 with a guanidine gradient. The final product was homogeneous and the single ultracentrifugal boundary had a sedimentation coefficient of 1.5 S, from which a molecular weight of 20000 was estimated. The amino-acid analysis was given as mol% for each residue. A basic protein with very similar composition was also found in bovine nerve tissue by two other groups [170, 183]. Both these bovine preparations had been studied as inducers of AE [112, 184]. The figures given for the porcine basic protein [253] were recalculated by KIBLER *et al.* [105] to show the relative numbers on a basis of 140 residues instead of the arbitrary 100, to make comparisons easier. This list of figures is shown in Table 4.2.

A bovine encephalitogenic protein analyzed by CHAO and ROBOZ-EINSTEIN [36] was purified from bovine spinal cord by NAKAO *et al.* [183–185], starting with a chloroform-methanol extraction. The sedimentation rate of the purified protein was 0.90 S, and a molecular weight of 12500 was estimated. The amino-acid composition was given for this encephalitogenic protein, and also for a peptide fragment (see below), as mol% [36]. The minimum molecular weight for the large protein was 10899. The moles of amino-acid residues were recalculated by KIBLER *et al.* [105] on the basis of 135 residues instead of 100, and these results are also shown in Table 4.2.

The basic protein of ENG *et al.* [58] was a purified product from human brain tissue. The amino-acid analysis has been recalculated on a basis of 141 residues, and is shown in Table 4.2.

Another study on the large encephalitogen and a comparison with a peptide fragment was reported by EYLAR and HASHIM [63], who used bovine spinal cord. In their preparation of basic protein, described later [66] but cited earlier in their publications [67], they concluded that this molecule is a single chain of 142 amino acids in a random coil configuration [67]. This tabulation is shown in Table 4.2 without further modification, since the total number fits in well with the other values calculated.

All the preparations tabulated in Table 4.2 showed surprising similarity in the numbers of each amino-acid residue per unit molecule. Thus, a good degree of clarification has apparently been achieved with regard to the high-molecular weight encephalitogen.

In addition to the low-molecular weight encephalitogen of KIBLER *et al.* [105] discussed above, two other preparations of low-molecular weight encephalitogen have been reported. CHAO and EINSTEIN [36] produced their preparation from the starting material described above, the encephalitogenic protein. It was obtained after the application of a purified acid protease, also taken from bovine brain tissue. The active fragment was purified and studied. It showed a sedimentation coefficient of 0.72 S. The amino-acid analysis indicated a minimum number of 58 residues, which corresponded to a molecular weight of 6243. These numbers, re-calculated to 68 residues, are given in Table 4.2. No work was reported on the amino-acid sequence.

One other similar preparation is that of EYLAR and HASHIM [63], which was prepared by digestion with pepsin of the large basic protein described above. These investigations have been described in a profusion of published reports [66, 80, 83, 84, 85]. In fact, two peptides were obtained, both of them highly active. The larger unit contained 26 residues, and its composition is given for comparison in Table 4.2. The smaller unit had only 16 residues, and the sequence has been determined. This is shown in Fig. 4.5. The 45-unit peptide of KIBLER and his colleagues has been described again by SHAPIRA *et al.* [225], who give a complete amino-acid analysis. A monkey encephalitogen has also been described [103].

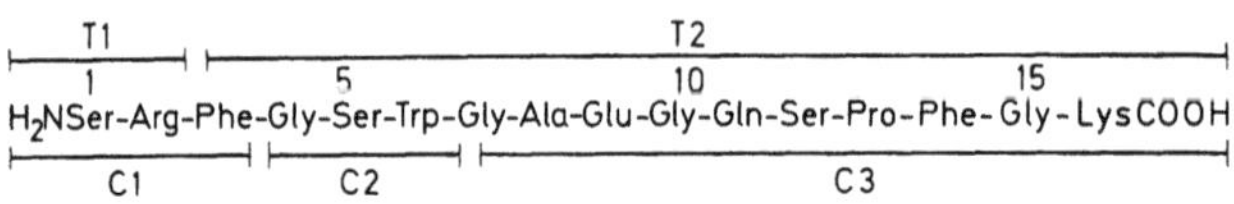

Fig. 4.5. Amino-acid sequence in the 16-residue encephalitogen molecule, according to EYLAR *et al.* [26]. Peptides obtained by trypsin (T) and chymotrypsin (C) digestion are indicated

More recently, EYLAR and his colleagues have examined the structures of the encephalitogens and their various fragmented peptides in considerable detail. Much of this work has recently been reviewed [60] and only some of the major points will be summarized here. First, we should note that these investigators have corrected the structure of the peptide of 16 residues mentioned above, attributing to it 14 instead of 16 residues and a slightly different arrangement: Ser-Arg-Phe-Ser-Trp-Gly-Ala-Glu-Gly-Gln-Lys-Pro-Gly-Phe; in addition, comparisons with other peptides, including synthetic ones, have led them to believe that a sequence of only 9 residues is actually responsible for the encephalitogenic activity, namely: Phe-Ser-Trp-Gly-Ala-Glu-Gly-Gln-Lys [62]. Secondly, the large encephalitogen, i.e. the basic protein, was carefully studied. They referred to it as the A1 protein, finding it comprised 30% of the myelin protein [66]. The complete amino-acid sequence has been determined for both bovine and human A1 proteins. The molecular weight of the bovine antigen is 18400, and it has 170 residues [59, 60]. There is only one tryptophan residue, and the disease-inducing site is a nine-residue sequence including the Trp unit (as mentioned above). The human antigen has a molecular weight of about 18600 and contains 172 residues. There are 11 positions in the sequences at which these antigens differ; otherwise, they are reported to be identical. The A1 protein seems to be an unfolded molecule with no secondary structure [25]. A peptide sequence of 45 amino acids, i.e. residues 44 to 89, can itself induce AE in the rabbit [68], while a major AE-inducing sequence for guinea pig and rabbit contains only 9 residues [62, 263]. Details relating to the three-dimensional structure of the whole molecule and to the effects of modification of one amino acid or another have also been studied, particularly the threonine and tryptophan residues [26, 64, 81, 243].

Another basic protein (termed P2 protein) has quite recently been isolated from the myelin of rabbit sciatic nerve and shown to be the antigen responsible for the induction of experimental allergic neuritis [24]. It has a molecular weight of about 11–12000 and contains 101 amino acids, as against 170 or 172 in the A1 protein.

d) Biological Properties of the Several Encephalitogen Molecules

LAMOUREUX *et al.* [129, 130] have examined the immunological activities of the encephalitogenic basic protein and polypeptide preparations prepared from bovine spinal cord or from guinea pig brain. In one study [129], they injected both outbred guinea pigs and inbred Wistar rats. The minimum antigenic dose required for the production of allergic encephalomyelitis in guinea pigs was extremely low, 1 μg for the protein and 50 ng for the polypeptide. In guinea pigs, the bovine protein induced encephalomyelitis, cutaneous manifestations of delayed hypersensitivity, and the production of circulating antibodies (tested by gel diffusion precipitation), while the bovine polypeptide produced encephalomyelitis and delayed hypersensitivity but no antibody reacting with the polypeptide, although there was antibody that could cross-react with the protein. Results with guinea pig preparations were similar. In the rats, the guinea pig materials were antigenically active and stimulated AE, but the bovine materials only stimulated a response of circulating antibody, whereas delayed hypersensitivity and encephalomyelitis were found only with very weak or questionable responses. The immunodiffusion reactions were found to be more pronounced at a slightly acid pH, such as 6.0 or 6.5, than at neutral and basic pH values of 7.3 or 8.6. Studies of cross-reactions in immunodiffusion and in delayed hypersensitivity seemed to indicate that a similar antigenic determinant was present in the compounds from these two animal species.

This group also made a more detailed study on the localization of a labeled preparation of encephalitogenic polypeptide. The distribution of this material within the body, and especially in the lymph nodes, of the guinea pig was studied after injection of a radioiodine-labeled purified bovine encephalitogen with Freund's complete adjuvant into the hind footpad. This led to quick enlargement of the popliteal lymph node. In two days there was a depletion of lymphocytes, the follicles had become confluent, and there was a proliferation of large cells throughout the node. At five days, the lymph-node architecture was disorganized and no germinal centers were recognizable. Similar, although milder, changes were present in regional nodes. In contrast, the injection of flagellin in Freund's complete adjuvant by a similar technique was followed by the preservation of lymph-node architecture and the accumulation of many lymphocytes in the germinal centers. When complete adjuvant was used with the encephalitogen, about 1% of the total radioactivity injected was concentrated in the popliteal lymph node 2–5 days after the injection. If the antigen was injected without Freund's complete adjuvant, however, there was no concentration of radioactivity in the lymph node, and the animals did not develop encephalomyelitis.

CASPARY and FIELD [34] have provided data in support of their opinion that radioiodine labeling is not sufficiently stable to eliminate possible errors in interpretation when used to trace the spread of injected encephalitogen in the living animal. They recommend a carbon-labeled encephalitogen, which they claim is highly stable even though it does not have a high specific activity. When using the carbon-labeled preparation they found a large amount of the encephalitogen in the blood lymphocytes after inoculation into the foot. It remains to be seen how the different patterns of antigen localization obtained in different laboratories will be reconciled.

LEVINE and SOWINSKI [147] have reported granulomatous inflammation in the liver subsequent to intrasplenic injection of neural tissue in adjuvant. They consider the liver to be a site of formation of encephalitogenic cells, but the significance of this concept and the mechanisms involved are not clear.

The effects of antilymphocyte serum (ALS) on the course and development of allergic encephalomyelitis in guinea pig have also been studied [135]. The serum completely suppressed the clinical and histological features of AE, and long-term suppression was obtained relatively easily, although tolerance was not established and the disease recurred later in some cases. Lesions appearing some time after ALS treatment were much more severe than the initial ones. The major factor in the suppression of AE by ALS was thought to be very slow development of the lesions, which caused the neurological signs shown by the animal to be less severe. However, the ultimate demyelination was no less than in animals not treated with ALS, and in some cases it was even greater. Thus, there was an increased chronicity of the lesion. The possible mechanisms of ALS action have been discussed with reference to the effects on the macrophages and lymphocytes [35].

Some effects of chemical modification of the basic protein have been explored by SWANBORG [243, 244]. Rabbit basic protein was prepared, which was highly encephalitogenic in guinea pigs and was shown by ultracentrifugation to be homogeneous with an extrapolated sedimentation coefficient of 1.8 S. It was diazotized, and sulfanyl and arsanyl groups were attached to the protein, giving an average of 3.5 azo groups per molecule. The product was no longer basic, although it retained the same sedimentation rate. It no longer induced AE, but did produce delayed hypersensitivity to basic protein, either modified or not [243]. Loss of encephalitogenic activity is related to the animal species involved, however, since modified bovine basic protein was not active in guinea pigs but was active in Lewis rats [245]. In another comparison, although the original basic protein of rabbit had only a weak immunogenic effect in rabbits, the modified protein was more active in stimulating the formation of hemagglutinating antibody [246].

e) Diversity of Antigenic Determinants

There have been decisive advances in the exploration of antibody responses to encephalitogenic substances and thus in the analysis of the antigenic determinants involved in recent years. A number of early studies described the antibody response during the course of AE, but many of these responses were rather weak, or late, or limited in function [69, 82, 165, 187]. HRUBY *et al.* [92] ascribe some of the earlier difficulties to the general weak antigenicity of basic proteins and the very narrow range of antigen concentrations used, and to the fact that acute and fatal encephalomyelitis has generally prevented experimental animals from surviving long enough for high titers of antibody to develop. Since the observation by ALVORD *et al.* [10] that encephalomyelitis could be inhibited by repeated injections of basic protein in Freund's incomplete adjuvant, this team has embarked on studies of the antibody responses. Multiple antigens are present in the basic protein, and although some of the antibodies are directed against trace contaminants in the preparation [15, 93], the antigenic determinants of the basic protein itself (and of its active fragments) obviously still need careful analysis [7, 8, 111], and a profusion of papers has been published and promised by this group. Titers of hemagglutinating antibody have now been found to be much higher in rabbits injected with rabbit (or bovine) basic protein than in the case of guinea pigs injected with guinea pig basic protein. This difference in responsiveness in the two homologous situations was at first considered surprising and no explanation was offered, but it should not cause any concern; it has long been an established concept—almost a dogma—that rabbits are especially capable of responding with antibody formation, whereas guinea pigs are especially liable to delayed hypersensitivity reactions. The expected sequential production of first 19 S and then 7 S antibodies was confirmed by the fact that the early antibody was sensitive to 2-mercaptoethanol, whereas the late antibody was resistant. The antibodies were stable in frozen storage, but their precipitating capacity was relatively unstable on storage at 4 °C. The instability varied in different antisera. Many of these observations suggest a complicated diversity of antibody responses to a number of distinctive antigenic determinant groups [92]. Later papers in the series [11, 78, 164] describe the detection of antibodies with cytophilic properties and the study of radiolabeled antibodies. Other authors have also used radioimmunoassay, immunofluorescence, and *in vitro* demyelinating activity to detect these antibodies [136, 172, 224].

f) Relationship of AE to Human Disease

It is by no means clear how human disease can be related to allergic encephalomyelitis as a model. Multiple sclerosis (MS) has been studied in a number of ways. LAMOUREUX *et al.* [128] have claimed that the cerebrospinal fluid in multiple sclerosis causes cytotoxicity in cultures of nervous tissue, and they therefore postulate that an autoimmune process is significant in the demyelination of multiple sclerosis. Antimyelin antibodies are detected by means of immunofluorescence tests in a high proportion of patients with MS but in few normal individuals [53]. Some MS patients also have demyelinating antibodies, detected by tests performed on living myelinated cultures of neonatal mouse cerebellum [52]. It is not clear whether an antigen similar to the encephalitogen in experimental animals is involved, although hypotheses of this sort have been proposed and discussed [57, 174]. BEHAN *et al.* [16] have quite recently found evidence of immune phenomena in two patients with demyelinating diseases. They observed lymphocyte transformation when stimulation was attempted with a purified myelin basic protein, although like LISAK *et al.* [1963] they were unable to detect circulating antibody to this protein.

Multiple sclerosis is an inflammatory disease of the nervous system in which immune responses seem to have a particular role. Pregnancy in women with this disease causes a considerable reduction in the severity of the ailment, which suggests hormonal influences, but the incidence of relapses is increased during the immediate postpartum period [177]. This raises the question as to whether there is a significant interaction between the manifestations of multiple sclerosis and the use of oral contraceptives. The effects of oral contraceptives have been studied in experimental allergic encephalomyelitis in an effort to clarify this question [13]. The administration of large oral doses of estrogen each day to rats developing encephalomyelitis did suppress the condition, whereas progestin failed to suppress it and in fact exacerbated it. Several oral contraceptive preparations containing estrogen and progestin in various ratios were also found to suppress allergic encephalomyelitis in a manner comparable to the effects of estrogen alone.

The exact nature of the relationship between AE and multiple sclerosis needs much further study [139, 177].

4. The Acidic Proteins

In sharp contrast to the extensive studies described above concerning the encephalitogenic properties and the chemical characterization of the causative factor as a basic protein, a different group of studies on brain-specific antigens and proteins has evolved in recent years; these studies are concerned with the properties of a highly acidic protein fraction. The existence of an acid protein fraction unique to vertebrate brain was first reported by MOORE and MCGREGOR [179] as a result of electrophoretic studies. The original method of isolation involved chromatography on DEAE cellulose followed by starch-gel electrophoresis of the fractions, which was said to reveal the presence of 70–100 protein bands, although the degree of chromatographic resolution might well be questioned, and the number of components may have been lower. Nonetheless, when similar studies were made on liver, it became apparent that at least two proteins were present in lower quantities in the liver than in the brain, or were not present in the liver at all. These were rather acidic substances, and probably of fairly low molecular weight, judging by their chromatographic and electrophoretic behavior. The faster-moving band of the two was present in the brain tissue of all species examined and apparently not in their liver tissue; at most, the concentration in liver was less than 1% of that in brain. The likelihood that a protein of this sort might be related to the unique function and organization of nervous tissue, aroused interest in purifying it for further study.

MOORE [178] then showed that it was possible to purify this protein, and because it was soluble in 100% saturated ammonium sulfate solution it was named the "S-100" protein. Purified preparations were made from bovine, porcine, and rabbit brain. The S-100 protein was present in the brain tissue of all species examined: cattle, hog, rat, rabbit, hamster, guinea pig, mouse, dog, monkey, man, turkey, eagle, alligator, black snake, turtle, pompano, and red snapper. It was easily detected in concentrated (20–30 mg per ml) extracts by means of POULIK'S [208] discontinuous method of starch gel electrophoresis. Fig. 4.6

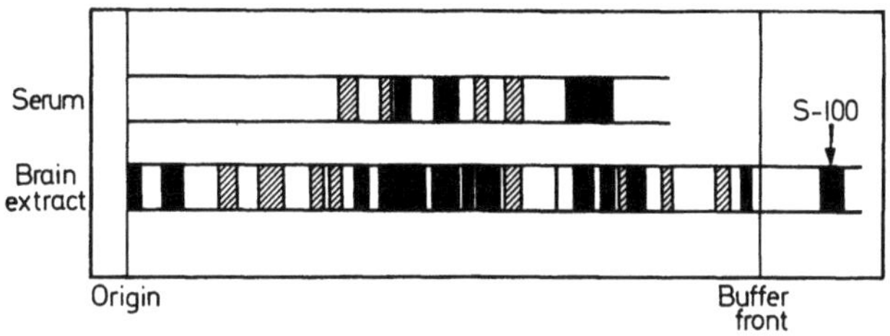

Fig. 4.6. Starch-gel electrophoretic patterns of rabbit brain extract and rabbit serum. The S-100 protein moves ahead of the borate buffer front in this system. (Sketch adapted from MOORE [100])

shows a typical pattern. The mobilities varied among the different species; the significance of this is unknown. A molecular weight of about 30000 was estimated for the bovine protein by gel filtration. It was found to be free of phosphorus, lipid, and carbohydrate. The electrophoretic properties and the amino-acid composition of rabbit brain S-100 and bovine brain S-100 were very similar. The acid nature of this protein was explained by the presence of a large number of acidic amino-acid residues. Rabbit antiserum to the bovine S-100 protein was prepared and was used in precipitation and complement-fixation tests performed after WASSERMAN and LEVINE [261]. Brain extract was the only tissue of those compared which gave positive results with the antiserum. The unique properties of this protein were summarized as follows: 1. it was distinct from other soluble proteins in being highly acidic and in having a high electrophoretic mobility on starch gel and being soluble in concentrated salt solution, 2. it was present in all parts of the nervous system, peripheral and central, including (in the rabbit) whole brain, gray matter, white matter, cerebrum, cerebellum, brain stem, spinal cord, sciatic nerve, and vagus nerve, 3. it was present in brain tissue of all species examined, 4. it was absent from organs other than the nervous system. On the basis of its distribution, MOORE concluded that it is a neuronal protein and not part of the myelin structure [178].

LEVINE and his colleagues undertook a number of studies with preparations of bovine S-100 protein [17, 42, 99], which revealed its unusual conformational properties. It is thermolabile but the confirmation is stabilized by EDTA, calcium ion, or 2-mercaptoethanol. LEVINE and co-workers studied rabbit antiserum and bovine S-100 protein and demonstrated the complete loss of antigenic activity when the protein was heated to 70 °C, and the protection from thermal denaturation provided by calcium ion and several other substances. Studies of the optical rotatory dispersion in various conditions were also made; these led to the conclusion that an alpha-helical structure is destroyed as the temperature is increased, and that some of this structure is restored in some conditions of cooling. Alternative polypeptide structures are formed at high temperatures.

A molecular weight of 21300 was determined by means of sedimentation equilibrium studies, and the existence of molecular subunits was indicated by electrophoresis in acrylamide gel in the presence of 0.1% sodium dodecyl sulfate. A molecular weight of 7000 was indicated in these conditions, suggesting that the S-100 protein, which has a native molecular weight of about 21000, is composed of three subunits each with molecular weight of 7000. These workers also showed that the protein is present in glial cells propagated in tissue culture.

Additional data on chemical properties, antigenic characteristics and functional behavior in regard to neurological activity are being actively studied, since little is yet known [27, 28, 40, 43–45, 79a, 79b, 88a, 235]. However, a new area of inquiry has been opened up, and this time the tissue-specificity has been demonstrated in biochemical terms before antigenic terms. As always, however, both approaches have come into play eventually.

A completely different acidic protein, immunologically unrelated to the S-100 protein, has been isolated from rat neural tissue. This component, termed antigen α by BENNETT and EDELMAN [18], has a unit molecular weight of about 39000 and occurs in various aggregated forms.

5. The Neutral Proteins

Other kinds of brain-specific protein have also been studied in aqueous extracts of brain tissue or in other ways. The group of substances with properties approximately in the neutral range is somewhat miscellaneous. For example, WARECKA and BAUER [260] studied aqueous extracts of brain homogenates and found two protein components that were not present in blood serum or cerebrospinal fluid. One of these proteins was present in other organs and thus was not brain-specific. The other protein, migrating at pH 8.6 as an α_2 globulin, corresponds to a component described by other authors as brain-specific. After absorption of an antiserum with liver or kidney extracts, reaction with this component in immunoelectrophoresis and in gel diffusion precipitation was not eliminated, which indicates brain-specificity. It stained for carbohydrate and was destroyed by treatment with neuraminidase. These findings suggest that the α_2 fraction was a glycoprotein rich in sialic acid. Other studies have been made in terms of the organ localization of antibrain antibodies [49, 50, 265]. However, the antigenic substances were very poorly defined in these investigations.

MACPHERSON and COSGROVE [167, 168] studied cerebrospinal fluid (CSF) and demonstrated two gamma-globulin components, one of which was specific for CSF and termed gamma c. Since the contents of CSF probably reflects the brain tissue, examination of this fluid is also of interest. HOCHWALD and THORBECKE [89] studied CSF and isolated two proteins which they called beta-trace and gamma-trace, which seemed characteristic of this tissue. Some antigens, however, were common to several tissues and fluids, including CSF, urine, and ascites and pleural fluids, as emphasized later by LATERRE *et al.* [133]. Additional evidence for distinctive gamma globulins in CSF was reported by YOKOYAMA and EINSTEIN [267].

MACPHERSON and co-workers [160, 169] reported the presence of twelve antigenic proteins in saline extracts of rat brain, one of which was both organ- and species restricted (OSR). In a later study [86], 17 antigens were detected in bovine brain extracts by means of gel diffusion and immunoelectrophoresis with antisera prepared by intensive immunization in rabbits. Ten of the antigens were found to be species-specific and shared by other bovine organs, five were organ-specific and common to the brains of other mammals, and two were both organ- and species-restricted. Compositional changes during animal maturation have also been described [167]. In later studies [87, 161], this term (OSR) was dropped, because the antigen was found in peripheral nerve as well as brain. A new term, species-restricted antigen of nervous tissue (SRANT) was introduced. Antigens of this type have been successfully purified from rat tissue [161] and bovine tissue [87]. However, the complexity of antigenic comparison is such that further clarification is impossible without much more analysis and extensive fractionation. Similar approaches were adopted by KOSINSKI and GRABAR [123], who described 11 antigens for rat brain, and RAJAM and BOGOCH [209] and RAJAM *et al.* [210], who reported 13 antigens for human gray matter; species comparisons were also made [211]. DAS and DAS [46] described 5 specific antigens for brain of rhesus monkey. ALVORD *et al.* [12] claimed that several neutral proteins of human or guinea pig brain reacted with dog sera, especially those from cases of canine distemper. It was not stated why dog brain proteins were not used. The various degrees of tissue specificity for each of these diverse components, and the biochemical nature of the more interesting ones, need much further study.

6. The Thermostable, Ethanol-Insoluble Proteins

Since the initial studies on the thermostable antigen of the adrenal tissues, some of which were described in Chapter 3, similar investigations have been conducted on brain tissue.

a) Antigenic Properties

Antisera were obtained by immunization of rabbits with thermostable ethanol-insoluble fractions of bovine, porcine, or human brain. These antisera made it possible to detect brain-specific antigens by several immunochemical methods [175, 176]. In double diffusion gel precipitation tests, the brain-specific component was demonstrated by one precipitation line. In immunoelectrophoresis at pH 8.2 the brain-specific line appeared in the anode part of the electrophoretic field. The antigen was entirely different from the thermostable ethanol-insoluble *adrenal*-specific antigen described earlier, and also from the brain lipid antigen described earlier in this chapter. Antisera to the thermostable antigens of porcine and bovine brain combined not only with brain preparations of the homologous species, but also with similar preparations from a heterologous species. Since the methods used in the extraction and preparation of these antigens were admittedly harsh, it appeared possible that artifacts were being studied, so that a demonstration that brain preparations obtained by very gentle methods also contained this tissue-specific antigen was called for. Accordingly, rabbits were injected with bovine brain suspension obtained by gentle homogenization with saline solution in a blender at low temperature. The antisera produced in this way did also contain antibodies against the brain-specific thermostable antigen [175].

Histological localization of this particular brain-specific antigen was also studied in bovine brain, spinal cord, and sciatic nerve, and in carefully dissected cerebral grey and white matter. The antigen was plentiful in the cerebral grey matter but completely absent from peripheral nerve; preparations from sciatic nerve were negative, and those from spinal cord showed only slight reactivity [175]. Comparisons were also made with the lipid thermostable brain-specific antigen, which is soluble in ethanol. The cross-reactions reported earlier between brain and testis in studies of lipid antigens (mentioned in Chapter 5) were not found in the studies on the thermostable, ethanol-insoluble antigens. This BE antigen may be similar to the antigens studied in the work of HENLE *et al.* [88]. When testing certain antisera against brain "particles", these workers had found both antibodies against the brain lipid antigens and antibodies that combined with thermostable and ethanol-insoluble antigens. They found cross-reactions between the antigens from mouse and cattle, however, which were more marked than the interspecies cross-reactions found in the later work [175].

b) Chemical Properties

The tissue-specific thermostable antigen preparations of bovine brain were quite heterogeneous chemically, containing nucleic acid, carbohydrate, protein, and possibly lipid constituents. Carbohydrate analyses revealed a content of 4.2% of protein-bound hexose and 0.4% of hexosamine as average values for this preparation. Ultracentrifugation revealed three major components, with extrapolated sedimentation coefficients of 8.60 S, 2.20 S, and 1.80 S. Electrophoretic analysis revealed 6 (or more) constituents. Because of the heterogeneity of the preparations, direct chemical characterization of the actual brain-specific antigen was not possible and degradative studies had to be performed with chymotrypsin and periodate as the destructive agents. On the basis of its thermostability, carbohydrate content of 4.6%, and destruction by dilute chymotrypsin but not by periodate, the brain-specific antigenic component was tentatively classified as a mucoprotein or glycoprotein [233].

There may be tissue-specific glycoprotein antigens, as well as species-specific antigens. It seems reasonably well established that the thermostable tissue-specific antigens of brain and of adrenal (Chap. 3) belong to this macromolecular category.

Reports on the production of AE with this type of preparation are contradictory. Although MILGROM *et al.* [175] reported negative results in rabbits, SWANBORG *et al.* [248] claimed positive results in guinea pig.

In purification studies by SWANBORG and SHULMAN [247] the fraction precipitating with 2.00 M ammonium sulfate contained most of the brain-specific activity,

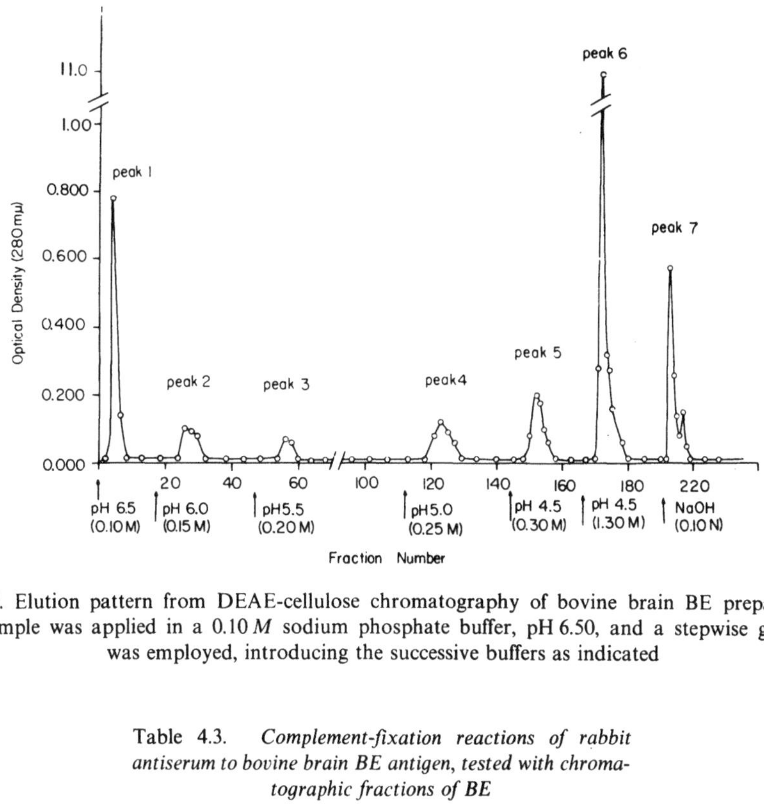

Fig. 4.7. Elution pattern from DEAE-cellulose chromatography of bovine brain BE preparation. The sample was applied in a 0.10 *M* sodium phosphate buffer, pH 6.50, and a stepwise gradient was employed, introducing the successive buffers as indicated

Table 4.3. *Complement-fixation reactions of rabbit antiserum to bovine brain BE antigen, tested with chromatographic fractions of BE*

Antigen	Concentration of undiluted antigen	Antigen titer[a]	Adjusted antigen titer[b]
Whole BE	0.30 %	243	16
Fractions:			
1	0.04	<3	<3
2	0.02	<3	<3
3	0.02	<3	<3
4	0.02	243	243
5	0.02	27	27
6	0.9	<3	<3
7	0.02	81	81

[a] Titer is highest dilution of antigen which still gives complete hemolysis.

[b] Adjusted to initial antigen concentration of 0.02 %.

as shown by complement-fixation titration. This globulin fraction was also shown to produce only two gel precipitation lines with antiserum as against the three produced with the supernatant and the original preparation.

The brain-specific antigen was better purified by means of stepwise elution in column chromatography on DEAE cellulose, with buffers of decreasing pH and increasing ionic strength. It was eluted primarily with a sodium phosphate buffer at pH 5.00 and concentration 0.25 M, giving a fraction designated as peak 4. This component showed ultracentrifugal and electrophoretic homogeneity, and complement-fixation titration revealed that it was very rich in specific antigenic activity [247]. The elution graph is shown in Fig. 4.7, and the antigen titration in Table 4.3. The brain-specific component was thus present in the slowest of the three ultracentrifugal peaks seen in the unfractionated preparation; it has a sedimentation coefficient of 1.8 S. Direct chemical analysis of this material supported the opinion that the antigen is a glycoprotein.

Chapter 5

The Reproductive System

Both male and female reproductive systems should be considered but far more work has been done on the male reproductive system, and more is known or amenable to study in the male than in the female system. As a result, much of this chapter will deal with the male, although the female is well represented in terms of her immune responses to male antigens, in addition to the study of female antigens and possible responses to them.

There are two quite different antigenic systems of the male reproductive tract, and it may even be necessary to subdivide each of these into several subsystems. Each of these antigenic systems includes antigens characteristic for several related tissues or organs; these antigens may also be capable of stimulating autoantibody formation. We are thus considering tissue-specific antigens, some of which are also autoantigens. In general terms, one of these two systems includes the specific antigenic activity of testis, epididymis, and the spermatozoa. This antigen (or group of antigens) is related to aspermatogenesis and testicular damage. The antigen (or group) related to the spermagglutinating activity found in the serum of some people may be the same or a different one. The second of the two systems is that of the prostate gland, the seminal vesicle, and the other accessory glands of reproduction. These organs share one or more antigens specific for the accessory glands. This system also includes the prostatic fluid and the seminal plasma, although some antigens of the first system can be detected in the seminal plasma.

An important goal is to delineate the number and the precise specificity of the antigens in each of these systems, and to determine which ones are autoantigens. The chemical nature of each of these antigens, the degree of antigenicity, and the relationship to experimental or clinical tissue damage must also be examined.

Several reviews dealing with many items related to the immunology of reproduction in more detail have recently appeared and can be consulted for diverse aspects and points of emphasis of the subject [269, 271–275]. A very extensive review of the biochemistry of these tissues and of reproductive interactions is given in the excellent monograph by MANN [157].

1. Spermatozoal and Testicular Antigens

The antigenicity of spermatozoa was first demonstrated in 1899 by means of immunization of animals of a foreign species, hence by the production of heteroantibodies, by LANDSTEINER [130] and by METCHNIKOFF [181]. In 1900,

METALNIKOFF [180] was the first to obtain autoantibodies to spermatozoa, in guinea pigs. He utilized an isoimmunization technic, injecting animals with material taken from other animals of the same species. The injected animals produced a factor that he called "Spermotoxin" (in analogy to "Cytotoxin"), which was demonstrable as sera of immunized animals immobilized spermatozoa in the presence of complement. A few years later, ADLER reported that autoimmunization also stimulated antibody formation, the animals producing autoantibodies after injection with their own sperm cells [1]. These initial discoveries were followed by a spate of studies of organ-specificity and species-specificity of spermatozoa and testicular homogenate as an alternative source of spermatozoal antigens. Sperm cells were found to contain both tissue-specific and species-specific antigens. It was later found that the only other tissue with which testis shared an antigen was brain; positive complement-fixation tests between an ethanol extract from testis and an antiserum elicited by injection of brain extracts were described [140]. It is not clear, however, that the alcohol-soluble antigen is the same antigen as the substance detected in the earlier studies, especially the component that was capable of being autoantigenic.

It is also important to note that the sperm cells contain at least two distinctive antigens, which are easily differentiated by their morphology. The realization that these antigens are characteristic of the head or tail parts of the cell was based on the observation that different sera produced agglutination of either the head-to-head or the tail-to-tail variety. HENLE *et al.* separated spermatozoa into heads and tails by means of ultrasonic treatment [92]. A head-specific and a tail-specific antigen were demonstrated, both of which were heat-labile, and also a third antigen, which was heat-stable, common to head and tail, and species-specific. Heteroantisera were used in these studies, so that it is not known whether *auto*antigenic activities are similarly separable. The various kinds of sperm antigens can be arranged in a number of groups, including sperm-specific antigens, blood-groups antigens, transplantation antigens, and spermatozoa-coating antigens. These will be discussed below; much more detail is given elsewhere [273, 275].

Studies on spermatozoal antigens and the autoantibodies that can arise can be divided into two main groups, which differ in several ways. One group involves production of aspermatogenesis and/or orchitis in experimental animals. The other group of studies involves a spontaneous human disorder in which antibodies against sperm appear but there is no histopathological picture such as production of testicular damage. Our knowledge of the varied ways in which sperm cells can be autoantigenic is still inadequate, although recent progress has emphasized the distinctive roles of several antigenic components. The two types of study will be discussed in the following two sections.

a) Experimental Aspermatogenesis

The natural occurrence of autoantibodies to sperm cells in serum in several kinds of mammal and bird was recorded as long ago as the twenties [215, 334]. Experimental induction of tissue damage was also attempted, for example, in the work of MCCARTNEY [168], who injected several male rats with rat semen and reported that atrophic changes and decreased sperm production resulted. Similar studies were reported by GUYER [82] and by KENNEDY [122]. This early work was rather inconclusive. Considerable progress was indicated by the reports of VOISIN and his group (1951) and FREUND and his group (1953). Voisin and colleagues showed that guinea pigs injected with testicular tissue of guinea pigs in certain adjuvants developed tissue damage in the testes, which they termed orchitis and epididymitis [326].

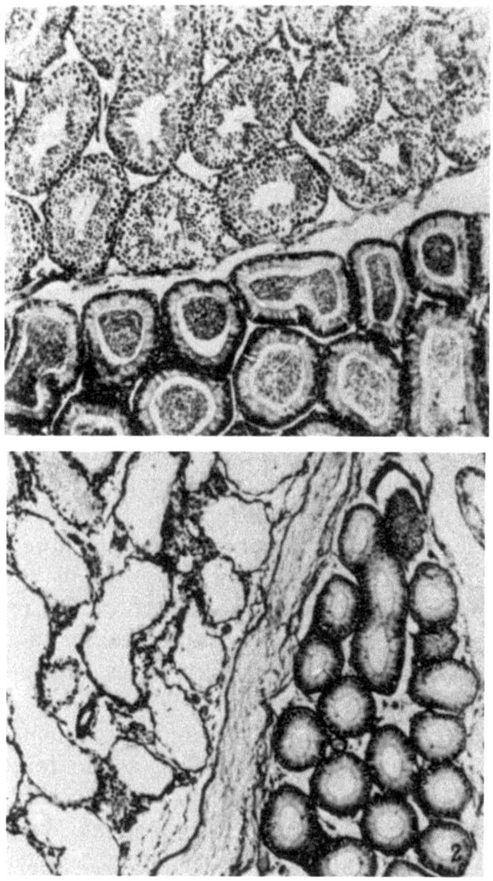

Fig. 5.1. Histological examination of guinea pig testis and epididymis. X90, approx. Upper picture: normal guinea pig, testis above and epididymis below. Lower picture: guinea pig injected with testicular suspension and adjuvants, showing 4+ injury, testis on left and epididymis on right. (Adapted from FREUND *et al.* [68])

FREUND and his colleagues [68] reported the study that made both the phenomenon and the adjuvant [70] famous. They showed that a suspension of testicular tissue from other animals of the same species, in combination with a paraffin oil and heat-killed tubercle baccilli, produced aspermatogenesis when injected in guinea pigs; this was apparent in cessation of sperm production and drastic changes in testicular histology. It was even possible to use the testis of the animal to be injected if hemiorchiectomy was performed. Typical degenerative changes are illustrated in Fig. 5.1. The injury does not involve inflammation, which makes it quite different from other experimental autoimmune diseases such as thyroiditis or allergic encephalomyelitis. The first injury is the inhibition of spermatozoal maturation; this is followed by the degeneration of spermatids, spermatocytes, and finally, spermatogonia. The Leydig cells are not affected. The seminal vesicles and prostate gland remain normal. Electron microscope studies have also been reported [153, 156].

The question of the existence of an inflammatory state has been much debated, as has the interpretation that the tissue damage is mediated primarily by a mechanism of delayed hypersensitivity. The necessity of Freund's complete adjuvant for production of the tissue lesions has been interpreted as indicating an essential role for delayed hypersensitivity in this lesion formation [333]. WAKSMAN (1959) claimed that the testicular damage involved specific sensitized cells and that cellular infiltration, particularly of polymorphonuclear leukocytes, was present [332]. This interpretation was challenged in 1963 by the report of BROWN, GLYNN, and HOLBOROW [35], who performed histologic examinations in groups of immunized guinea pigs at frequent intervals after injection. They reported that as the lesion developed, the only cellular infiltration to be seen was a secondary phenomenon and that the damage was seen in the complete absence of any such infiltration in any part of the testis or epididymis. It is generally agreed that inflammation—the invasion of the tissue by mononuclear cells—is not a feature of this particular autoimmune disease, but the more recent studies of LEVINE and SOWINSKI [139], JOHNSON [111], and TUNG *et al.* [316–318] have shown that the phenomenon is more complex than previously thought, and that inflammatory processes do play an important role, depending on certain factors such as the nature of the immunizing antigen preparation. The observations also differ considerably in different anatomic regions, such as the seminiferous tubule, rete testis, and epididymis. A more detailed review and discussion has been presented elsewhere [273].

These injections of testicular material also stimulated the formation of specific antibodies against testicular tissue and against spermatozoa. FREUND *et al.* [69] gave convincing evidence that the response was a specific immune response, showing it to be tissue-specific, since neither liver nor kidney of guinea pig could induce such a response, and also species-specific, since the response was not produced in guinea pig by testis from rabbit. This phenomenon, termed experimental (allergic) aspermatogenesis, autoimmune aspermatogenesis, or allergic orchitis, has been used as a model for autoimmune responses in general and especially for various types of experimental autoimmune diseases. The use of imcomplete adjuvant leads only to the production of antibodies, but the use of complete adjuvant leads to the additional production of atrophic tissue damage when whole tissue homogenate is used. These responses can also be induced by injection of various purified preparations derived from testicular tissue, or by injection of suspensions of epididymal sperm. An aspermatogenic factor was thus recognized in the testicular tissue and the sperm cells. Much study has been devoted to the role of the adjuvant, and alternative adjuvants have been widely investigated by KATSH *et al.* [113, 115, 116, 120, 121] and BISHOP *et al.* [25–27], among other.

Similar studies have been performed in other species [163, 164, 218], but the guinea pig seems to illustrate this phenomenon particularly well. There was reasonable success in rats [69]. LAURENCE *et al.* showed that it is possible to transfer the disease within strains of rats by means of leukocytes [134, 135]. EYQUEM and KRIEG have extended the possibilities of producing testicular lesions by direct injections of Freund's adjuvant into a testis of rabbits and monkeys [56]. MANCINI and his co-workers [154] studied patients suffering from prostate carcinoma. These men were injected with an autologous testicular homogenate, plus adjuvant. Testicular lesions and circulating antibodies were produced, *i.e.*, the results were very similar to those described for guinea pigs. Other work has been done in monkeys [5, 191], including a study of biopsy samples [39] taken at various intervals.

Many studies have been aimed at elucidation of the chemical nature of the aspermatogenic material. FREUND *et al.* [71] partially purified this tissue-specific antigen by making an acetic-acid extract of testicular tissue, precipitating it in 30% saturated ammonium sulfate, and using trichloroacetic acid and mixtures of chloroform and butyl alcohol. The product was at least 100 times more active than the crude extract in inducing aspermatogenesis. It was quite thermostable, a property of considerable interest in view of other thermostable antigens of tissues that have been studied in recent years, such as those of adrenal [182–184, 291]. They detected a considerable proportion of carbohydrate material in their product. Many subsequent reports have emphasized its carbohydrate character, but there has been no proof that the final product is not still a mixture of substances. BROWN *et al.* [35, 37] used phenol extraction and other procedures, which also yielded a very active preparation with a high carbohydrate content. Amino-acid and carbohydrate analyses of preparations containing high degrees of aspermatogenic activity have been published by KATSH and by BISHOP and their co-workers [26, 126], but again the reports do not state the degree of molecular purity of the preparations.

Chemical analyses have been reported recently by VOISIN and his group [327], who claim that there is more than one aspermatogenic factor. They claim that there are four such factors and have termed them S, P, Z, and T. All but compound Z have been obtained in moderately well-purified condition, and each of them seems to have quite different antigenic and biochemical properties. They also show different degrees of pathogenicity in terms of the ease of inducing experimental aspermatogenesis, or, as VOISIN *et al.* prefer to term it, autoimmune aspermatogenic orchitis (AIAO). Further studies on these components can be expected to clarify the chemical and immunopathologic confusion, eventually.

The fractionation procedure started with the treatment of an extract of guinea pig spermatozoa with 5% trichloroacetic acid. The supernatant contained mostly antigen S, with some antigen P. The sediment contained mostly P, and it was agitated with chloroform to give a better preparation of P in the aqueous phase. Each of the preparations was filtered on a column of Sephadex G-100, giving S and P preparations free from each other. The major properties of these and the other two antigens can be summarized as follows [327, 328].

Antigen S is a glycoprotein which is very rich in sugar. It is thermostable, water soluble, and soluble in trichloroacetic acid. It is sensitive to proteolytic enzymes and to periodic acid. VOISIN *et al.* describe this component as highly autoantigenic. It elicits hypersensitivity of the delayed, anaphylactic, and Arthus types, and also antibodies giving anaphylaxis and passive hemagglutination, but not precipitation or spermotoxicity. It is potently orchitogenic and aspermatogenic.

Antigen P is a protein which is poor in sugar. It is thermostable and water soluble, but it is precipitated by trichloroacetic acid. It it less sensitive than S to the action of periodic acid and proteases. It elicits hypersensitivity of the three types. It provokes the formation of antibodies that are able to precipitate and to give anaphylaxis, but not to be spermotoxic. It can also induce lesions of AIAO.

Antigen T may be a proteolipid. It is thermolabile and water insoluble, and it is destroyed by trichloroactic acid. It elicits the formation of spermotoxic antibodies and can bring about testicular lesions of the AIAO type.

Antigen Z is a labile and nonabundant component. It is thermolabile, water soluble, and soluble in trichloroacetic acid. It has not been much studied.

The immune responses induced by purified S or P were studied either at various times after immunization with one dose (chronological study), or at a given time after immunization with various doses (quantitative study), or by varying both parameters (but only for early responses). Examination of some typical experiments will allow an appreciation of the profound differences between these factors, which used to be considered together as a single agent producing this general activity. The following details were reported recently by VOISIN and TOULLET [328].

Ten guinea pigs were immunized with a quantity of S equivalent to 10^8 spermatozoa in complete adjuvant. Five more guinea pigs received complete adjuvant alone, and five animals received nothing; these last 10 animals thus served as controls. On each of days 7, 10, 14, 17, and 21, two experimental and two control guinea pigs were studied for their immune responses, as judged in the skin, serum, and testes. Table 5.1 shows that delayed hypersensitivity appeared first (day 7), and this was followed by anaphylactic hypersensitivity (day 10), the most sensitive sign of the presence of antibodies; on day 14, other signs of the presence of antibody (Arthus hypersensitivity, hemagglutinating antibodies) appeared and, at the same time, the lesions of AIAO appeared, accompanied by increased vascular permeability in the testis. No responses were noticed in the 10 controls.

In two other experiments, 18 guinea pigs were immunized with various doses of antigen S (corresponding to 5×10^4, 5×10^5, 5×10^6, 1×10^7, and 1×10^8 spermatozoa). The immune responses of these animals were studied on days 28 and 29. The smallest dose (5×10^4) gave no sign of any immune response, but the next higher doses (5×10^5 and 5×10^6) induced some responses of the delayed type and of anaphylactic hypersensitivity, along with occasional lesions, although no Arthus hypersensitivity and no circulating antibody was detected.

Table 5.1. *Immune responses in experimental aspermatogenesis. Reactions to autoantigen S, tested in guinea pigs*

Type of Reaction	Days After Immunization				
	7	10	14	17	21
Skin Reactivity					
Delayed	2/2	2/2	2/2	2/2	1/2
Anaphylactic	0/2	1/2	2/2	2/2	2/2
Arthus	0/2	0/2	1[a]/2	0/2	2/2
Serum Activity					
Hemagglutinating antibodies	0/2	0/2	1[a]/2	0/2	2/2
Testis Damage					
Lesions	0/2	0/2	1[a]/2	2/2	2/2
Increased vascular permeability	0/2	0/2	1[a]/2	2/2	1/2

All animals were immunized with a quantity of autoantigen S equivalent to 10^7 spermatozoa.
The figures express the actual proportions of animals with a positive reaction.
[a] Same animal.

The two maximal doses (10^7 and 10^8 sperm) induced the best results, showing lesions in most animals, and positive results in all the skin and serum tests.

It was thus seen that the presence of delayed hypersensitivity to autoantigen S is not sufficient to induce AIAO; the presence of serum-mediated immune responses (anaphylaxis, Arthus, serum antibodies) seems to be more related to the appearance of AIAO. Of the 11 animals that developed AIAO, 9 had both delayed and anaphylactic hypersensitivity, while of the 27 animals not having both types of hypersensitivity, only 2 (one with anaphylaxis, the other with delayed hypersensitivity) showed AIAO.

A similar study, both chronological and quantitative, was made of autoantigen P. Twenty-four guinea pigs received one of 3 doses (corresponding to 1.2×10^7, 6×10^7, or 30×10^7 sperm) of P, and were studied after one of 6 intervals following immunization (6, 9, 14, 21, 28, or 56 days) for immune reactions (skin hypersensitivity of the three types, precipitating antibodies, specifically increased vascular permeability, and lesions in the testes). Increasing the dose of antigen accelerated the appearance of the various signs of immune reactions, and the delayed reactions appeared later (day 21 to 56, according to the dose) than anaphylactic reactions (day 14 to 28, according to the dose), and also later than testicular lesions (with the 6×10^7 dose). Autoantigens S and P thus differ in that all the immune responses to P develop later than those to S, and the delayed hypersensitivity response is so much delayed that it is the last response to P, whereas it is the first response to S. It is also worthwhile to note that, in contrast to antigen S, antigen P induces complement-fixing antibodies. Of the 7 animals that developed AIAO, 6 had both delayed and anaphylactic hypersensitivity, while of the 6 animals which did not have both types of hypersensitivity, only 1 (with anaphylaxis) showed AIAO.

From these data, it should be emphasized, as had already been suggested [327], that there is an essential coexistence of two types of hypersensitivity—the delayed type, depending on the action of sensitized cells, and the anaphylactic type, depending on the action of circulating antibody. It was similarly argued recently by BROWN *et al.* [36] that testicular lesions developed best in the experimental conditions where delayed hypersensitivity and serum antibodies both occur. VOISIN *et al.* [328] proposed that the major role of the cells is to make the target tissue accessible to the action of the antibodies (and complement, perhaps) by increasing the vascular permeability and tissue permeability. Furthermore, POKORNÁ has recently shown that aspermatogenesis can be passively transferred in mice through the antiserum or other noncellular material [216, 217]. She used either immune serum or effective material obtained from the aspermatogenic mice by treatment of cells from spleen, lymph node, or peritoneal exudate. These cells were washed thoroughly and then incubated for an hour at 56°, as if to elute cytophilic antibody from cells. The supernatant from this incubation was considered an eluate; it was active in the disease transfer.

Other means of inducing aspermatogenesis and/or orchitis have been described by various workers [225, 230, 301, 347].

b) Human Spermagglutinins

We can now turn our attention to antibodies that form against spermatozoa in certain human individuals. The past fifteen years have seen a number of reports on the occurrence of spermagglutinating activity in the blood serum of certain men and women. This activity has generally been attributed to the existence of specific antibodies against the sperm cells, and it has also been claimed that a correlation exists between this activity and the condition of unexplained infertility. Studies on the male indicate clearly that such an antibody is an autoantibody. In the female, while it is tempting to term it an isoantibody, we must recognize that the only grouping of individuals within the general population for the distribution of the corresponding antigen is that of the sex difference for sperm production. It is not really proven that no sperm-like antigen is present in female urogenital tissue. It may be better to avoid the term isoantibody, and thus avoid any implications of genetic control and presence of a certain antigen.

In 1954 WILSON [346] and RÜMKE and his colleagues [245] reported that spermagglutinins occur in the serum and in seminal plasma of 2–3% of men suffering from unexplained sterility. For example, autoagglutination in the semen was seen in 10 of 15 patients showing serum activity, and might well have been seen in the others, had the density and motility of the sperm been sufficient [246]. Later studies of RÜMKE and HELLINGA [255] investigated several thousand infertile patients and showed that 3% of them had spermagglutinins in titers of 1:32 or more, while a large group of fertile men had no such activity. They detected this activity by means of one of two technics of macroagglutination in small test tubes, many details of which had been worked out by KIBRICK *et al.* [123, 124]. In the Kibrick method [124], motile sperm cells from a fresh ejaculate are suspended in a 10% gelatin solution in saline. The use of gelatin and the conditions of concentration and temperature may minimize the problem of nonspecific agglutination sufficiently. In other studies, immunofluorescent methods were applied to these investigations [58, 247].

The criteria of immunological specificity must be positively established. The early efforts at direct visual observation of agglutination of sperm suspensions met with great difficulties because the suspensions in normal serum or even in buffer solution sometimes developed spontaneous agglutination, which was difficult to distinguish from agglutination by antibody. MUDD was the first to study this problem seriously [192, 193]; he recommended that the tubes be centrifuged and then shaken to resuspend the sediment; shaking should be continued until a reasonably homogeneous suspension was obtained in the control tubes [192]. This procedure failed at times, because the loose clumps of antibody-bound spermatozoa were also easily broken by agitation. On this basis KIBRICK *et al.* [123, 124] developed their improved methods, suggesting first the use of narrow-bore tubes [123] and then a gelatin medium [124]. This gelatin agglutination method has been applied by a number of workers, as noted above; it has usually been used for human sperm [59, 64, 245, 247, 255], but occasionally for sperm from other animals [202]. This method is both sensitive and specific, but motile sperm must be used. Newer methods of spermagglutination testing have been proposed which do not require motile sperm and are quite simple [284, 285, 351]. These procedures have been described in considerable detail [276, 276b, 276c].

We still do not know why the spermatozoa have to be motile for successful and sensitive testing for antibody; motile spermatozoa are also required for the microscope method, to be discussed below. TYLER suggested [319]: "Sperm-suspensions are useful test-antigens in that agglutinative reaction is easily read macroscopically as well as microscopically and the motility of the spermatozoa favors quick reaction without the necessity of shaking". KIBRICK *et al.* [96, 97] published several statements, but some points are really contradictory. For example, "The long whiplike tail and flattened pear-shaped head lend themselves to the formation of loose entangling floccules. The more active the spermatozoa, the more rapid is the formation of the floccules", [123, p. 422]; but, "The size and motility of the spermatozoa, however, may enable the organisms to overcome the agglutinative forces, especially in the presence of small amounts of antibody, and the resultant agglutinates may be so weakly bound as to be easily disrupted by mild jarring or shaking", [123, p. 422]; and, "In the presence of small amounts of antibody, actively motile spermatozoa apparently may overcome the cohesive agglutinative forces and by breaking away reduce the size of the floccules, thus limiting the sensitivity of the test", [124, p. 431]. The only point emerging clearly from all this is that the relationships are difficult to understand.

It has been suggested that autoantibodies to sperm might result from occlusion of the efferent duct of the testis, either the epididymis or the vas deferens. Direct experimental proof of this mechanism [209] has not yet been extensively developed, but several preliminary reports have appeared. Investigations have been undertaken in recent years, making use of patients who have undergone voluntary vasectomy for the purpose of sterilization. The first of these studies included control studies of pre-vasectomy sera, and serum samples were obtained at various intervals. Just over half the group of men developed antibody against sperm, as detected by the Kibrick test [300, 351]. This finding has been confirmed by two reports from different laboratories where different antibody procedures were used [6, 41]. Again, about 50 to 60% of the men in each group developed antibody activity of this sort [276a]. More data are needed, however, based on many more men and on more samples for each one, along with information on any cross-reactions of these antibodies with antigens of other tissues. Spermagglutinins and other such activities have been reported in experimental animals after vasectomy or vasoligation [34, 256].

Although there are reports to the contrary [214], the recent studies by FJÄLLBRANT [59–61, 63] again showed a correlation of spermagglutination with infertility. He also reported a good correlation between the level of sperm antibodies in the man's serum and the deficiency of penetrating ability of his spermatozoa into cervical mucus [62]. Reports and reviews of this general subject have been published by RÜMKE and colleagues [87a, 111a, 248–254] and by SHULMAN [272, 273, 275, 276c, 286, 295, 296].

It is by no means clear whether the antigen or antigens of spermatozoa that elicit autoantibody formation in these men are analogous to any of those that cause aspermatogenesis and testicular tissue damage in guinea pigs immunized with testicular material. It seems likely that the antigens are different, since there is no indication of testicular damage in men with autosensitization to spermatozoa. The spermatozoal autoantigenicity may arise from absorption of fluid secretions from various components of the reproductive tract. Some sperm proteins have been partially purified [40, 74, 75, 344, 345], and the ultrastructure of the cell has been studied [14, 15, 221]. Cellular interactions between spermatozoa and cervical epithelium have been described [231]. The various antigens in or on the sperm cell have been much discussed [28, 30, 32, 33, 88, 107, 155, 204, 219, 220, 226–229], as has the question of sperm-specific antigens [21, 106–108, 141, 178]. It is important to note that epididymal and ejaculated spermatozoa differ in antigenic properties, and the development of better methods of obtaining ejaculated sperm has been an important subject of study [72, 73, 131, 161]. WEIL and RODENBURG [335, 341, 342] have shown that a protein of the seminal plasma, arising as a secretion of the seminal vesicle, in rabbit and in human and referred to as the spermatozoa-coating antigen (SCA), coats the sperm cells as they traverse the urethra and thus modifies their antigenic properties, so that there is no longer any cross-reaction with extracts of testis or epididymis. The antigens of seminal plasma, including this SCA fraction, will be discussed below.

Most studies on the human female including examination of spermagglutinins in sera from women have been prompted by investigation of sterility [49, 66, 68, 194, 261, 313]. FRANKLIN and DUKES [49, 66, 67] and SCHWIMMER *et al.* [261] have claimed a remarkably high incidence of spermagglutinating activity in females with unexplained sterility. The first group reported positive results in about 80% of women with unexplained sterility. The second laboratory reported approximately 40% positive in such women; this is still rather high for a clear interpretation of the findings, especially since they also found 20% positive in their control groups. In these studies, a particular method of microagglutination was used. However, we have considerable grounds for questioning the degree of specificity of the agglutination, since the method had not been well evaluated with regard to various immunological factors, and it is not clear how correct is the interpretation that all the cases of agglutinating activity are based on specific antibody against sperm cells. One group using this microscope method found that 7–8% of *men* from infertile couples had spermagglutinating activity [261], exactly twice the incidence reported by RÜMKE [245, 246] and by FJÄLLBRANT [59], who both had used the Kibrick test. The first clearly described microscope method was used in the sperm studies of HENLE *et al.* [90–92]; he referred to a "slide agglutination reaction" [92]. Very similar procedures were used by SNELL [303] in studies on mouse spermagglutinins, and by FLOCKS *et al.* [64] in studies on rabbit antibodies to human spermatozoa. The results of these earlier studies indicated quite different concentrations and times of incubation from the more recent studies of women's sera [65, 66]. More detailed study and comparison of these and other alternative procedures for microscope observation of agglutination would be highly desirable. A wide variety of cluster patterns is seen in these microscope inspections; one typical pattern, illustrating a mild degree of head-to-head agglutination, is shown in Fig. 5.2.

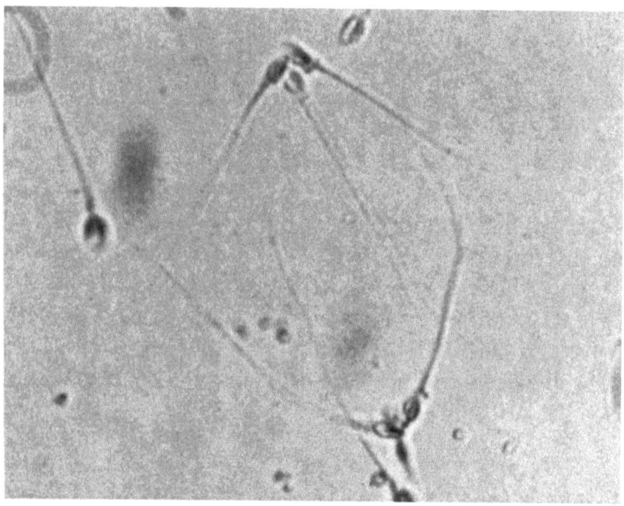

Fig. 5.2. Microscope view of human sperm cells showing agglutination (head-to-head) resulting from action of human (male) serum containing spermagglutinating autoantibody. X800, approx

Reduction of fertility in female animals following immunization with seminal or testicular material has been described by several workers. An early study by ISOJIMA *et al.* [105] was then followed by other reports [7, 8]. Early studies were also made by KATSH *et al.* [114–118] and by BEHRMAN and NAKAYAMA

[19]. BEHRMAN and OTANI emphasized the production of sperm antibodies as a result of transvaginal immunization in experimental animals [20]; the possibility of vaginal immunization was first described by MCCARTNEY [168]. Conflicting reports on the immunological control of fertility have recently been published by MCLAREN [170, 171] and EDWARDS [52]. On the other hand, reduced fertility has been described as a definite consequence of immunization in a number of reports [33, 125, 172–175, 177–179, 203]. These and other papers [91, 117, 119, 320] should stimulate much more work on the immunologic approach. The subject has been reviewed recently by ISOJIMA [104] and by SHULMAN [272]. Clearer results are to be expected in the future on the precise levels of sperm antibodies in human serum, especially in women, but it will still be necessary to consider the significance of positive results. Even genuinely positive activity in the serum may be considered to have no bearing on a woman's fertility, unless these antibodies are at the same sites as the spermatozoa, deposited there by antibody transport or by local secretion. EDWARDS [53] has reviewed some factors affecting the passage of antibody molecules across various membranes. A number of studies have been directed at the detection of antibody in the cervical mucus or some similar adjacent tissue or mucus [250, 312]. Many of these studies involved searching for antibody by exploring the presence of the blood group antibodies, while others were based on detecting the antigenic characteristics of the immunoglobulins. This topic is discussed later, in connection with the studies on the tissues of the female reproductive system.

ABO incompatibility between parents has been postulated as a cause of reduced fertility in the offspring. The suggested involvement of the ABO and even other blood group systems has attracted much interest and some controversy, but a detailed discussion is beyond the scope of this book, and other sources should be consulted [78, 85, 109, 137, 138, 165, 208, 306, 307, 314]. On the basis of family and statistical studies MATSUNAGA and ITOH [165] and BEHRMAN *et al.* [18] proposed that blood group antibodies were present in the cervical mucus and the entering sperm cells were blocked or immobilized. More recently, a number of reports have disagreed with this hypothesis, and the possibilities now are thought to be more complicated. The subject has been more thoroughly reviewed by BOETTCHER [30], ISOJIMA [104], and KRIEG [128]. The immunological relationships between mother and fetus have also been studied [32, 176, 305, 329] and will be discussed below.

2. Antigens of the Male Accessory Glands of Reproduction

a) Prostate Gland and Prostatic Fluid

The term prostate specificity is often used as a convenient and brief way of referring to the tissue specificity of a group of related and adjacent organs; these include the seminal vesicle, the prostate gland, the coagulating gland (seen especially in rodents), and the bulbo-urethral (*or* Cowper's) gland, in other words, the group of glands collectively termed the male accessory glands of reproduction.

Since the prostate gland is by far the best known and the most commonly mentioned of these glands, especially in connection with the human reproductive system, we shall use it as a brief reference to the group as a whole, especially with regard to antigenic components. In recent years it has been made quite clear from studies in three species, man, rabbit, and dog, that the property of tissue specificity can be associated with this glandular group, and some of the evidence will be surveyed below. The results can be grouped by species studied for convenience.

The first antigenic studies on these particular urogenital tissues were reported by FLOCKS and his co-workers in 1960 and 1962 [64, 65]. They reported double-diffusion experiments which indicated that rabbit antisera against human prostatic tissue could be prepared and that the antibodies were specific for the prostate. The evidence seemed to indicate the existence of antibodies against at least two antigens of the prostate. However, 8 of 10 of their antisera contained antibodies to other human organs and tissues, although not against extracts of dog or rat prostate tissue. In other words, while the antisera were restricted to the species insofar as was tested, they did not show the strict organ-specificity that might have been expected from preliminary immunization in a different species of animal. This was not pursued further to differentiate between prostate-specific antigens and ubiquitous antigens.

α) *Human Prostatic Fluid*

The immunologic properties of human prostatic fluid have been described in tests with antisera from intensively immunized rabbits [12, 13]. At least four or five antigens were distinctive for this fluid, and three or four other antigens were shared with the blood serum [13]. Immunoelectrophoresis and immunofluorescence were used to characterize these antigens and to distinguish them from serum antigens. In addition, various tissues showed one or two lines of precipitation with an antiserum that had been absorbed with human plasma [12], although these were not the major lines of prostatic fluid or extract. These tissues included seminal vesicle, testis, kidney, liver, and lung. However, bladder and adrenal gave no reaction. The method of passive hemagglutination also revealed the existence of one or several prostatic fluid-specific antigens. These antigens were found in male urine, but not in female urine; the proteins in male urine may represent prostatic secretion, and their appearance may vary from time to time [12].

The biochemical nature of the substances responsible for this tissue specificity has been studied. Human prostatic fluid has been revealed as a complex mixture when examined electrophoretically [290, 304], ultracentrifugally [281], and enzymatically [283, 288, 289]. There have been many studies on the phosphatases and other enzymes, only a few of which can be cited here [10, 11, 46–48, 50, 51, 100, 102, 147, 148, 150, 200, 201, 232, 237, 238], but the more recent approach has been to measure these enzymes by a combination of enzymatic and antigenic properties [46–48, 170, 171, 190, 213, 283, 288, 289]. Prostatic fluid and the closely related seminal plasma will be compared and discussed below.

β) Canine Prostatic Fluid

The dog has a simpler type of prostatic fluid and a simpler glandular system. Canine prostatic fluid has generally been obtained by means of pilocarpine stimulation, utilizing surgically treated animals in which the prostate and urethra are isolated from the rest of the urological system by a method developed by HUGGINS and MASON and their colleagues [101, 159]. These dogs can be stimulated to elaborate essentially pure prostatic fluid and to yield prodigious quantities of this material—40 to 60 ml per hour. A number of studies have been made on the ions, enzymes, and other biochemical constituents of canine prostatic fluid [101, 151, 237–239].

Antigenic analyses have revealed that canine prostatic fluid contains strong antigenic activity, judging from the antibody responses in rabbits [349]. A significant part of this antigenic mixture represents prostate-specific antigens, shown by passive hemagglutination and gel diffusion precipitation. There was no cross-reaction with other canine tissues, such as bladder, testis, kidney, liver, spleen, heart, muscle, and brain. This is illustrated in Fig. 5.3 by gel diffusion. Reactions

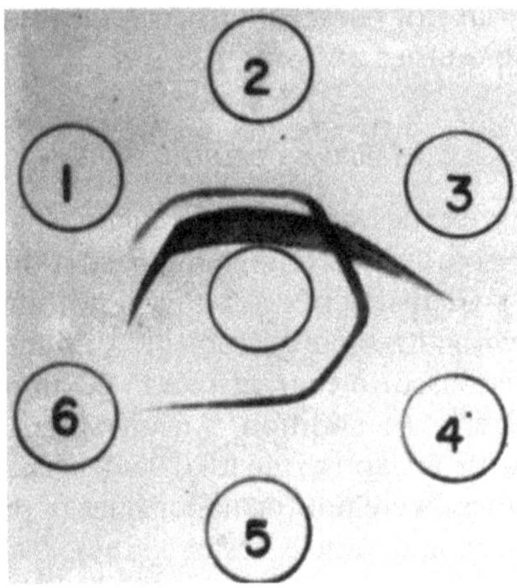

Fig. 5.3. Double diffusion gel precipitation. Central well: rabbit anti-canine prostatic fluid. Peripheral wells: (1) canine prostatic fluid, 1:10 dilution, (2) canine prostate gland extract, (3) canine bladder extract, (4) canine kidney extract, (5) canine serum, 1:50 dilution, (6) saline

occurred with prostate extract or seminal plasma, but these reflected the prostatic fluid component in these tissues. The lack of reaction of other tissues cannot be ascribed to any failure in coating the cells, because of the identical information provided by inhibition of hemagglutination, as shown in Table 5.2. Thus this is a tissue-specific antigen which is a major component in the mixture and should thus be easy to purify and characterize. Recent reports have described the purification and study of this major antigen and of a minor antigen, and also interactions between them [2, 277].

The influence of anti-prostate antibodies introduced by passive transfer has been explored following the injection of rabbit anti-canine prostatic fluid into normal dogs. Degenerative changes in the recipient's prostate gland were described, and a number of immunological interactions were studied [149, 210], but the reactions are very complex and far from clarified.

Table 5.2. *Tanned cell hemagglutination inhibition test*

Inhibition of reaction between rabbit anti-canine prostatic fluid[a] and human erythrocytes coated with canine prostatic fluid, using as inhibitors various tissue extracts and fluids from canine and other species

	Inhibitor			
Dilution of the inhibiting specimen	Canine prostatic fluid	Canine seminal plasma	Canine serum[b]	Human prostatic fluid[c]
1: 2	–	–	+	+
4	–	–	+	+
8	–	–	+	+
16	–	–	+	+
32	–	–	+	+
64	–	–	+	+
128	–	–	+	+
256	–	–	+	+
512	–	–	+	+
1024	–	–	+	+
2048	–	–	+	+
4096	–	–	+	+
8192	–	–	+	+
16384	–	–	+	+
32768	–	+	+	+
65536	–	+	+	+
131072	+	+	+	+
262144	+	+	+	+

[a] Absorbed with canine serum.
[b] Other canine preparations tested were pooled extracts of bladder, testis, kidney, heart, and brain; these were all completely negative as inhibitors.
[c] Other species preparations tested were pooled extracts of monkey, rabbit, and guinea pig prostate gland; these were all completely negative as inhibitors.

γ) Rabbit Prostatic Tissues

i) The Accessory Glands

The tissue specificity of the prostate-related antigens has also been examined in rabbit, although most of these studies have been performed on tissue extracts rather than on prostatic fluid, and most of the studies have been related to the formation of autoantibodies. Nonetheless, an antiserum containing autoantibodies can be used to establish the existence of tissue-specific antigens, and this reagent has been used as an alternative to the type of heteroantibody used to study the human and the dog systems. Fig. 5.4 shows the anatomical arrangement of the urogenital system of rabbit as a labeled sketch. Extracts were prepared from the prostate gland itself or from the total cluster of the four accessory glands, and rabbits were then immunized with homogenates of tissue incorporated into complete Freund's adjuvant with additional killed tubercle bacilli—a preparation that has been termed fortified adjuvant [297]. The series of blood samples were then examined by means of passive hemagglutination and gel diffusion and antibody responses were obtained after several weeks of injections; the antibodies were in fact autoantibodies. These antisera were then used for tissue and species comparisons. Strong reactions were produced in each of the accessory tissues, even with an antiserum obtained from a rabbit immunized with an extract of prostate gland carefully separated from the other tissues. This strongly suggested a common antigen in all these related tissues. A reaction was also obtained with this rabbit's own autologous prostate. Inhibition was *not* produced by bladder, liver, serum, or testis of rabbit. In other experiments, prostatic fluid from human or dog origin did not react, indicating the species specificity of the antigen. Gel diffusion experiments gave results in complete concurrence with these. Negative results were obtained with rabbit liver, kidney, adrenal, heart, thyroid, testis, bladder, uterus, and vagina. The gel diffusion experiments indicated that this reaction might involve two antigens. Many of the results have been published in some detail [264, 297, 299].

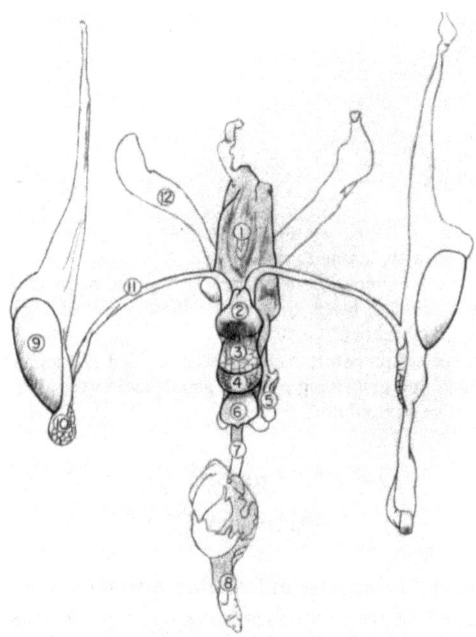

Fig. 5.4. Sketch of the urogenital system in the male rabbit. The structures are: (1) bladder, (2) seminal vesicle, (3) coagulating gland, (4) prostate gland, (5) paraprostate gland, (6) bulbo-urethral gland, (7) urethra, (8) penis, (9) testis, (10) epididymis, (11) vas deferens, (12) fat

ii) Stimulation by Cryosurgery

A different approach to the experimental production of autoantibodies to the accessory glands has been developed in recent years. This method involves intensive freezing of the tissue *in situ*. This cryosurgical procedure is the basis of cryo-immunology [110, 265–268, 278, 282, 298, 348]. Cryo-immunization may also prove useful as a model for studies on the mechanisms of spontaneous autoantibody formation [267, 268, 301].

iii) The Antigens Shared with Seminal Plasma

There are two possible explanations for the positive reaction of seminal plasma with the antiserum to accessory glands antigen(s). One is that the earliest portions of the semen itself, as manufactured in the testis and epididymis, contain the antigen, in which case the semen is a source of contamination for the tissue extracts that are prepared from the prostate gland and the other tissues and the antigen should then be referred to properly as a semen antigen. An alternative possibility is that the semen does not originally contain the component but acquires it as it courses through the urethra, and the secretions from the accessory glands are added to the seminal plasma. The autoantigen would then be a component of these accessory tissues of reproduction.

The experiments concerning this question utilized extracts of rabbit epididymis and of vas deferens. The results with rabbit epididymis extracts were negative, although they did contain adequate antigen, as seen from their several strong lines of precipitation when tested with a guinea pig antiserum against rabbit epididymis extract [299]. The vas deferens was divided into three separate portions and separate extracts were made. Subsequent testing showed negative results for the third that had been next to the epididymis and also for the middle third but positive results for the third that had been next to the urethra [299]. The antigen being studied was not characteristic of seminal plasma but a unique constituent of the group of accessory glands of reproduction. In the light of data from RÜMKE and HEKMAN [87], described in detail below, it should be pointed out that these autoantibody sera were not tested against rabbit milk or spleen; they found an interesting cross-reaction between these two tissues and seminal plasma. Similar testing with the autoantibody should be attempted in future studies.

b) Seminal Plasma

α) Immunogenicity of Seminal Plasma

The antigenic properties of seminal plasma were first studied by WEIL and his associates in pioneer investigations. They demonstrated a number of strong antigens in rabbit [337], and three antigens (or groups of antigens) in human seminal plasma [340]. Similar studies were published in the same year by PERNOT *et al.* [211, 212], describing the seminal plasma of guinea pigs and of bulls. We shall discuss the work of WEIL'S group.

The antisera that had been prepared against human seminal plasma or against whole semen or washed spermatozoa reacted in complement fixation or in precipitation with seminal plasma in quite high titers and also reacted with well-washed spermatozoa [340]. This cross-reaction with ejaculated spermatozoa was the first hint that at least one of the dominant antigenic components of the spermatozoa might derive from the fluid constituents of the semen rather than from the spermatozoa themselves. Later work showed the existence of an antigen of seminal plasma which they termed the spermatozoa-coating antigen (SCA). This was found in both rabbit [335] and man [341]. They showed, for example, that antisera against ejaculated spermatozoa, while showing strong positive reactions with ejaculated spermatozoa, did not react at all when tested with epididymal spermatozoa. Secondly, antisera against seminal plasma also gave strong positive reactions with ejaculated spermatozoa and were negative with epididymal spermatozoa. These studies indicated quite strongly that: 1. the antigenic natures of epididymal spermatozoa and ejaculated spermatozoa are significantly different, 2. the epididymal spermatozoa acquire an additional antigen property while they pass through the urethra, and 3. there is a component of the seminal plasma that interacts with and coats these spermatozoa. WEIL and his co-workers gave good evidence that this spermatozoa-coating antigen originated in the seminal vesicle [342]. This was a portion of their study of seminal plasma antigenicity [336, 338, 339].

In a more recent study [233, 294], in which the approach to isoimmunization was again undertaken, but from somewhat different points of view, rabbits were injected with three different types of preparation for comparison; whole semen, seminal plasma, and extract of epididymis. The epididymis material did not elicit autoantibody, but the seminal plasma and semen injections did. This provided autoantibodies as reagents for the evaluation of tissue specificity. In hemagglutination tests some tissues gave negative results when tested with this autoantibody; these included testis, epididymis, kidney, and serum, while the results with extracts of the accessory glands and the seminal plasma were positive. This strong degree of cross-reaction between the seminal plasma and the accessory glands of reproduction was not surprising, since it had already been shown that at least some antigens are common to semen and accessory reproductive tissue, although absent from blood and from other tissues of the body.

Some clarification was obtained from gel diffusion studies. When the anti-seminal plasma was tested in gel diffusion against rabbit seminal plasma, one band of precipitation was seen for each early bleeding, but after several injections an additional line appeared. The first line, or main line, was shown to merge in a reaction of identity with the line that was characteristic of the organs in the accessory glands complex, so this must represent the characteristic antigen of the accessory glands discussed above, and studied in the semen. The other, fainter line, was found to be associated with an antigen of seminal plasma that was not connected with the accessory glands and was apparently characteristic of seminal plasma itself. It was shown in other experiments to be present in extracts of epididymis. As mentioned earlier, epididymis constituents did not cross-react with accessory glands constituents. Seminal plasma was also seen to contain two distinctive antigens in this type of immunization, one of which is shared by the accessory glands but not the epididymis, while the other is shared by the epididymis but not the accessory glands [294].

These studies in the rabbit suggest that human seminal plasma constituents might also have the propensity for stimulating autoantibody formation and thus leading to pathologic conditions.

β) Composition of Human Seminal Plasma

i) Physicochemical Properties

The physicochemical analysis of the protein components of seminal plasma from various species has been widely described in the literature. Some technics have utilized the ultracentrifuge [31, 132], and others have been based on optical, *i.e.*, moving boundary, electrophoresis [80, 133, 242–244]. Many studies have utilized zone electrophoresis, commonly on filter paper [38, 54, 185, 207, 224] and more recently immunoelectrophoresis has been used with increasing frequency [93, 98, 124, 185, 211, 212, 262].

One disadvantage of many of these reports was that the condition of the semen sample was left undescribed. There was apparently no uniform opinion on the effects of storage. Some workers did realize that electrophoresis should be performed as soon as possible in view of the labile character of the material. In 1955, for example, SCHNEIDER demonstrated a continuing qualitative change in the electrophoretic pattern with time as a sample was stored [257].

These questions of composition and lability were reopened in a study that made use of filter paper electrophoresis [279]. A total of 9 components were revealed, component 7 accounting for about 60% of the pattern. When samples were refrigerated at 4 °C, the percentage of component 7 declined continuously, while that of component 5 steadily rose. These changes with time of storage suggested the presence of proteolysis initiated by some seminal plasma enzyme. It seemed unlikely that both the enzyme and the substrate would be elaborated by the same tissue. Accordingly, several ejaculates were obtained in the form of split fractions. The two fractions of a donation did contain different electrophoretic components, but even more important, each pattern was more stable on cold storage. It was concluded that these split fractions could therefore be better starting materials for isolation and purification of the major constituents [279].

ii) Antigenic Analysis

The degree of heterogeneity of human seminal plasma can also be evaluated by means of antigenic analysis. One of the earliest studies of this sort was conducted by HEKTOEN and his colleagues, the group that had done so much work on the tissue-specific properties of the thyroid gland. Although work can be cited from as long ago as 1901, the early reports generally described whole semen rather than the separated elements, and the reactions to sperm cells and to seminal plasma proteins cannot be differentiated. In the work of HEKTOEN *et al.* [89], we seem to have the first fairly clear separation of these two elements. They obtained rabbit antiserum against human seminal proteins, which seemed to be specific in its reaction in fluid precipitation. They also showed that an antiserum to human blood serum yielded precipitation reactions with semen, and this might well have been a very early indication of the presence of the serum components in semen, a subject much discussed in more recent work.

Serological studies of human seminal plasma, employing fluid precipitation, were reported by Ross in 1946 [241]. Rabbit antiserum against human seminal plasma was used; various degrees of precipitation were obtained, and component antigens were distinguished by means of fractionation.

Herrmann and Schirren [98], who used rabbit antiserum, concluded from immunoelectrophoresis studies that there were 8 to 9 protein fractions in human seminal plasma.

Klopstock *et al.* [127] reported their finding of 7–10 different protein fractions in immunoelectrophoretic analysis of human seminal plasma. They claimed that most of these samples contained a γ-globulin identical to serum γ-globulin, though it was missing from others. Their pictures do not show a completely clear resolution of these various components.

Rozin *et al.* [244] described five arcs as components of seminal plasma. However, they only utilized a rabbit anti-whole blood serum, and thus only studied serum components.

Searcy *et al.* [262] showed that four arcs were obtained when anti-human serum was used, and at least 7 when anti-human seminal plasma was used. Fjällbrant [60] used gel diffusion and described 16 lines of precipitation with seminal plasma tested against antiserum to semen, 6 of which were also given by human blood plasma. Unfortunately, no pictures were shown with this abstract. Rao and Sadri [169] claimed that buffalo seminal plasma contained at least 16 antigens; they used rabbit antiserum in gel diffusion in their studies.

Eyquem *et al.* [55] found 13 antigenic components by means of goat antiserum but stated that some of these antigens are also found in human serum, including γ-globulin, two β-globulins, one α-globulin, and albumin.

Quinlivan [222, 223] found three to five precipitation lines in double-diffusion studies on human seminal plasma and its antiserum.

Behrman and Amano [4, 17] reported several studies on the antigenic properties of human seminal plasma. Their major effort was devoted to an attempt to separate the components by CM-cellulose chromatography. They claimed to find fifteen precipitation lines for human seminal plasma, at least 5 of which were produced in reaction with human serum. The pictures shown, however, do not clarify the precise pattern very well.

Studies have also been made of blood group substances in the seminal fluid. It has been well documented for years that ABO blood group substances appear in seminal plasma, and Lewis substance has also been detected. The Le^a and Le^b substances occur in seminal fluid, paralleling their occurrence on the subject's red cells [146].

This brief survey shows that many reports have appeared in recent literature on the analysis of human seminal plasma by the use of antisera, but some of these reports suffer from technical or theoretical defects. It has not always been realized that not all immunized animals will produce equally full collections of antibody responses, and the use of only one antiserum against each antigenic material has led to inadequate studies. Furthermore, the extent of antibody responses to components of blood serum and to components that are common to other tissues of the body has not always been studied. In addition to these theoretical problems, there have been only limited efforts, in the frequent use of gel diffusion methods, to study variations in concentration of seminal plasma or of antiserum, as well as the geometry, time of incubation, and temperature. In some reports, commercial antisera have been put to use, with no studies of the sensitivity or the degree of specificity of these reagents.

In a recent study by SHULMAN and BRONSON [280], rabbit antisera to human seminal plasma gave precipitation with normal human serum and revealed several such lines of reaction, indicating the presence of a number of serum components in the seminal plasma which had been used for immunization. (The pre-immunization rabbit sera gave no reactions.) The exact number of apparent cross-reacting components varied with the individual rabbit and with the particular blood sample; in addition, the number of lines indicated varied considerably with the geometry of the arrangement of wells. A total of 6 lines was distinguished for human serum itself. The number of lines, apart from serum lines, was quite different under varying conditions of geometry and dilution, suggesting a total of 8–11 distinctive components [280]. Similar patterns have been described by RAO and her co-workers [226–229].

Immunoelectrophoresis, with an antiserum selected for its ability to show many well-separated lines was then applied for a clearer resolution. This often revealed as many as 11 or 12 distinctive arcs. The exact number varied from one sample to another, but analysis of numerous experiments revealed a rather typical pattern of precipitation. A schematic diagram is shown in Fig. 5.5. The

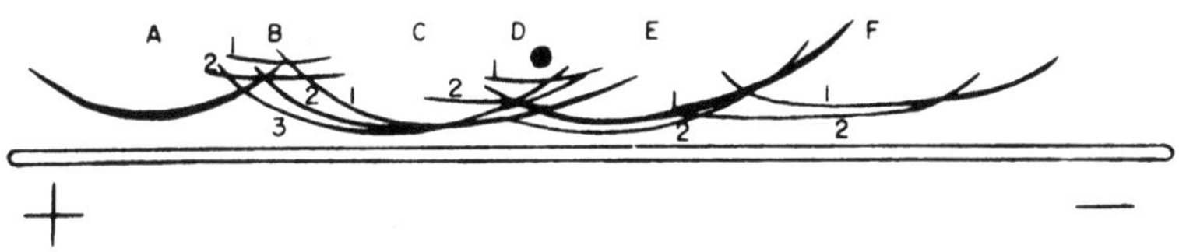

Fig. 5.5. Immunoelectrophoresis, idealized sketch. Human seminal plasma analyzed with rabbit antiserum. (From SHULMAN and BRONSON [280])

major arcs were indicated by the letters A, C, E, and F. The lines for C and E were actually groups of lines with very similar mobilities. The individual components were therefore distinguished as C_1, C_2, C_3, and E_1, E_2. A faint additional pair was frequently seen in the F-region, and these were termed F_1 and (fainter) F_2. In addition to these eight components, there were several lines at a much greater distance from the antibody trough; these were located near the fast end and the slow end of the C group of arcs. They have therefore been designated as the B and D groups. Since two members of each of these minor groups were detected, it was concluded that there was a minimum of 12 reproducibly detected components in seminal plasma, as recently described [280]. An immunoelectrophoretic pattern for rabbit seminal plasma was recently published by MENGE *et al.* [178], and this pattern is rather similar in many details to the pattern obtained for human material. An antigenic analysis of this sort has also been made of guinea pig seminal plasma [158, 211].

The presence of serum albumin in seminal plasma is best proven by an experiment according to the method of OSSERMAN [199], wherein one trough contains instead of antiserum an antigen, for example, 0.01% human serum albumin; the parallel trough contains the usual antiserum to human seminal plasma. In one such study, a horizontal line of precipitation was seen between the troughs, resulting from migration of the serum albumin toward its corresponding antibody in the antiserum; the line showed a perfect and complete reaction of fusion with the arc that had been designated component A, in the pattern for seminal plasma components [280].

RÜMKE and HEKMAN [86] have recently presented an immunoelectrophoretic pattern for human seminal plasma that is very similar to the one described above. Their study was prompted partly by interest in the spermatozoa-coating antigen (SCA) of WEIL. Their pattern is shown in Fig. 5.6, as taken from a

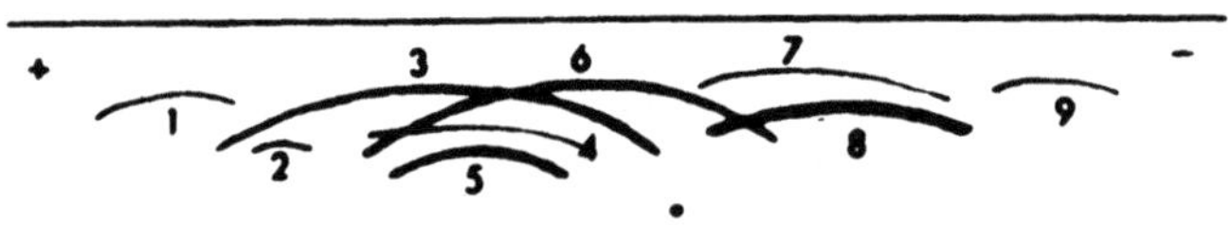

Fig. 5.6. Immunoelectrophoresis, idealized sketch. Human seminal plasma analyzed by rabbit antiserum. (From HEKMAN and RÜMKE [87])

more recent report [87]. There are only 9 components, but it should be noted that the antiserum used here had been absorbed with human serum. The SCA was definitely shown to be one of the faster-migrating components and not the major component. In fact, they found the SCA to be component 5, and this would seem to be the same as D_1 in our own system (Fig. 5.5). This SCA fraction and our major fraction, C_2 (see below), are thus of interest for further purification and characterization, as possible components of the antigenic stimulus involved in autoantibody formation. HEKMAN and RÜMKE [87] showed that seminal vesicle components corresponded to lines 5 and 6 in their pattern, and that three antigens, for lines 3, 7, and 8, came from the prostate gland.

Further studies have been made on the purification and properties of the SCA by WEIL *et al.* [145, 343] and by BOETTCHER and colleagues [29, 236]. The latter group showed that the SCA is an iron-binding protein of seminal plasma, and that it shares antigenic groups with lactoferrin but not transferrin; they proposed to name it scaferrin [236].

HERRMANN and SCHIRREN also described quite a similar immunoelectrophoretic pattern for human seminal plasma [98]. In much more recent work, a number of organ-specific proteins were described in the seminal plasma, as well as certain blood plasma proteins and other proteins [95]. A group of 8 characteristic proteins have been described in some detail. This includes two aminopeptidases, both secreted by the prostate gland, which have been studied in terms of antigenic structure, electrophoretic mobility, and molecular weight [94]. The presence of certain γ-globulins has been studied by several gel diffusion procedures, and γG, γA, and two kinds of molecular fragments of γ-globulin were detected [96]. Antigenic studies of seminal plasma have also been reported by BANDHAUER [9], and ZIMMERMANN *et al.* [354].

Most of the studies described involved the use of heteroantibodies. Although RÜMKE [245, 247] and others [255, 346] showed that autoantibodies to semen can occur in the human, these antibodies are directed against sperm cells, and do not provide any evidence that autoantibodies against antigens of the seminal plasma occur in man. However, the recent demonstration that rabbits can be immunized to produce autoantibodies against components of rabbit seminal plasma [233, 294], has prompted more thorough investigation of the possible role of human seminal plasma as an autoantigenic stimulus. This will necessitate much more knowledge than we now have about the diverse antigenic constituents of human seminal plasma in general. The multiplicity of protein components contained in this fluid will need further sorting out, and the individually defined substances should then receive more precise characterization.

HALPERN *et al.* [83] have shown that human antibodies against constituents of human seminal plasma can definitely occur. This case of antibody formation to such antigens is not of central import here, because it was a reaginic antibody, which caused anaphylactic-like reactions in the woman involved, in addition to being detectable by the usual skin-testing procedures. However, the very fact that seminal plasma was apparently antigenic under these conditions indicates that much more investigation is necessary on the genetic and other parameters that may control the possible formation of non-reaginic antibody to immunization with this material. These workers [83] also performed some fractionation studies and the allergenic activity was associated with a glycoprotein fraction of seminal plasma which was rich in sialic acid and gave a single immunoelectrophoretic line as against six lines seen for whole seminal plasma. While a precise comparison of the given pattern and that described above is difficult, it seems probable that their allergen is found in our group of E components [280]. Reports by STEVENS *et al.* [309, 310] have suggested the presence of human autoantibodies to antigens of seminal plasma. A reaginic antibody to human seminal plasma has again been described and more thoroughly studied by LEVINE *et al.* [136a].

These multitudinous components of human seminal plasma were separated by starch block electrophoresis, using preparations from split ejaculates [297]. There was reasonably good resolution into 6 peaks, arbitrarily designated by numbers. Fraction 3 was the major component, and only this fraction has been further studied in any detail. It was analyzed repeatedly by immunochemical procedures, and found to be a much more homogeneous product than the original whole seminal plasma, as judged by filter paper electrophoresis, analytical ultracentrifugation, and especially by gel diffusion analysis. The ultracentrifugal result showed a single component with no sign of faster peaks. This single sedimenting peak had a sedimentation coefficient of 1.0 S. The immunoelectrophoretic method was also used to confirm the improved homogeneity and to show the identification of this isolated component by the OSSERMAN technique [197]. The single horizontal line of precipitation showed a deviation into an arc which was a component of the C group, probably C_2, of whole seminal plasma. Thus, this major immunoelectrophoretic component has been identified as corresponding to the tallest peak in the zonal electrophoretic pattern [279, 280]. Gel filtration has also been used for fractionation of these antigens [142, 287, 353]. A 1.1 S protein was also described by HERRMANN [95], as was a 3.72 S protein. This 3.72 S component has now been purified, and some of its properties have been described by HERRMANN and HERMANN [97].

c) Seminal Vesicular Fluid

In studies on the guinea pig, components of the seminal vesicle have been analyzed. Fig. 5.7 shows a drawing of the anatomy of this gland, a remarkably large structure in this species. A number of electrophoretic, ultracentrifugal,

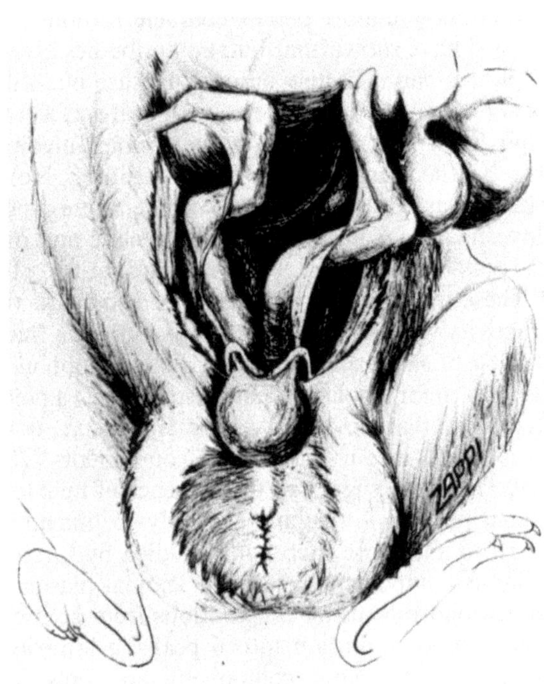

Fig. 5.7. Sketch of the seminal vesicles, in their abdominal setting, in the guinea pig

and antigenic characterizations have been made on the vesicular fluid, as well as some biochemical and physiological studies.

In an effort to discover one or more tissue-specific antigens of the fluid of the guinea pig seminal vesicle, with the attendant possibility of discovering antigens against which autoantibodies might be stimulated, it was shown that guinea pigs could produce antibodies to vesicular fluid, as a result of isoimmunization [270, 292, 293]. The same phenomenon was discovered by VULCHANOV, with quite high antibody titers [330, 331]. Zone electrophoresis of vesicular fluid on membranes of cellulose acetate revealed stained patterns that were very consistent in appearance, showing three major and three minor components. Fig. 5.8 shows a typical electrophoretic pattern of vesicular fluid, with migration

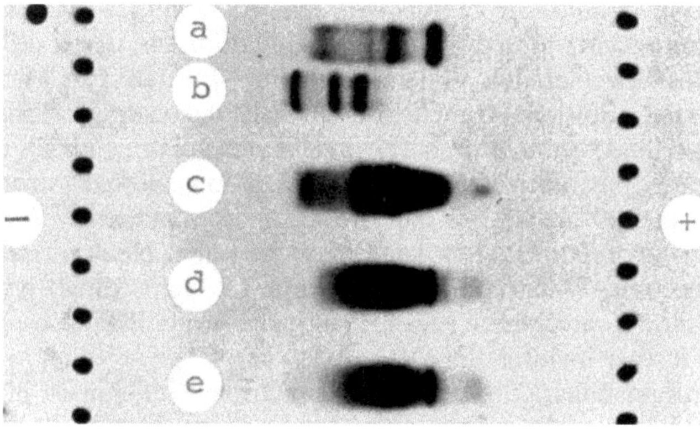

Fig. 5.8. Electrophoresis on cellulose acetate membrane, of seminal vesicular fluid and related materials, all from guinea pig; pH 8.6. Line a, serum; line b, vesicular fluid; line c, seminal plasma; line d, seminal vesicle extract; line e, prostate-coagulating gland extract

towards the anode. The vesicular fluid is compared with guinea pig serum, seminal plasma, extract of whole seminal vesicle, and prostate-coagulating gland. The major components have been termed I, II, and III, starting with the one closest to the anode. Minor components could also be seen when large sample sizes were applied. A number of ultracentrifugal examinations showed that this material looked quite homogeneous, the single symmetrical peak having a sedimentation coefficient of about 1.5 S.

Starch block electrophoresis at pH 8.6 was used to separate the three major components. The isolated fractions were reasonably pure, judging from the patterns in cellulose acetate electrophoresis performed on each isolated sample and compared with the pattern for the whole material. Immunochemical studies

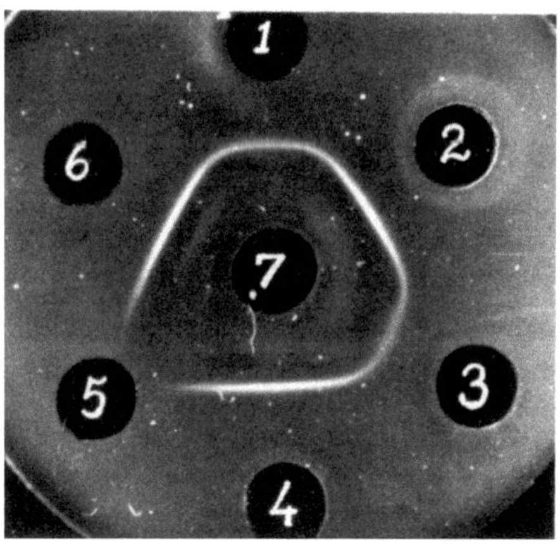

Fig. 5.9. Double diffusion gel precipitation. Central well: rabbit anti-guinea pig vesicular fluid. Peripheral wells: (1) component II of vesicular fluid, (2) seminal plasma, (3) prostate-coagulating gland extract, (4) seminal vesicle extract, (5) saline, (6) whole vesicular fluid

were carried out by injecting rabbits with the whole guinea pig vesicular fluid; each rabbit antiserum showed a strong precipitation line in gel diffusion when tested with the vesicular fluid. These results are illustrated in Fig. 5.9, which also shows certain additional comparisons, namely, the reactions of this antiserum with vesicular fluid, seminal plasma, prostate-coagulating gland extract, and seminal vesicle extract. Each of these tissue preparations showed a strong precipitation line and they all merged to indicate a common antigen. Well 6 contained a preparation of component II, isolated from the starch block. It clearly showed a positive reaction. When components I and III were tested, however, they completely failed to precipitate [293]. These interesting differences in properties will demand further investigations.

These antisera failed to give any precipitation with guinea pig serum, or with other guinea pig organ extracts tested at various dilutions. These included testis, epididymis, and kidney—all of these were completely negative. The only organ extracts which contained antigenic material in common with the vesicular fluid were seminal plasma, prostate-coagulating gland, and seminal vesicle extract, as already mentioned. Similar studies have been reported on the vesicular fluid of the rabbit [198].

3. Proteins and Antigens of the Female Reproductive Tract

Many reports have appeared on studies of the composition of uterine fluid and related fluids. Most of them seem to be on rat fluid, which is thus often termed cornual fluid. Most early studies described the composition in terms of electrophoretic patterns, whereas later work has added various methods of antigenic analysis. There has been much interest in the study of cervical fluid or cervical mucosa, and especially recently, because of the upsurge of interest in the question of possible antibody activity against components of semen, either the sperm cells *per se* or the blood group substances. Studies have also been made on the components of tubal, oviductal, and follicular fluids. In addition, a large area of observations, and also speculations, exists in regard to the immunological aspects of the mother-fetus interaction. All these matters will be briefly discussed below.

a) Uterine Fluid

JUNGE and BLANDAU [112] reported in 1958 that the cornual fluid of the rat, filling and distending the organ during heat, could be aspirated to give about 0.5 ml per animal, and could be examined by electrophoresis. The total protein concentration was estimated at about 0.3%, or about 5% of the normal serum level. They found four major components in quite low concentration, as seen by moving-boundary electrophoresis, and they saw a component with unusual mobility, compared to blood serum, by means of filter paper electrophoresis. Whether any of these components are similar to the proteins of serum was left unanswered.

ALBERS and NEVES e CASTRO [3] continued this kind of study, applying antigenic analysis based on gel diffusion and immunoelectrophoretic methods, using antisera from immunized rabbits. In this way, they found five components in rat uterine fluid, but considered only one was specific for this fluid, whereas the other four were common to rat serum.

RINGLER reported that this fluid shows six electrophoretic components, significantly different from those of plasma, and that six components were also seen by sedimentation analysis, but no details were given [234]. Additional studies reported the presence of four electrophoretic peaks which seemed to correspond to components of rat serum, and also a protein fraction which had a mobility greater than that of albumin. It was generally concluded that the uterine luminal fluid is a mixture of an ultrafiltrate of plasma along with a secretion from the uterus [235]. HOMBURGER *et al.* [99] found four protein bands in paper electrophoresis of mouse uterine fluid, the fastest moving of which seemed to be the same as mouse serum albumin.

Some of the more recent work on rat uterine fluid has been done by MOYER and his colleagues [129], who used acrylamide gel and acrylamide gel-Ouchterlony methods. They demonstrated nine protein components by the gel electrophoresis technic above and at least four precipitating antigens were revealed by use of rabbit antiserum to rat serum. It was thus concluded that at least four proteins of uterine fluid are also to be found in rat serum, and that five other proteins may well be native to the uterine fluid. Further evidence was thus added to strengthen the concept that uterine fluid is at least in part a secretory product of the endometrium. Rabbit uterine fluid has also been studied [311].

b) Tubal and Oviductal Fluids

MASTROIANNI and colleagues have studied the components of rabbit tubal fluid [160, 308, 350]. Immunochemical and other studies have been made on bovine and porcine follicular fluid [45, 263].

The possibility of autoimmune responses to ovarian tissue or to ova has been explored, although with limited rewards. LEVI [136] discussed the antigenicity of ovarian cancer. VALLOTTON and FORBES [324, 325] described autoimmune conditions in relation to gonadal dysgenesis and to various chromosomal disorders. Experimental anti-ovary sera have been studied [305].

Several studies have appeared on the study of human fallopian fluid [152, 186]. A very recent report by LIPPES *et al.* [143] has opened the way to improved surgical technics for the continuous collection of fallopian tube fluid. A number of studies have been made on a large group of women. Electrophoretic and immunoelectrophoretic patterns were described, and the distributions of various ionic constituents, glucose, and several enzymes were measured. The major immunoglobulin was γG, and the distribution of immunoglobulin was similar to that in serum rather than resembling that of other secreted fluids.

The oviductal fluid has been examined in various species including rabbits [57, 84, 323] and monkeys [162].

c) Cervical Mucus

Studies on the cervical mucus are based on the fundamental knowledge concerning the structure and composition of the material. The biochemistry of cervical mucus has been the subject of many studies, which have explored both the chemical and structural aspects of this gel. This complex subject is beyond the scope of this review; a more detailed discussion has been presented elsewhere [273, 275]. Valuable reports on the composition have been presented by SCHUMACHER [258–260], ODEBLAD [195–197], GIBBONS [78–80], MOGHISSI [187–189], DAVAJAN and NAKAMURA [42–44] and their colleagues. Long filaments of mucus derive from single glands or clefts, and these filaments are the structures that contribute to the formation of cervical mucus. The composition of the mucus is quite heterogeneous. ODEBLAD [196] spoke of a "mosaic pattern", as the qualitative differences between the secretions of different areas of the cervix. A sample of mucus in bulk will give average values of the diffusible components, since the water and soluble molecules can diffuse within the structural network of the mucus gel. The components of this heterogeneous material include some cellular elements, but primarily the material is a gel, that is, a semisolid structure (a three-dimensional network) with a fluid permeating it, and this fluid may be looked on as cervical plasma. Some writers refer to two types of chemical components, high-viscosity and low-viscosity components. High-viscosity components are the structural units of glycoprotein, and low-viscosity components, the dissolved substances in the plasma, notably soluble proteins and other constituents. The only glycoprotein structures are cross-linked and the degree of cross-linking determines the viscosity and elasticity of the mucus.

The cervical plasma contains many soluble substances, including a number of proteins. MOGHISSI and NEUHAUS [187] described the presence of albumin, transferrin, γ-globulin, and several other components. Other proteins include prealbumin, orosomucoid, α_1-antitrypsin, haptoglobin, and certain components of the complement system, as described by SCHUMACHER and colleagues [260]. Studies on the question of antibodies within this mucus have been reported with increasing frequency in recent years. This work has included the detection of blood groups antibodies. The presence of isohemagglutinins has often been shown in the uterine fluids, and especially in the cervical mucus. In fact, studies in the human system have included the search for antibody activity against the AB0 blood group system in cervical [307] and follicular [85] fluids, as well as in uterine fluid [76]. The antibodies were found in all three kinds of material. More work has been done with cervical fluid, especially with regard to the possible implication of these agglutinins in infertility. Quite a detailed study was reported very recently by SOLISH [306], who studied the occurrence and the titers of cervical isoagglutinins in 204 infertile women and 93 fertile women. The presence of A and B antigens on the spermatozoa *per se* is itself much debated [219, 208]. Solish found the agglutinins more frequently in fertile women, the reverse of what might be expected if these antibodies really diminished fertility on account of AB0 incompatibility. Data of 1403 women of various ethnic groups were given to show the relationships of occurrence and titer to ethnic origin.

A very different, very attractive approach is the detection of the immunoglobulins, *i.e.*, of the antibody molecules, by detection of their antigenic characteristics rather than their antibody functions. This is easily possible, since the immunoglobulins do have distinctive antigenic natures, but unfortunately, it may not be apparent what antigen it is that the antibody is directed against. In 1969 HULKA and OMRAN published data on immunoglobulin levels and measured the ratios of the concentrations of γG to γA in cervical mucus [103]. They also showed that the transport piece (TP) of γA was present in cervical glandular epithelium and mucus.

LIPPES *et al.* [144] in 1970 reported the presence of immunoglobulins and of transport piece in the endometrium, fallopian tubes, and cervix. Another recent investigation has studied these questions in greater detail [315]. The presence of γA, γG, γM, and TP has been examined by immunofluorescence in various tissues of the human female reproductive tract, including the uterus, the endometrium, the cervix, and the vagina. Predominant immunoglobulin in all these tissues was found to be γG. It was localized predominantly in the interstitial connective tissue, where it was apparent as diffuse noncellular staining. It was also seen along the basement membranes. The localization of γA was the same, but the intensity of staining was less. The staining for γM was very light. Most of these tissues also contained TP. The point of special interest is the occurrence of these structures in the cervix. All three immunoglobulins, as well as TP, were situated mainly in the lumina of cervical glands. In addition, small numbers of lymphoid cells that stained for γG and γA were seen in the stroma. The amount of γG in these interstitial tissues is relatively larger than that seen in other secretory organs. Furthermore, there were no large numbers of immunoglobulin-producing plasma cells in these tissues, another difference from the situation in other exocrine gland tissues.

All these studies are disappointing in that no clear results have yet indicated the actual level or titer of any antibody activity, or how the titer may vary during the days of the menstrual cycle, or even whether there are antibodies against spermatozoa, as against blood groups antibodies or any other kind of immunoglobulin activity. However, recent studies have shown that sperm antibody can definitely be detected in cervical mucus from at least some infertile women [276d, 283a].

d) Maternal-Fetal Interactions

The placenta has been studied from the aspect of its immunological role [169, 322]. The broadest point of interest has been the puzzling question of the lack of a graft-rejection phenomenon. It is many years since it was first pointed out that the fetus and its placenta constitute a homograft (or rather an allograft), since they contain (foreign) histocompatibility antigens derived from the father; they should therefore be rejected as with all other grafts placed in a foreign body which do not derive from a source of identical genetic constitution. Clearly, mechanisms permitting the embryo and fetus to survive for a long and sufficient time have evolved: this enigma remains one of the major unsolved problems of transplantation immunology. Many of the arguments, theories, and experimental studies on this question have been discussed in a number of reports and reviews some of which can be consulted for further information [16, 22–24, 81, 206, 302, 321]. Some suggested explanations are: 1. the fetus is antigenically immature, 2. the immunologic reactivity of the mother is weakened during pregnancy, 3. the uterus is an immunologically privileged site, 4. there is a physiologic barrier between mother and fetus, 5. local steroid production is immunologically protective. There is sufficient evidence to eliminate the first two concepts completely. The fourth concept is one of the currently favored ideas and proposes that the trophoblast furnishes this barrier. Other theories have been proposed; one rather attractive new idea is based on immunologic enhancement, a concept that a host animal may provide an immune environment of a sort that actually enhances certain experimental tumor growths, for example, rather than inhibiting them. This idea has been proposed as a basis for explaining the protection given to the fetal allograft [81]; it may very well become an important part of the eventual explanation.

Chapter 6

The Eye

The eye is composed of a variety of tissues, so that several distinctive tissue-specific antigens exist as characteristic components of the individual eye structures. These different antigens can also be important in terms of possibilities for autoimmunization and for pathologic function that may result from antigen-antibody interactions. We will consider the specific localization of each antigen with respect to each ocular component, as well as comparing each component with diverse organs of the body. It will be convenient to consider each of the major eye structures as a separate unit in the following discussion.

1. Antigens of the Lens

The phenomenon of tissue-specificity (*or* organ-specificity as it was then more frequently termed) was first observed by UHLENHUTH in studies on the lens of the eye [99]. He injected rabbits intravenously with saline homogenates of bovine lens, and obtained antisera which precipitated a homogenate of lens but failed to precipitate extracts of other organs of the body. The same antisera did, however, give strong reactions with extracts of lens from other species of mammal. This double meaning of specificity of a particular tissue component—the failure to share the component with other tissues of the same body and simultaneously the presence of identical or sufficiently similar antigenic components in the analogous tissue of other species—had been the hallmark of the most classic type of tissue-specificity for over half a century. It implies that there are closely similar antigenic structures in the corresponding organ in these various species. Attention was thus drawn to the exact chemical structures at the basis of these antigenic comparisons. For many years it was thought that this antigenic property of lens was due to a lipid component, but it became clear in the 1920's and 1930's that a group of protein components called "crystallines" were prominently present and were probably connected with the antigenic characteristics.

It was thought earlier that there were three soluble lens proteins, the α-, β-, and γ-crystallines, and in fact these were separated by several early workers, including HEKTOEN and SCHULHOF, who had done such important work on the tissue-specificity of the thyroid gland [47]. Originally, each of these three fractions was thought to possess distinctive antigenic properties. In more recent years, however, the picture has become complicated—and the word has generally become "crystallins". This complexity has been recognized primarily because more modern antigenic methods of characterization of these heterogeneous protein mixtures are now used, largely based on the use of Freund's complete adjuvant for the production of more potent heteroantisera and the use of immunoelectrophoresis with its very high resolving power. There are at least ten antigenic components in the lenses of various mammals. Much of this work has been reviewed by HALBERT and MANSKI [40–43, 69–74], with special emphasis on the evolutionary viewpoint. The specificity of lens among the vertebrates, for example, was found to be based on the antigenic similarity of at least 6 lens components [41]. Some authors have tried to associate this kind of antibody response with the development of cataract [42, 100]. These lens antigens have also been studied by means of cytotoxicity of the antisera in tissue culture experiments [26–28].

High-voltage agar electrophoresis has made it possible to distinguish at least 16 protein fractions [34]. Nonetheless, careful analyses by means of gel diffusion have justified the original division into three main classes, which may well have some fundamental biological significance. MANSKI *et al.* [71] have stressed the importance of applying both immunochemical and physicochemical methods to such analyses.

Continuous-flow paper electrophoresis was used for the study of rabbit lens proteins by WOOD *et al.* [110]. They obtained five major components and examined the solubility, light absorption, isoelectric point, and ultracentrifugal properties of each. Their fraction 5 (with the highest mobility of the group, at pH 8.9) showed a sedimentation coefficient of 19.2 S, and for several reasons it was thought to correspond to the α-crystallin of earlier workers. The molecular weight was roughly estimated as 1 to 1.5×10^6. Earlier reports had suggested a molecular weight of 1.2×10^6 for α-crystallin [36]. Fractions 1, 3, and 4 had sedimentation rates of about 3.9 S and an approximate molecular weight of 60–80000 was estimated, which was close to the value reported earlier for β-crystallin [53]. Their fraction 2 had a sedimentation coefficient of 2.1 S, which corresponds to an approximate molecular weight of 20000. These workers also claimed that the individual globulins had been obtained in crystalline form; this claim has apparently not been confirmed [110].

Human lens proteins were examined in extracts by means of gel diffusion and immunoelectrophoresis by DUPREE *et al.* [25]. In gel diffusion tests with rabbit antisera, 7 precipitation lines became visible at different times during the experiment. Immunoelectrophoresis also revealed a pattern of 7 precipitin bands. These components seemed to be specific for lens, at least insofar as human serum was concerned, since the lens antiserum gave no reaction with human serum and anti-human serum gave no reaction with lens extract. These specificity tests were limited to the use of immunoelectrophoresis, however, which may not be as sensitive as gel diffusion; no other specificity tests, such as tests with other body tissues, were conducted. Ultracentrifugal analysis of lens extracts revealed four distinct components with sedimentation rates of approximately 17.0–19.7 S (10–20% of the total protein), 8.4–10.6 S (16–26%), 5.6–6.3 S (12.4–22.2%), and 1.2–2.7 S (38.8–52.1%). These can be compared to results obtained for chick lens, as described below. DUPREE *et al.* [25] propose that the 19 S component corresponds to α-crystallin and gives rise to 2 precipitin bands, the 2 S component corresponds to γ-crystallin and gives rise to 3 precipitin bands, and the 10 S and 6 S components both correspond to β-crystallin and each gives rise to at least one precipitin band. There may well be some uncertainties with regard to all these identifications.

MAISEL and LANGMAN [67] performed studies on chick lens extract with a rabbit antiserum. They associated the α-crystallin with an ultracentrifugal component of 17.3–17.8 S, β-crystallin with an 8.9–9.5 S peak, and γ-crystallin with a 4.2–4.3 S peak. Each crystallin fraction contributed several gel diffusion components. In later studies LANGMAN and MAISEL [55] isolated the three main proteins of the chick lens and estimated the molecular weights: α-crystallin, 1000000; β-crystallin, 200000 to 300000; γ-crystallin, 60000. Later work described several molecular subunits of α-crystallin [86].

Many ultracentrifugal analyses on the soluble components of the lens have been reported. More recent studies have been especially concerned with the nature of the α-crystallin complex. SPECTOR and KATZ [94] reported a detailed study on bovine lens α-crystallin, which they considered was a heterogeneous system composed of a number of different-sized molecular species. They performed several types of sedimentation equilibrium studies to estimate the molecular weight and also the heterogeneity of their purified preparations. At neutral pH they obtained a weight average molecular weight of approximately 1.0×10^6. They showed that under various conditions of pH or of added reagent the α-crystallin molecules dissociated into half or quarter units, and there were general deaggregation phenomena. In a later study, SPECTOR *et al.* [95] indicated that α-crystallin molecules seemed to be formed as aggregates from molecular subunits with a molecular weight of approximately 20000. Under normal conditions the average aggregate contains approximately 50 of these subunits, which are held together by non-covalent forces, and this is the reason for the average molecular weight of approximately 1×10^6. It would be of interest to explore the packing arrangements and architectural structure of the molecular complex to learn more about how these units fit into the structure of the lens itself. Their experiments suggest three different packing arrangements of the subunits, and these are discussed as they are influenced by various environmental situations. The conformation seems to involve no significant amount of alpha helix structure, but does involve the anti-parallel beta structure for about half the total, with a random coil comprising the remainder. Polyacrylamide gel electrophoresis in the presence of urea revealed subunits of molecular weight 19000. In more recent studies [14] these authors found that this protein contains at least four different subunits, which were first characterized as differing in their content of crysteine residues. One of these peptides was sufficiently pure for sequence studies, and a total of some 30 residues have been identified and positioned. Other reports on the subunit construction of the crystallins have been published by CLAYTON [21], CORRAN and WALEY [23], SHAPIRO [91], TRUMAN *et al.* [98], and MANSKI and co-workers [74a, 114, 115].

To summarize the work described above, α-crystallin sediments at a rate between 15 and 19 S, corresponding to a molecular weight about 1000000–1500000 [94]. The β-fraction has a molecular weight about 60000–300000. The γ-fraction consists of smaller proteins, with molecular weights apparently ranging about 15000–60000. These fractions also differ in antigenicity. In the absence of any adjuvant, α-crystallin is the most potent antigenic component in the homologous species [47]; in the presence of adjuvant, this antigen is the first one to stimulate antibody production in isoimmunization [30].

During embryogenesis in the chicken, the α-crystallin is the first of the lens proteins to be demonstrable. The β- and γ-antigens appear later in embryogenesis. Although these fractions are widely present in vertebrate lenses, only closely related species show appreciable antigenic similarity in these fractions [43]. In aging and in cataractous lenses the amount of soluble protein decreases and that of insoluble protein increases. It has been proposed that much of the insoluble protein, the albuminoid, in human and bovine lens is formed from the α-crystallin component [18]. Although α-crystallin persists in the adult lens [35] and is structurally very similar to albuminoid, some structural differences have been noted [80].

SPIRO and FUKUSHI [37, 96] have reported a thorough analysis of the composition of the carbohydrate units of the bovine lens capsule. Since the study involved the capsule and not the lens body, it is not of major importance here; furthermore, the protein definition is not too clear. We shall give only a brief summary of their work. The lens capsule has been considered as a basement membrane, and in fact, there are points of similarity between the lens and the basement membrane of the kidney glomerulus, as each contains a similar quantity of carbohydrate. The amino-acid composition of the lens capsule classes it as a collagen protein. Digestion and fractionation procedures led to the isolation of several glycopeptides containing disaccharide units linked to hydroxylysine, glycopeptides containing heteropolysaccharide units, and combinations of these kinds of units [96]. Thus glucosylgalactosylhydroxylysine was a predominant unit; the number of amino-acid residues ranged from 37 per 1000 for calf anterior capsule to 45 per 1000 for cow anterior capsule [96]. Many other structural details can be found in the original report [37, 96]. DENDUCHIS and KEFALIDES [24] have also emphasized the resemblance of lens capsule to glomerular basement membrane. They described a collagen-like component and two non-collagen-like glycoproteins, and examined the antigenic relationships among these substances.

MAISEL [61–66] has studied various components of the eye of chick by gel diffusion and electrophoretic analysis; he used rabbit antisera prepared by injection with Freund's adjuvant. He points out [62] that the term "organ specificity" seems to be inappropriate in several ways it may have been applied to lens antigen. One point of the argument is that the lens is a single tissue rather than an organ, since it is made primarily of long lens fibers cemented together to form a transparent structure. These fibers are derived from epithelial cells of the ectodermal surface of the embryo and they are surrounded by a thick capsule of intercellular substances. Secondly and more important, the antigens of the lens are not, in general, restricted to lens tissue and are also found in cornea, iris, retina, aqueous humor, brain, and skin, although absent from serum, liver, kidney, skeletal muscle, heart, stomach, spleen, sclera, choroid, testis, and ovary. Earlier investigators had also found some similar degree of common antigen among the eye tissues. For example, KODAMA [52] had indicated that lens antigens of guinea pig are also present in cornea, uvea, retina, and vitreous humor. BURKE *et al.* [17] had indicated a sharing of chick lens antigens with brain and retina. RAO *et al.* [87] had detected bovine lens antigens in aqueous humor and vitreous humor. LANGMAN and PRESCOTT [56] and MAISEL and LANGMAN [68] had revealed lens antigens in the chick cornea, iris, and pigment retina. FLICKINGER and STONE [33] had observed cross-reactions between frog lens and frog oocytes, neurulae, pigment retina, and aqueous humor. The more detailed analyses that MAISEL now reported [62] showed that the antigens shared by several tissues are not equally distributed or always immunologically identical with the lens components. For example, the antigen characteristic of lens α-crystallin was found in cornea, iris, and pigment retina of the chick eye, but not in nervous retina, brain, or skin. On the other hand, β-crystallin antigen of the lens is not found in the cornea, but is found in the pigment retina and the iris; this component was also found in brain and nervous retina in some cases, suggesting the sharing of some antigenic groupings in brain and nervous retina. Thirdly, the lens γ-crystallin antigens were shared by all the tissues mentioned above. Similar observations of antigenic cross-reactions between lens and epidermis among other tissues have recently been reported by RATHBUN *et al.* [88], who were apparently unaware of the work of MAISEL.

Even the classic expectation of lens organ specificity in terms of a common antigen in the lens obtained from various unrelated animals must be tempered with modification. It seems that lens antigens among vertebrates are generally present in the iris and in some cases at least in the pigment retina and the cornea. There is, however, a distinct kind of specificity of the lens antigen, inasmuch as all the tissues mentioned for shared occurrence derive from the primitive ectoderm. Furthermore, no reaction has been obtained between lens antiserum and tissues that derive from endodermal or mesodermal origins. Maisel therefore proposed that the lens antigens would be better described as tissue-specific for ectodermal derivatives, and he proposes to call them "ectodermal" rather than "lens-specific" antigens [62].

Since the lens antigen is present in aqueous humor, the question of autoimmunization to lens proteins may arise. Lens proteins were formerly thought to be inaccessible to the antibody-producing system, but it must now be admitted that as lens antigen is found in aqueous humor it could quite possibly diffuse into the bloodstream. It has been speculated therefore that autoimmune disease of the lens, which can lead to the development of endophthalmitis phacoanaphylactica, might follow the release of α-crystallin into the aqueous humor and the subsequent release of this intact molecule into the circulation during a period of increased permeability of the blood-aqueous barrier [62].

Studies by MEHTA *et al.* [79] suggest that the β- and γ-antigens are also found in various bovine and human organs. They attempted to distinguish between species-specific and organ-specific antigens by absorbing the rabbit antiserum with bovine lens by the use of bovine liver extract. They found that the unabsorbed anti-bovine lens serum gave cross-reacting precipitations with other tissue extracts, such as liver, kidney, spleen, and brain, with 2–4 precipitation lines as against six for lens. They used absorbed antiserum and found that bovine lens contained two antigens which bovine liver did not in the α-mobility range and a third antigen in the β-γ range. Although earlier workers had reported rabbit anti-lens serum as not reacting with extracts of other tissues of the body, MEHTA *et al.* [79] did obtain reactions of this sort, and they suggested that the contradiction might be due to their antisera having a stronger response to the β- and γ-crystallins which are more common to homologous tissues. The discrepancy is not completely resolved, however. They discuss the distinction between organ-specific and tissue-specific antigens, but this contrast is probably not useful.

CLAYTON *et al.* [19, 20] have examined the question of tissue specificity, and have applied several immunochemical procedures in their recent very detailed study [20]. In testing a number of tissues, such as iris, retina, cornea, brain, liver, kidney, muscle, ovary, oviduct, skin, lysed blood, and lens, they found that all these tissues contained some antigenic determinants similar to those found in the lens, and that all the major classes of lens proteins contained cross-reacting groups. They emphasized the importance of concentration differences for antigenic determinants in different tissues. Thus the nature of the cross-reactions varied in a complex manner among the various tissues; none of the lens antigens was found in all other tissues tested. Furthermore, the cross-reacting material in the non-lens tissues was not always identical in molecular form to that obtained from the lens [20].

The necessity for intensive re-investigation of the extent to which lens antigens truly are tissue-specific and species-specific is obvious. It is unfortunate that many studies of lens proteins have involved the use of antisera that were not absorbed, so that it is impossible to say whether the antigens tested in these studies are tissue-specific. This question has recently been re-opened in a study utilizing newer methods of analysis [15a].

2. Antigens of the Cornea

The cornea is a remarkable tissue in that it is frequently transplanted with almost perfect success between unrelated members of an animal species, and not only survives, but retains the transparency of its structure. Little information is available on the tissue-specific antigens of the cornea. Heterologous cornea can be antigenic in rabbits, which is due in part to cornea-specific antigens. WACKER and DODD [102] used rabbits immunized with corneal suspensions from rabbit, guinea pig, cattle, or man to give a convincing demonstration of the antigenicity of corneal tissue. The procedures included emulsification in complete Freund's adjuvant or with staphylococcus toxin adjuvant. The corneal tissue was antigenic when it originated from a different species of animal and the antibody produced was capable of reacting with ocular tissue from the rabbit as well as from the heterologous species. This antibody response could *not* be obtained, however, by injection with homologous ocular tissue. All these observations were equally true of uveal tissue. They did not find any evidence for gross pathological changes in the ocular tissue of animals stimulated to produce antibodies in this way, although they did see allergic encephalomyelitis and abnormal alopecia.

They also found an agglutinin in non-immunized rabbit, chicken, guinea pig, and human sera. This agglutinin, which may not be an antibody, caused positive reactions with tanned erythrocytes coated with rabbit corneal extract. Titers as high as 1:320 were obtained, but agglutination by the serum was not obtained with cells coated with extracts of other tissues. The authors concluded that this serum component was not the same as the Kidd-Friedewald factor [50, 51], which is a naturally occurring antibody for rabbit tissue and is found in normal rabbit serum. The Kidd-Friedewald antibody is demonstrated by the complement-fixation method. It shows several characteristic properties: 1. it reacts with extracts of several different rabbit tissues, notably kidney; 2. it is absent from serum taken from rabbits less than 24 days old; 3. it is destroyed by heating at 65 °C for 30 minutes; 4. the corresponding antigen of tissue is readily destroyed by heating at 65° for 30 minutes. In constrast, the serum component reacting with rabbit cornea could not be demonstrated by the complement-fixation test, and it reacted specifically in tanned-cell hemagglutination tests only with rabbit corneal tissue. Furthermore, it was present in serum from rabbits only 14 days old, it was unaffected by heating at 65° for 30 minutes, and the activity of rabbit corneal tissue was not affected by heating at 65° for 30 minutes. Rabbit corneal tissue suspension does not fix complement with normal rabbit serum, again indicating the absence of the Kidd-Friedewald antigen. This natural agglutinating activity was also demonstrated in the normal serum from guinea pig, chicken, and man, and it is possible that this activity is not due to an antibody at all, but to some change induced in the cells by the rabbit corneal extract which makes them non-specifically agglutinable by normal serum.

Antisera against rabbit cornea have been produced in the duck [39]. An antigen specific for cornea was suggested by gel diffusion studies, although there seemed to be some cross-reaction with kidney tissue. The cornea also contains some lens antigen [52, 56, 68], as already mentioned, but little is known of the various relationships between these common antigenic structures and the really specific components of cornea.

The success of corneal homografts requires some explanation. This problem has generally been discussed under two headings, the degree of vascularity of the recipient bed and the nature of the transplanted tissue [75]. The cornea is avascular and this characteristic seems to be the main factor involved in the success of a transplant of other corneal tissue. Aqueous humor contains antibodies, however, including the appropriate isoagglutinins in the human [82]. It has even been claimed that antibody formation can occur directly in the eye [76, 109]. Perhaps in some situations an incompatible graft interacts with antibodies and leads to opacification even in the absence of vascularization. The structure of the cornea may be one explanation for its resistance to rejection; since it is poorly endowed with cells and the transplantation antigens are cellular components, it probably contains much less antigen than other tissues. There may also be physical blockage in terms of the geometric relationship between the cells and the mucopolysaccharides of the stroma tissue.

After corneal grafting, when the donor material was from a person whose blood group was incompatible with that of the recipient, an immune response was observed only as a rise in the serum isoagglutinin titer and then only in the type of graft involving perforating keratoplasty and not lamellar keratoplasty [82]. In perforating keratoplasty an immune reaction might be obtained because the graft comes into direct contact with aqueous humor; in the other type of graft, the graft is smaller in volume and has no direct contact with the aqueous humor [82]. Even a transplant involving ABO incompatibility does not have any adverse consequences in corneal homografting unless the antibodies are present in very high titers, in which case rejection occurs [83]. The sharing of some corneal antigens with leukocytes was shown by NELKEN and NELKEN [81]. The effects of antilymphocyte serum as an immunosuppressive agent in modifying the corneal homograft reactions that do occur in experimental animals under appropriate conditions, have been studied by WALTMAN *et al.* [107, 108]. It was found that this serum, given early or late, markedly inhibited the rejection phenomenon.

KHODADOUST and SILVERSTEIN [49] showed that corneal grafts are secure so long as they remain avascular, because of a reduced ability to sensitize the host and also because of a reduced ability of the host, even if otherwise sensitized, to reject the tissue. If the graft becomes vascularized, rejection is quite probable but still not inevitable. They concluded that the degree of vascularization in a corneal bed cannot be as intimate as in a dermal bed which is the case in a skin graft rejection.

Of the antigens that may occur in the cornea, the immunoglobulins of blood serum merit particular interest. While it is true that these proteins cannot contribute to the tissue-specific antigens of this eye component, their localization can shed more light on such matters as vascularity, transparency, and local antibody responsiveness in the cornea and in all eye tissues and structures; in addition, the presence and distribution of the immunoglobulins would be indicative of a distribution of antibody in these structures. For these reasons, ALLANSMITH and colleagues [1, 3, 3a, 3b] studied the localization of immunoglobulin G in these tissues, and found this protein under the epithelium of the cornea and the conjunctiva. KAWERAU and OTT [48] found IgG in fluid extracted from the corneal stroma of cattle, pig, and man. In a more recent and detailed study, ALLANSMITH *et al.* [2] explored the distribution of this protein throughout the eye structures, and the results can be summarized here for the cornea and for the other components. The technic used was immunofluorescence, and rabbit eye was the object of study. IgG proved to be a normal constituent of the stroma of the cornea and of the conjunctiva, as well as of the sclera, choroid, and ciliary processes and the connective tissue of the extraocular muscles. Within the cornea, it was present throughout the stroma, extending from the basement membrane of the epithelium to Descemet's membrane, and being more dense near the limbus. In the sclera, it seemed less dense than in the structures just mentioned, but was again dense near the limbus. There was no sign of this protein in the trabecular meshwork. The ciliary body contained an uneven distribution, showing a high concentration near and in the processes and much less near the iris. In the iris itself there was no trace of the immunoglobulin. The choroid showed positive results, which stopped at Bruch's membrane and did not appear in the pigment epithelium of the retina. The lens contained no IgG, even though all parts of its structure were explored. The retina showed none of this protein, and the extrinsic ocular muscles showed none of it, except for the connective tissue, as has been mentioned.

The presence of this globulin is presumably due to the rich blood supply, except in the case of the cornea. Although the cornea is avascular, some blood proteins do permeate it by means of diffusion if their molecular weights are not too high. It has been estimated from several studies that molecules with molecular weights up to 500000 could diffuse through the corneal structure [77, 78]. The iris, which has a rich vascular network, contained none of these serum proteins, although they were present in the other components of the uveal tract. ALLANSMITH and NEWMAN postulated that the explanation rests on the peculiar features of the blood-vessel construction in these tissues [2].

Since immunoglobulin is present in certain eye structures, antibody activity may occur. Antigen may arrive by the same routes, so that some diseases of the eye, especially inflammatory responses, may become more clear on the basis of local antigen-antibody reaction. The various hypersensitivity responses of the cornea after preliminary sensitization by foreign antigen have been discussed with reference to protein escape rates, immunologic memory, and corneal disease [89, 90].

3. Antigens of the Uvea

The earliest studies on the tissue-specific antigen of the uvea suggested that the pigment was the most likely candidate for this immunological characteristic. In more recent years, however, it has been proposed that the tissue-specific antigen is not the pigment itself but the matrix of the pigment granule [13, 21a, 102]. These studies were combined with explorations of experimental autoimmune uveitis[3]. As an example, rabbits immunized with suitable emulsions of bovine uvea prepared in Freund's adjuvant produce antibodies against uvea preparations, including rabbit uvea. WACKER and DODD [102] found that the injection of rabbits with homologous uvea failed to produce any demonstrable immune response, but the injection of heterologous uveal tissue did produce an antibody response even to rabbit uvea. Again, as with cornea, it was suggested that the failure of homologous material to stimulate antibody production, although an antibody reaction to the homologous tissue could be induced by the use of heterologous extract, indicated that these uveal antigens are haptens and that they owe their antigenicity to the attachment to protein of a foreign species. These antigens from the uvea were found to be quite labile.

In this same investigation, a reaction was discovered between normal rabbit serum and uvea in complement-fixation tests; a natural antibody was thought to be involved.

These general findings were in essential agreement with earlier studies by ELSCHNIG [30, 31] and by WOODS [111, 112], who had reported the presence of an antigen considered to be the pigment material in uvea. The work of

[3] This experimental disease has also been called "experimental allergic uveitis", "homoimmune uveitis", and "isoimmune uveitis".

WACKER and DODD demonstrated that albino uvea also contained such an antigen and thus raised the question as to whether the pigment or some other component of the uvea is actually the source of the organ-specific component, and even whether more than one kind of such an antigen is present.

Studies were conducted by ARONSON and colleagues [13] on experimental allergic uveitis. Skin hypersensitivity was developed in guinea pigs immunized with homologous uveal tract material combined with complete Freund's adjuvant, although there was no difference between animals according to whether they were injected with pigmented uveal tract or with albino uveal tract. Clinical and histological uveitis was produced. However, they also obtained similar reactions for the spleen extract, although not for whole blood, and they suggested that there is a common antigen in these several tissues that obscures the specific factor active in uveitis.

It was shown by WACKER *et al.* [106] that antisera from guinea pigs immunized with homologous uvea in adjuvant react by complement-fixation with an antigen in saline homogenates of guinea pig uvea: this antigen appears to be both tissue-specific and species-specific. These workers also showed that uveitis could be produced in guinea pigs by suitable immunization with homologous retina, as well as uvea [103].

ARONSON *et al.* [5, 9, 10] described the role of homologous and heterologous uvea and also retinovitreous antigens in the stimulation of experimental uveitis in both guinea pig and rabbit. Uveitis was produced in either species by injection of homologous extracts in complete Freund's adjuvant. The inflammation was much more severe in the guinea pig than in the rabbit. In both species, lymphoid infiltration of the corona of the ciliary body was the mildest and probably the earliest lesion [6]. It was not possible to determine whether the antigen was common to both the uvea and the retinovitreous, or whether dissection was incomplete [5], in which case, the precise site of the antigen—uvea or retina—will need further study. In terms of circulating antibody, generally demonstrated by gel diffusion precipitation, the guinea pig again was a much better responder. Antibody was rarely seen in the rabbit after multiple injections of homologous antigen (in close agreement with the negative results of WACKER and DODD [102]), but a majority of guinea pigs showed a single precipitin band, and some showed two bands. On the other hand, uveitis failed to develop in response to immunization with heterologous antigen, although circulating antibody was produced. One exception cited was that 20% of guinea pigs injected with human uvea did develop histologic uveitis; in contrast, no animals responded to injection of retinovitreous antigen from human, bovine, porcine, or lapine origin with inflammation. Inflammatory response in the guinea pig has also been obtained by direct injection into the vitreous humor [93]. In more recent work, strain 13 guinea pigs were used. Over 40% of them showed two bands to uvea and three bands to retinovitreous material (the stimulating preparation). One of the bands shows common reactivity with lens antigen. These animals develop a chronic, progressive uveitis reminiscent of sympathetic ophthalmia [7].

Comparisons have been made for similar isoimmunizations with retina material by WACKER *et al.* [101, 104, 105, 105a]. The guinea pigs thus treated developed uveitis, bearing a resemblance to the disease induced by immunization with uveal tissue. However, certain points of difference were noted, and the question as to whether there are two models of experimental uveitis or only one is still open.

ARONSON *et al.* have extracted an antigen from human uvea [12], which gives a single line of precipitation with serum obtained from patients with (endogenous or exogenous) uveitis. Previous reports have described immune responses in patients with uveitis by several criteria, such as skin tests, complement fixation, hemagglutination, and precipitation [46, 59, 113]. In the present study [12], precipitation in gel was much more sensitive and useful, as the antibody was concentrated and each serum sample was precipitated at 40% saturation with ammonium sulfate and the globulin fraction re-dissolved to give a concentration 3.5 times higher than in the original serum. With this type of globulin preparation, testing with specially prepared human uveal antigen [8] gave a positive result with 45 of 91 patients with uveitis (39 of 75 endogenous and 6 of 16 exogenous), in 10 of 43 cases of other ocular diseases, and in no cases of 136 monocular disease control patients. A larger series was later reported with similar results; 63% of 307 patients with uveitis showed positive results in precipitation testing, as did 49% of 119 patients with other ocular diseases, whereas this was found for only 2 people out of 300 with no known eye disease [11]. A somewhat lower, but nonetheless significant, incidence was reported by LUNTZ [60]. Indeed, if we consider only sympathetic ophthalmia (as a form of exogenous uveitis), we may note that 8 of 9 cases (or 87%) were positive.

The antigen used in these tests is not stable. It can be prepared from homogenized uvea after the bulk of the protein has been removed by precipitation and the lipid has been extracted. A similar antigen can be isolated from the uvea of guinea pig which reacts in gel diffusion with an antibody found in sera from guinea pigs with autoimmune uveitis [4, 12].

In a quite different approach, EPSTEIN *et al.* [32] have found that about 30–50% (depending on the precise form of the disease) of patients with uveitis have antibody to double-stranded RNA. These findings are similar to the results for patients with systemic lupus erythematosus. Further studies in this direction may be helpful in clarifying the pathogenesis of these diseases.

In addition to the tissue-specific antigens, the uveal system also contains the α-, β-, and γ-crystallins in the iris [55], as well as antigen of the basement membrane in the choroid [84]. One can also find species-specific and Kidd-Friedewald antigens [102]. There may also be an antigen common to prostate and joint diseases [85]. There is still a lot to learn about the relative importance of all these shared antigens and tissue-specific antigens[4].

---

[4] In a completely different area of immunity related to the eye, HALL and O'CONNOR [44, 45] have studied the effects of immunization by the intravitreal route. A rapid onset of uveitis occurred in the rabbits. However, these investigators were not concerned with the uvea as a source of antigens, but rather with its capability to provide a response to a foreign antigen challenge, as had also been true of the earlier work of SILVERSTEIN and colleagues [92, 93]. They considered that the eye can act as a kind of accessory lymph node. They discussed the response mechanisms in terms of the X, Y, Z scheme of antibody-forming cells of ŠTERZL and SILVERSTEIN [97].

Treatment of autoimmune disease is a difficult problem. Recent reports have claimed some success with the use of cyclophosphamide in Behcet's disease, in a condition involving uveitis [16], and in peripheral uveitis [38].

4. Other Antigens of the Eye

Several additional antigenic systems may be mentioned very briefly, without any claim of completeness.

The protein mixtures in the aqueous and vitreous humors have been analyzed, along with the specificity properties of the antigenic components. COOPER *et al.* [22] showed that human and bovine vitreous contained many serum proteins, but that they also contained many non-serum antigens (at least 5 in human and 9 in bovine systems). Some of these antigens were absent from other body tissues, as well; more detailed studies are now needed, however. In sheep, human, and bovine vitreous, a number of these antigens were related, indicating in this way also, their tissue-specific properties. BASH *et al.* [15] produced autoantibodies in sheep against sheep vitreous. These antibodies were shown to be tissue-specific in both senses. No ocular lesions developed in these animals.

The proteins of human aqueous humor have been analyzed by means of disc electrophoresis by KRAUSE and RAUNIO [54]. The total protein content and its composition were discussed in terms of the pathologic conditions.

A group of patients with optic neuritis were tested for hypersensitivity to encephalitogenic protein (prepared from myelin), and several of the patients showed a positive reaction apparent as lymphoblast transformation [58]. The authors felt these findings showed an immunologic relationship to certain disorders of the central nervous system; the data are very few, however.

Experimental chorioretinitis has been induced in monkeys by immunization with monkey retinal tissue, as described by LERNER *et al.* [57]. The authors considered these eye lesions to represent a tissue-specific autoimmune disease.

Chapter 7

The Kidney

The numerous investigations on kidney antigens can be considered conveniently in two broad categories. The first of these relates to studies on tissue specificity, in which various kinds of antisera are used as reagents for the analysis of characteristic antigens. The second category relates to experimental and clinical studies on glomerulonephritis and the immunological factors that might be involved in the etiology of such conditions. As far as tissue specificity is concerned, the kidney occupies a somewhat anomalous position. Kidney extracts have often been used as control samples in the evaluation of other organ extracts, to provide the background data of non-specificity. These studies suggest that the kidney antigens are ubiquitous components of the body tissues in general. This has been illustrated in Chapter 2 in several discussions on the specificity of the thyroid. Nonetheless, there are several tissue-specific antigens among the kidney components [3, 168, 200]. A thermostable antigen has been reported that is kidney-specific [73] and similar in physicochemical properties to antigens of adrenal and brain, which are discussed in Chapters 3 and 4. In general, kidney-specific antigens are more readily observed under conditions of isoimmunization, and possibly also if the morphological elements of this organ are studied separately. It is important to keep in mind that the glomeruli are quite distinctive structures, as are also their basement membranes. The other structure of major importance is the tubule, with its tubular cells, in both descending and ascending forms. An excellent portrayal of kidney fine structure has been given by RHODIN [153]. Other structural studies may also be of interest [1, 98, 148].

Although we shall try to discuss the specific antigens of kidney in the two categories mentioned above, there will necessarily be some overlap. We shall begin with a discussion of the salient features of Masugi nephritis.

1. The Experimental Production of Nephritis by Antiserum —Masugi Nephritis

In 1933, MASUGI reported the experimental disease now called Masugi nephritis which has become a standard reference for the concept of nephrotoxic serum in general. He injected rabbits with tissue homogenates prepared from rat kidney, and found that the anti-kidney serum was nephrotoxic when injected intravenously in normal rats [114]. Injection of such sera results in albuminuria and histologically detectable renal damage in most animals. The capillaries in the affected glomeruli dilate widely within the first few hours, but by 24–48 hours after the injection this is much reduced by swelling of the endothelial cells. These initial experiments have been followed by innumerable similar studies directed at elucidating the site and nature of the renal antigens that play a role in this reaction and the pathogenesis of the lesions formed. Masugi nephritis is very similar to some forms of human kidney disease. The disease involves the capillaries of the glomerulus, and in severe cases both the efferent and the afferent vessels. MASUGI also discovered that rabbit kidney homogenate given to ducks elicited antibodies which caused diffuse glomerulonephritis in rabbits when the serum was given intravenously [115]. Many investigators attempted to define the species specificity and organ specificity of these effects and also the nature and localization of the responsible antigen, often termed the nephrotoxic antigen [9, 10, 50, 69]. However, we should turn at this point to studies directed at clarification of the mechanisms involved in the production of nephritis.

Work by KAY [78] on the action of duck anti-rabbit kidney sera indicated that the renal lesions were not a direct result of interaction between the antiserum and the antigen present in the rabbit's kidney. If this interaction were responsible, the renal lesions would be expected to appear within the first 24 hours, whereas no sign of renal damage was observed until the 5th day or later. KAY [78, 79] suggested the following sequence of events leading up to the glomerulonephritis found in rabbits after injection of a heterologous (duck) nephrotoxic antiserum:

1. Duck antibodies to rabbit kidney plus the antigen present in rabbit kidney form a harmless complex *in situ*.
2. Normal duck proteins, being antigenic in the rabbit, stimulate the production of rabbit antibody to duck protein.
3. The rabbit antibody reacts with the duck antibody protein which has become attached to kidney antigen, and this interaction is the immediate cause of the renal lesions.

If the antigen-antibody reaction occurs in the circulating rabbit blood there is no significant reaction, but if the duck antibody has been bound to rabbit kidney antigen, nephritis results, the localization of the reaction in the renal glomeruli being favored by the previous localization there of the duck serum proteins. These arguments were based on observations in rabbits injected with duck nephrotoxic serum. In general, however, nephrotoxic antibodies do not give a harmless reaction in combination with kidney antigen, as HAMMER and DIXON [59] later demonstrated. KAY also proposed a model for the cause of human nephritis which will be discussed below.

In confirmation of KAY'S findings, PRESSMAN, KORNGOLD, and HEYMANN [149] found that with duck anti-rat kidney sera a latent period is observed even though the experiment is performed in rats. However, MASUGI [114] had found that when *rabbit* anti-kidney sera were injected into rats, there was no comparable latent period. There is thus a significant difference between the actions of duck and rabbit antisera even though the same recipient, *i.e.*, rat, is used. Both kinds of antisera (duck and rabbit) were shown to localize in the glomeruli, and the difference in latent period consequently was attributed to the inability of duck antisera to fix complement. If complement is essential for damage to the glomerular components, the injury is delayed by the requirement for production of a complement-fixing antibody, which is fulfilled by rat (or rabbit) antibody to the duck serum globulins. When rabbit nephrotoxic sera are used in rats, no such latent period is necessary, since the nephrotoxic sera are able to fix mammalian complement themselves, being of mammalian origin. These mechanisms have been reviewed by LANGE *et al.* [97].

2. The Antigens of the Glomerulus; the Nephrotoxic Antigens

There have been many attempts to identify the antigen(s) responsible for Masugi glomerulonephritis. The nephrotoxic component was shown to be located in the glomerulus by the ability of glomerular fractions to absorb the activity from a rabbit anti-kidney serum [171]. The first direct evidence that glomeruli are antigenic was given by GREENSPON and KRAKOWER in 1950 in the first of a series of papers on this subject [57]. Isolated glomeruli from dog kidney were injected along with alumina-gel adjuvant into rabbits, and led to the production of potent nephrotoxic serum.

More recently, well-purified glomeruli have been isolated, not by this original method of repeated centrifuging of the sieved tissue homogenate, but by infusion of a suspension of iron oxide particles into the kidney; the particles lodge in the glomeruli, which are removed from the sieved homogenate with an electromagnet [27, 169].

In contrast, other cortical components, which did not contain glomeruli, failed to stimulate this antibody response when administered by a similar technique. Shortly afterwards the antigenic activity was shown to be localized actually in the glomerular basement membrane (GBM) [83, 84]; the other glomerular components, such as the endothelial or parietal epithelial cells, were essentially inactive [55]. Further studies were directed at chemical characterization of the nephrotoxic antigen and yielded a fractionated product which was homogeneous and free of cell membranes and also of nucleoprotein [56, 86]; the nephrotoxic activity was readily destroyed by proteolytic enzymes. A number of studies suggested that the nephrotoxic antigen is a protein-polysaccharide complex characteristically located in the GBM and usually not soluble [26, 53, 54, 107, 128, 130, 140, 143, 146, 164, 166]. It may well be, however, that some cellular constituent might also contain nephrotoxic antigens. Electron microscopy has suggested a multiple origin of the GBM, so that one component may be secreted by the glomerular epithelial cells while others arise from connective tissue and capillary endothelium [2, 39, 88].

Localization of the antibodies has been studied by various means, including autoradiography and immunofluorescent procedures [154, 155, 161, 194]. The binding of antibody to the glomerulus persists for many months [161]. ANDRES *et al.* [2] used electron microscopy to show that most of the antibody was found in the true basement membrane (lamina densa), although some of it was also present in the cytoplasm of epithelial cells in foot processes and sometimes in the endothelial capillary cytoplasm. At least some of the antigen may thus be transported from the glomerular epithelial cells, which have a well-formed endoplasmic reticulum, into the GBM. KRAKOWER and GREENSPON [85] showed some correlation in various tissues between the content of this nephrotoxic antigenic activity and the degree of vascularity. However, the content of this antigen was strikingly higher in glomerular capillaries than in those of other organs. They suggested that this might be connected with the hydrostatic pressures on the glomerular structures.

We have seen the importance of the basement membrane and of the capillary endothelium, as well as of the epithelial cells. Other membrane studies [38, 161, 201] had indicated that the active material was a trypsin-resistant mucoprotein, which may also involve a component related to reticulin [29]. The GBM may have at least two connective tissue antigens, one distributed like reticulin (according to argyrophilic staining patterns) and another shared by vascular and non-vascular basement membranes [126, 159]. It has also been claimed that collagen preparations can absorb out the antibody activity, although the antigen cannot be completely identical to collagen [109, 163]. The collagen of kidney has been further characterized antigenically by ROTHBARD and WATSON [154, 155].

Although other identifications have been claimed from time to time, the current situation seems best summarized by the concept that the nephrotoxic antigen of GBM has three main components, originating in connective tissue, glomerular epithelium, and capillary endothelium. The mesenchymal component may be related to reticulin or its glycoprotein [170]. The epithelial component may be related to the mucoprotein of Reichert's membrane [127]. The endothelial cells may contribute a mucopolysaccharide to the GBM complex. GBM antigens have been found in normal human urine and serum [118–121]. A number of chemical analyses have been reported [5, 90, 129, 165, 172–174].

3. The Antigens of the Tubule

Some of the earliest work on the organ specificity of kidney and its subcellular particles was that by FURTH and KABAT [48] and HENLE *et al.* [60]. HILL and CRUICKSHANK [68] were the first to distinguish between antigens of the tubular cell cytoplasm and antigens of the basement membrane of glomeruli and tubules. This was accomplished by the use of rabbit antisera to rat kidney, and immunofluorescence with these antisera. After absorption with rat lung, the sera stained only the cytoplasm of renal tubule cells; the staining was uniform throughout the cell, present in all tubules, and specific (not absorbed by liver antigens). Antisera to glomeruli stained only with glomeruli and gave no reaction with tubules, except for their basement membranes.

A number of subsequent studies have been reported on kidney-specific antigens, in which many, if not all, of the antigens are probably of tubular origin. WEILER [197] prepared antisera in rabbits by injection of mitochondria and microsomes from hamster kidney. After suitable absorption treatment these antisera showed antibody activity only against kidney tubular cytoplasm. The immunofluorescence was not intense on the brush border of the proximal convoluted tubules, although there was some activity in the collecting tubules and the Henle loops [198]. Similar observations have been made by others [45, 131, 132], showing especially that antisera to microsomal fractions of kidney are tissue-specific and gave antibody staining in the tubule cells in various species of mammals and birds, and some fish, but not in reptiles, amphibia, or other fish. OKADA and SATO [133, 138] prepared purified microsomal fractions from kidney tissue of chicken. These antigens are thought to be mainly a lipid-protein complex from the membranes of the endoplasmic reticulum and seem to appear during development of the mesonephros [43, 44, 134–137, 139]. Autoantibodies prepared by JOHNSON *et al.* [74] by immunization with rat kidney also stained only with certain renal tubule cells.

Recently EDGINGTON *et al.* [34–36, 51] have reported the purification of a pathogenic antigen from the renal tubular epithelium (RTE). The authors studied its capacity to induce nephritis of the immune complex type, which is discussed more fully below; this antigen was termed "nephritogenic", and the difference in pathogenic mechanism between this antigen and the nephrotoxic antigen was emphasized. Their assay for the nephritogenicity of an antigen preparation was based on the urinary protein output of suitably injected rats [34]. They also suggested that this (RTE) antigen was derived from the brush-border cells of the proximal convoluted tubule of the kidney [34]. Although not noted, this seems to be quite consistent with the earlier emphasis by WEILER [198] on the specific antigenic activity associated with these cells. Three RTE-specific antigens, termed RTE-α_3, RTE-α_4, and RTE-α_5, were identified and isolated from rat kidney preparations and tested for nephritogenic activity. The first two were negative [36]; only the RTE-α_5 antigen was found to have this activity [35]. As a result of further fractionation, this antigen was judged to be a high-molecular weight lipoprotein molecule with a sedimentation coefficient of 28.6 S and an electrophoretic mobility similar to that of serum α-globulin. The RTE-α_5 was considered to be a subunit of the cell membrane, probably of the plasma membrane of the brush border or the intracellular membranes of certain tubular epithelial cells of the kidney [35].

4. The Formation of Autoantibodies Against Kidney Antigens

a) Early Studies

The possibility of stimulating the formation of autoantibodies against one or more components of the kidney has been explored by various means. Some of these investigations have been associated with the formation of a disease response, often, though not always, glomerulonephritis, in which case the antibody response was frequently considered less important and sometimes even incidental. In other situations, however, damage to the tissue was not explored, and the activity of autoantigens of kidney as such was the main subject of study. In 1939 SCHWENTKER and COMPLOIER [158] injected rabbits with rabbit kidney mixed with staphylococcal or streptococcal toxin and obtained antibody which reacted with normal rabbit kidney as determined by complement fixation. There was no mention of glomerulonephritis. In 1941, PARKS and SHANKS [142] attempted to produce lesions by direct injection of a suspension of various organisms or culture filtrates into the renal artery of rabbits. The rabbits were killed 24–30 hours later. The kidneys of these rabbits were homogenized and injected into other rabbits intraperitoneally. Antibody was obtained to extracts of the injected kidneys. The antibodies were not nephrotoxic to the antibody-producing rabbit. In another experiment, a kidney was damaged by tying off the renal artery, and after some time, a homogenate of this kidney was injected intraperitoneally into other rabbits. This method also yielded precipitating non-toxic antibody. In these early experiments with streptococcal adjuvants, there may have been some danger of eliciting an antibody response that could cross-react with some kidney antigen in a similar way to the analogous human situations described below.

b) Isoimmunization in Rabbits and Rats by the Use of Streptococcal Adjuvants

Undoubtedly the first work that really involved an autoimmune response to kidney tissue was performed by the CAVELTIS in 1945 [17]. They injected rabbits with a mixture of rabbit organ extracts and a suspension of streptococci, using as many as 40 intraperitoneal injections. The antisera contained antibodies to kidney, liver, brain, erythrocytes, and serum. The antibody titers were measured by both latex agglutination and precipitation tests. When absorbed with rabbit liver or serum, only the antikidney antibody remained, showing reasonable titers of activity. Streptococci themselves had only slight antigenicity when used in control immunizations. Kidney damage in the immunized rabbits was not reported in this report. In a second paper, CAVELTI and CAVELTI [18] used the same kind of procedure with rats and reported renal lesions. In a complementary report [19], they stated that the rats recovered from the acute phase of nephritis, but if it was severe enough, chronic obliterative nephritis occurred. The antibodies were determined by means of a collodion particle agglutination method [16]. The same strains of streptococci were used as adjuvants in rabbits and rats, in these investigations, yet immunized rats showed renal lesions, while rabbits did not [15]. These findings in rabbits appear to parallel the earlier findings of PARKS and SHANKS and those of SCHWENTKER and COMPLOIER; these two teams obtained the same results using staphylococcal or streptococcal filtrates.

c) Isoimmunization in Rats by the Use of Freund's Adjuvant

Many attempts to reproduce the CAVELTI work failed and the original findings fell into some disrepute and were forgotten. HEYMANN and his group were probably the next to be successful in this general area, and re-established that kidney autoimmune responses could be induced. They emphasized the importance of the route of injection. Subcutaneous injections, even into the footpads, always gave negative results, but the results of intraperitoneal injections were consistently positive. They studied rats, using either homologous or heterologous material for immunization. Their interest lay almost exclusively in the experimental induction of renal disease (which they usually refer to as nephrosis), rather than in any detailed analysis of the response of circulating antibody. For example, HEYMANN *et al.* [63] performed unilateral nephrectomies on rats. The tissue obtained was homogenized, mixed with complete Freund's adjuvant, and injected intraperitoneally into the same rat. After several injections, a nephrotic syndrome was observed. Histological examination revealed that the basement membrane of the kidney was thickened and the endothelial cytoplasm was swollen. In later experiments, in which an incomplete adjuvant was used, no renal disease resulted [64]. The histologic appearance was a great contrast to that after injection of nephrotoxic sera. Neither the glomerular cell changes nor the closed capillary lumina so conspicuous in nephrotoxic nephritis developed. The striking feature was considerable thickening of the basement membrane, suggesting a parallel with human membranous glomerulonephritis. Membranous glomerulonephritis is a disease of the renal glomeruli, characterized by the loss of the foot processes of the epithelial cells and by thickening of the basement membrane. It is the most frequent cause of the nephrotic syndrome, the three basic features of which are marked proteinuria, hypoproteinemia and generalized edema. Another important renal disease situation is that of lipoid nephrosis. It is generally agreed that the terms membranous glomerulonephritis and lipoid nephrosis both refer to the same condition. Lipoid nephrosis is usually used for early stages of the disorder and membranous glomerulonephritis for the more advanced stages.

Immunization with rat liver suspensions by a similar method also resulted in nephrosis, even though the incidence was considerably lower than in the animals immunized with kidney suspensions. HUNTER *et al.* [72] reported that rat liver contained an antigen apparently also present in rat kidney, as shown by immunoelectrophoresis. Two of five rat antikidney sera cross-reacted with rabbit and guinea pig kidney. HESS *et al.* [61] and HEYMANN *et al.* [65] showed that experimental nephrosis could be transferred by injection of spleen cells from actively immunized animals into healthy recipient rats rendered tolerant to the donor's tissues. These experiments lent support to the opinion that experimental rat nephrosis was an autoimmune disease. HEYMANN *et al.* [67] showed that when heterologous kidney and Freund's adjuvant were injected intraperitoneally in rats, the same incidence of disease as in the autologous experiment was found; kidney suspensions from guinea pig, rabbit, and man were used in these studies. The homologous tissue gave better resistance to kidney disease. The authors suggested that the findings supported the hypothesis of an autoimmune response [67]. The results of immunofluorescent studies indicated that the autoimmune mechanism in rats causes membranous glomerulonephritis and a nephrotic syndrome involving a different group of antigens from those responsible for the heterologous nephrotoxic rabbit antisera, as in Masugi nephritis [67]. Studies by HESS *et al.* [62] confirmed many of these findings and also indicated that the mitochondrial fraction of rat kidney is the one involved in production of nephrotic disease in rats. All this pioneering work was to be more fully explained later on the basis of a tubular cell antigen and its initiation of antigen-antibody complex formation leading to kidney damage.

d) Isoimmunization in Rabbits and Guinea Pigs by the Use of Freund's Adjuvants

MILGROM *et al.* [125] studied the humoral antibodies resulting from immunization with kidney suspensions within the same species. Rabbits and guinea pigs were selected for these experiments as these species are generally found to be better producers of humoral antibodies than rats; an additional reason for using rabbits was that CENTENO *et al.* [22] had found that immunization of rabbits with rabbit adrenal tissue could give rise not only to adrenal-specific antibodies, but also to antibodies which reacted with extracts of rabbit kidney. In this study [125], nine rabbits were immunized with a suspension of pooled rabbit kidney in Freund's adjuvant enriched with additional forms of tubercle bacilli. Seven of these rabbits formed large amounts of antibody to kidney. Antisera from some of these rabbits were tested in gel diffusion, and two lines developed. This, the very first antigenic analysis, revealed that one of the antigens was common to all the organ extracts tested, while the other was indicated only for the kidney extract, whether homologous or autologous. This specific line thus revealed the kidney specificity and also the autoimmune nature of the antibody response. Similar studies were performed with either homologous or autologous material in 12 guinea pigs. All the animals developed potent antibody responses, but in many cases the antibodies were not organ-specific, although they were species-specific. It was concluded that immunization with kidney leads to the formation of both organ- and species-specific autoantibodies in rabbits, while in guinea pigs, only a species-specific autoantibody is formed.

In subsequent studies, CENTENO *et al.* [23] followed the course of immunization by immunodiffusion and by analyses of urine for proteinuria. Pronounced proteinuria was detected at some stage of immunization in 5 of the 9 rabbits, early in the course in three of them and late in the other two. There was no apparent correlation between proteinuria and antibody response, nor between early proteinuria and increased kidney size and tissue damage. In one rabbit, which showed extensive early proteinuria but a poor antibody response, the kidney was four times the normal size, and amyloidosis was detected in histological preparations. Calcification was found in renal foci, suggesting bouts of necrosis which may have occurred at times during immunization. Further studies have been reported on the purification and properties of the kidney-specific antigens [20] and on a non-kidney-specific antigen [167].

It became clear that several antigens in the kidney tissue were capable of functioning as autoantigens [21], and that they should be purified to allow better correlation with the respective antibody activities. SHULMAN and WYPYCH [168] have recently reported that isoimmunization of rabbits with kidney extracts and Freund's adjuvant leads to responses to a multiplicity of autoantigens. If a large number of kidneys are pooled, isoantigens can also be detected. These immunization procedures result in antisera that generally possess multiple specificities with varying proportions of the antibodies. If the most useful antisera are selected, lines of precipitation corresponding to each separate antigen can be unambiguously shown in immunoprecipitation. A typical precipitation pattern is shown in Fig. 7.1, indicating all twelve combinations for the four antisera taken three at a time in reaction with a kidney extract. A total of five antigens was found for kidney, three of which were kidney-specific and two of which were shared with liver. A sixth antigen, not seen for liver, may be only a minor constituent of kidney and was not detected directly in the kidney extract. It was important that fresh concentrated extracts of kidney homogenate be used. The detection of isoantigens also requires concentrated extracts prepared from individual kidneys [168].

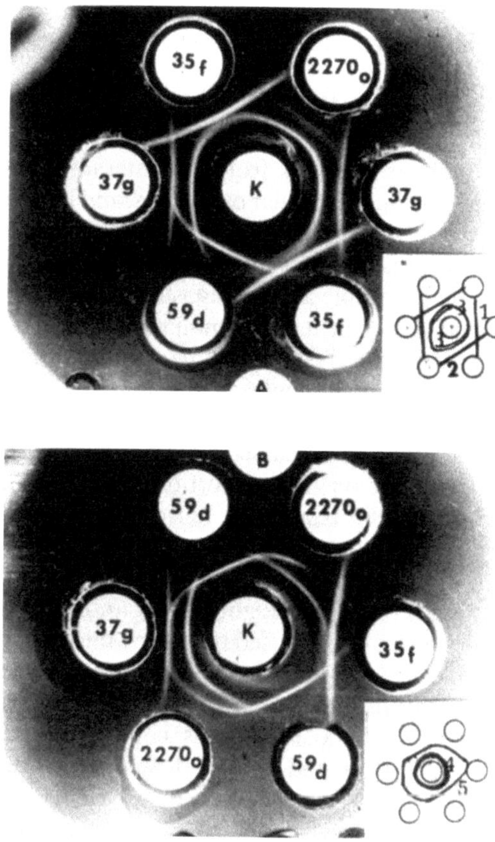

Fig. 7.1. Double diffusion gel precipitation. A comparison of the reactions of four different rabbit antisera to rabbit kidney with a saline extract of kidney. The sera are grouped so that each can be compared with every one of the other three at least twice in the two plates

Further studies [200], involved attempts to fractionate kidney extracts in order to isolate and characterize these various antigens. Zone electrophoresis followed by gel filtration was used to obtain a number of fractions. Antigens 1 and 3 of the kidney-specific antigens were separated in different protein fractions, associated predominantly with 7 S and 4 S components.

The use of precisely identified and isolated fractions of tissue should allow substantial advances in the study of disease mechanisms. DIXON and his associates

[35, 51] have shown that immunization of rats with rat renal-tubular antigen, described below, seems to cause lesions some distance from the natural site for the antigen, and that the immune complexes in the glomerular lesions contain quantities of the antigen far in excess of those used for the immunization. This makes it necessary to postulate an autologous source of the antigen in order to maintain the disease. The number and variety of these autologous antigens needs further study.

5. Experimental Glomerulonephritis

All the major forms of immunologically-based kidney disease involve damage to the glomerulus and these forms can be described in terms of two clear-cut mechanisms [24]. One of these results from the interaction of antibodies and the antigenic components of the glomerular capillaries, and is generally exemplified by nephrotoxic serum nephritis (NSN). The other form results from the accumulation of antigen-antibody complexes of any sort, not necessarily related to the kidney antigens at all; these complexes are deposited in the glomerular capillary walls, giving rise to what has been termed immune-complex nephritis. The two forms are histologically different. The NSN type shows linear, smooth deposits along the basement membrane. In contrast, the immune-complex type shows lumpy, granular deposits along this membrane.

The Masugi type of nephritis discussed above can result from this second kind of mechanism, depending on the proportions of various components and other factors, but is usually the result and the classic example of NSN [118, 192]. The standard examples of immune-complex nephritis are acute and chronic serum sickness. It is also true that nephritis can be produced by immunization of animals with homologous or heterologous renal antigens, but in many such cases, the disease can be shown to be caused mainly by one of the two mechanisms mentioned above. The complexity of, and evidence for, a great many factors involved in these mechanisms and phenomena have been much clarified in recent years by the work of DIXON and his colleagues; they have recently reviewed the subject [189, 191] and only a few points will be summarized here.

a) Nephrotoxic Serum Nephritis

There are two stages in the form of glomerulonephritis induced by heterologous (passively-transferred) antibody. The first stage, the "heterologous" or "anti-kidney" stage, occurs immediately after injection of the foreign antiserum (or fractionated antibody); it results from the reaction of this antibody with antigens in the glomerular capillary wall. The second, "autologous" or "anti-immunoglobulin", stage develops some days later, after the host animal has produced an antibody response to the injected foreign immunoglobulin. The immunoglobulin has now changed its role to that of antigen implanted in the glomerular structure and the host antibodies are mainly responsible for tissue damage. During the first stage, the foreign antibodies bind to antigens of the glomerulus, and the main antigenic structure is the basement membrane, as has been discussed above. Although the same or a very similar antigen occurs in several other tissues, and some of the antibody is bound in liver, lung, spleen, muscle, and other tissues, the only significant injury occurs in the kidney. The antibody bound in the other organs is either too low in concentration or too weakly bound. Cross-reacting antibodies produced by immunization with heart, spleen, or muscle are also effective in producing nephritis, providing they bind to the glomerulus [77]. The most important parameter in the subsequent course of disease during this anti-kidney stage is the quantity of antibody bound. UNANUE and DIXON [187] have measured the minimum amount of antibody needed for injury in various species; in rat this is approximately 75 µg per g of kidney, in rabbit, 12 µg, and in sheep, 5 µg. This can also be expressed as the amount of antibody per unit of glomerular filtration surface; it was thus calculated that about half the filtration surface was covered by antibody molecules. The fixing of antibody is then followed by the fixation of complement. This can be seen from the fall measured in serum levels of complement [175]. The significance of complement levels has been reported in several studies [103, 157, 193]. Complement binding can also be demonstrated by appropriate immunofluorescence studies of the glomerulus [59, 82, 186], and it is followed by the accumulation of polymorphonuclear leukocytes, presumably attracted to the site by action of the fifth, sixth, and seventh components of complement [196]. If the invasion of these cells is prevented, nephritis does not occur. The exact mechanisms whereby these cells cause the damage is not completely clear; it may involve the release of certain hydrolytic enzymes [25]. The second stage of the disease develops after the production of circulating antibodies to the foreign protein and represents a continuation of the disease, as was originally proposed by KAY [78]. These antibodies are deposited in the glomerulus, along with the originally deposited antibody [59, 141]. Further development of disease, however, is possible with much less of the original foreign antibody. During this phase, complement is again deposited [186], although it is not clear whether this step is essential. The final deterioration of the tissue components seems to result from the continuing formation of deposits of material along the capillary wall [40, 41]. Cellular immunity has been explored [52, 70, 144].

b) Immune-Complex Nephritis

The form of glomerulonephritis induced by deposition of circulating immune complexes can be considered in both acute and chronic forms [12, 31, 32, 147]. BENACERRAF *et al.* [6] and MCCLUSKEY *et al.* [116] were the first to propose that such complexes could cause kidney disease. They injected soluble antigen-antibody complexes intravenously into rats and mice, producing serum sickness and acute glomerulonephritis. They used an antigen excess for rabbit anti-ovalbumin and rabbit anti-BSA, among others. Although severe glomerulonephritis was produced, there was no apparent change in the basement membrane, and the nephritis regressed after injections ceased. DIXON *et al.* [32] injected BGG, BSA, HGG, or HSA into rabbits and elicited various levels of antibody and glomerulonephritis. If much antibody was produced, the disease was acute and self-limiting, and there was immunity to further damage. In contrast, if the antibody level was just enough to neutralize the antigen, a chronic disease resulted, and complexes were found deposited along the renal capillary basement membrane. BSA and BGG were said to be more toxic to the rabbits then were HSA and HGG, suggesting that human proteins are better antigens in rabbits and therefore elicit a high titer of antibody, which is protective. Hence, the work of BENACERRAF *et al.* [6, 116] showed that complexes in the presence of antigen excess would initiate glomerulonephritis. DIXON *et al.* [32] showed that antibody excess would prevent disease, and suggested that weak antigens would be more likely to induce kidney disease, since they elicit a poor antibody response. In general, the glomeruli contain antigen, antibody, and complement, arranged in granular, irregular deposits quite different in shape from the uniform, linear deposits seen in NSN. The glomeruli show membranous thickening and accumulation of PMNs. The important parameters in the induction of tissue injury include the size of the immune complex, the activity of the reticulo-endothelial system, and the participation of vasoactive substances [31]. If the soluble complexes are formed in antigen excess, they will largely localize in the glomeruli; if they are formed in the equivalence zone or in antibody excess, they will be mostly taken up by the cells of the reticulo-endothelial system.

c) Nephritis Following Injection of Kidney Components

Glomerulonephritis can also be induced by immunization with either heterologous or homologous kidney preparations [11, 30, 101, 188, 190]. Although the disease responses can largely be ascribed to mechanisms of the two kinds described above, the immunizing kidney antigens probably do play some distinctive role. More clarification of this possibility is still badly needed. The immunization of rats with rat materials was introduced largely by the work of HEYMANN *et al.* [66], as described above. Later work showed that the antigens that are effective in these conditions are not the glomerular basement membrane components, but the tubular cell components [51, 62]. The localization of the deposits seen in the glomerulus resembled that seen in immune-complex disease [33, 40]. It has now been suggested that experimental glomerulonephritis is an autologous immune complex (AIC) disease [34]. It becomes manifest as a chronic progressive form of membranous glomerulonephritis with the standard hallmarks of antigen-antibody complex-induced nephritis, including the deposition of γ-globulin and complement along the glomerular capillary walls in granular form and electron-opaque deposits along the subepithelial aspects of the GBM. In the rats immunized with a crude tubular fraction or with the purified antigen (RTE-α_5) described above, an autologous material identical to or cross-reactive with the nephritogenic antigen was found to be localized in the glomerular deposit along with the host γ-globulin and complement [35]. The tiny amount of antigen used seemed insufficient to account for the amount of RTE antigen found deposited in the glomeruli. Furthermore, AIC nephritis can be induced with heterologous antigen in rats, and in this form autologous antigen is found along the glomerular capillary walls, as well as the usual γ-globulin and complement. Autologous antigen is thought to be an important source of antigen for the antigen-antibody-complement deposits found in this renal disease [51]. There is also a circulating antibody response to renal tubular but not to glomerular antigens in rats with AIC nephritis, as demonstrated by GRUPE and KAPLAN [58]. Although this disease is certainly an autoimmune one, the glomerulonephritis originates in an autoimmune response not to a glomerular component, but to a tubular component, which is nonetheless autologous. The great variety of pathogenic mechanisms which appear among the immunity-based diseases must be stressed [37, 51].

Effective isoimmunization and autoantibody formation have been described in rabbits [125]. In this situation, the effective material is the GBM, and antibody is localized in the diseased animal's glomeruli [185]. The other example of major interest is the sheep, which responds to immunization with heterologous or homologous GBM preparation in complete Freund's adjuvant with severe glomerulonephritis, as shown by the studies of STEBLAY and colleagues [176, 178]. Examples reviewed include rat, rabbit, human, or dog GBM injected into sheep with Freund's adjuvant, causing a fulminating and fatal glomerulonephritis. Proof of the suggestion that the disease is an autoimmune one will depend ultimately on its passive transfer by serum antibody or sensitized cells [178]. Serum transfer has been reported [100]. The importance of the adjuvant was emphasized by the observation that two sheep immunized with human GBM without adjuvant failed to develop any disease, even after 20 injections. The same investigators have also noted that no disease is produced when autologous kidney is used [179]. The deposition of antibody in the glomerulus is uniform and linear, just as in the NSN condition. The presence of circulating autoantibodies can also be shown [99]. STEBLAY and LEPPER [180] also immunized rabbits with purified human GBM or dog GBM; either kind of rabbit antiserum produced glomerulonephritis in dogs. The conditions were indistinguishable by clinical, chemical, or pathological criteria. They also studied these rabbit antisera by complement fixation, and found the same degrees of cross-reaction between the dog and human GBM antigens. It seems that dog and human GBM contain common determinants, representing a rather striking exception to the fairly good species specificity of nephrotoxic sera. STEBLAY [179] also reported that sheep antibody to human kidney tissue can produce disease in rabbits. Similar studies on induction of nephritis in goats and monkeys have also been described [177, 199].

6. Human Glomerulonephritis

The possible causes of this human disease have been sought in numerous investigations, many of which have indicated an involvement with streptococcal infection, the disease frequently being recorded in patients who have previously had a streptococcal infection of the upper respiratory tract or skin. Autoimmune mechanisms have also been postulated. Although progress has been made in the clarification of this problem, some recent reviewers have been quite negative about earlier claims and theories [156]; this pessimistic viewpoint may well be exaggerated, however.

The kidney diseases relevant to immunology can be described briefly. It is convenient to distinguish several major groups. First, there are certain diseases of the glomerulus, secondly, the disorders grouped together as the nephrotic syndrome, and thirdly, the forms of nephrosis. The first group contains the major forms of glomerulonephritis, which includes several forms of diffuse inflammatory disease manifested mainly in the glomeruli. Two major forms of acute or subacute disease are poststreptococcal proliferative glomerulonephritis (also termed acute or subacute (poststreptococcal) glomerulonephritis *or* Ellis Type 1 nephritis) and membranous glomerulonephritis (also termed Ellis Type 2 nephritis). Membranous glomerulonephritis has already been discussed above. A third condition is chronic glomerulonephritis. There is one especially interesting form of glomerulonephritis, "Goodpasture's syndrome", in which the patient's serum may show antibodies to glomerular basement membrane. Similarities to experimental NSN disease are seen. The nephrotic syndrome refers to a group of symptoms that can be caused by a variety of disease conditions, the four most important being: 1. membranous glomerulonephritis (*or* lipoid nephrosis), 2. chronic glomerulonephritis, 3. poststreptococcal proliferative glomerulonephritis, and 4. nodular glomerulosclerosis. This last condition (also called diabetic glomerulosclerosis) is believed to be a specific lesion of diabetes. The nephrotic syndrome involves diseases of the glomeruli. In contrast, the third group, *i.e.*, the diseases known as nephrosis, affect primarily the tubules, and major examples are: 1. cholemic nephrosis, 2. glycogen nephrosis, and 3. hemoglobinuric nephrosis.

a) Antibodies to Kidney Antigens

In the search for antibodies against kidney constituents, the first major study was that of LANGE *et al.* [91], who used polystyrene latex coated with kidney antigen. In 1949 they were able to show the presence of antibodies to these antigens in the sera of patients with acute and chronic glomerulonephritis. Then PFEIFFER and BRUCH [145], using coated collodion particles, were able to show positive results in sera from both acute and chronic disease, with higher titers for the latter group. WAGNER *et al.* [195] found positive results for patients with eclampsia and preeclampsia. This technic of collodion particle agglutination is difficult and sometimes unreliable, and there have since been contradictory reports. The more recent and better technic of tanned-cell hemagglutination has, however, now been applied to this purpose, and in 1958 LIU and MCCRORY [106] showed by this method that antibodies to kidney were present in 71% of cases of acute glomerulonephritis and 89% of cases with a nephrotic syndrome, thus confirming the findings of LANGE *et al.* [91, 95].

GAJDUSEK in 1958 [49] used complement fixation for the detection of antibody to kidney, placenta, and liver in the sera of patients with nephritis, lupus, and infectious hepatitis. He found strong reactions to kidney and placenta. In addition, 20–50% of sera from acute rheumatic fever, glomerulonephritis, and nephrotic nephritis reacted with kidney, liver, or both. KRAMER *et al.* [87] also found that about half of a group of patients with membranous, subacute, or chronic glomerulonephritis had sera which gave positive results in complement fixation with human kidney suspension.

MELLORS and ORTEGA [123] used fluorescence methods with rabbit antibody to human gamma globulin. The globulin was localized in glomerular lesions in human glomerulonephritis. FREEDMAN and MARKOWITZ [47] showed complement was present in the lesion. BERNS *et al.* [7] demonstrated the binding of insulin to the lesions of glomerulosclerosis of diabetic etiology. LIPPMAN *et al.* [105] proved that sera from glomerulonephritis patients, but not sera from patients with other conditions, inhibited the growth of certain chick embryo tissues. These included kidney, heart, and brain, but not liver, bladder, and spleen. LOEWI [108] found that rabbit antibodies to rat kidney could kill cultures of rat kidney cells. KASUKAWA *et al.* [75, 76] have described some serological properties of such sera, and their reactions with tissue cultures.

LANGE *et al.* [92] recorded other findings that were of significance for the understanding of this disease. The levels of complement were decreased in nephritis during the acute episodes, and returned to normal on remission [96].

LERNER *et al.* [102] started a study on the possible role of anti-GBM antibodies in human glomerulonephritis. They were seeking a mechanism similar to that in experimental glomerulonephritis, induced either by injection of nephrotoxic serum or by immunization with homologous or heterologous GBM. They pointed out that while human γ-globulin was often localized in human nephritic kidneys, it had never been identified as an antibody to GBM or any other specific glomerular antigen. This cannot be expected if streptococcal intervention is involved, but the many non-streptococcal cases leave this question open. These authors did find anti-GBM antibodies in the serum or the kidney tissue or both in nine human subjects with glomerulonephritis in a study on approximately 100 patients [102]. They succeeded in eluting this antibody activity; transfer of either the serum or the eluted antibody to monkeys caused them to develop glomerulonephritis. Among the patients, the anti-GBM antibodies were found in cases with Goodpasture's nephritis and in some cases of subacute and chronic glomerulonephritis. It is important to note that these workers did not put forward any argument for the occurrence of anti-GBM antibodies in acute disease; this lends support to certain interpretations (discussed below) on the role of streptococcal involvement in the acute form of the disease. They point out that a mechanism of autoimmunization is quite possible in cases in which anti-GBM antibodies are present.

b) Streptococcal Antigens

RAMMELKAMP and WEAVER [152] noted in 1953 that streptococci of Lancefield types 12 and 4 were the most prevalent types in acute glomerulonephritis of streptococcal origin. It was then found that the infectivity of these organisms depends on the presence of an M protein, and that infection with these strains leads to a type-specific immunity [150]. It was also reported that the so-called nephritogenic strains of Group A, types 12, 4, 3, 25, and Red Lake are susceptible to lysis when infected by the appropriate bacteriophage [151]. The lysis of such cells with release of various antigens may lead to the formation of immune complexes, leading in turn to a form of glomerulonephritis suggestive of the model investigated by BENACERRAF *et al.* [6, 116] and by DIXON *et al.* [31].

The diffusion chamber experiments of KELLY and WINN [81] and MARKOWITZ *et al.* [110] yielded evidence for the involvement of soluble antigens. Many other studies have associated streptococcal antigens with human glomerulonephritis [4, 8, 13, 71, 94, 104, 110–113, 182–184, 202].

FISCHEL [42] noted that one antibody in serum from subjects with this disease is directed against exotoxins of streptococci and another against the C polysaccharide, while still another is directed against human kidney antigen. An experimental model has recently been achieved by BECKER and MURPHY [4], who infected rabbits with Group A streptococci, and induced a human-like glomerulonephritis.

In 1941, KAY *et al.* [80] had proposed the following mechanism:

1. Streptococcal toxin and human kidney interact to form a new antigenic determinant.

2. The new combination, together with the antibody it elicits, produces nephritis. Their postulates were actually based on events observed in rabbits injected with duck nephrotoxic serum.

In 1951, LANGE *et al.* [92], in an effort to explain the human disease, proposed an initially non-immune alteration of kidney structure, a concept that could be extended to other tissues. They postulated the following sequence of events:

1. In the absence of the proper antibiotic, toxins from infectious organisms cause alterations in kidney proteins, and an antigen is formed.

2. The host produces antibodies to these altered components. When the antibodies bind to antigen, the complex binds complement to initiate nephritis.

3. Any process that either depresses antibody synthesis, such as radiation, nitrogen mustard therapy, ACTH, or cortisone therapy, or competes for complement, as in some other disease states, causes a remission of nephritis.

The models of KAY *et al.* [80] and of LANGE *et al.* [92] for the incidence of human glomerulonephritis both insisted that renal components are altered in some way, implying that the disease has the character of an autoimmune reaction. The findings of LANGE *et al.* [91], LIU and MCCRORY [106], and KRAMER *et al.* [87] supported a role for autoantibodies, rather than an action of non-kidney antigen-antibody complexes. These conclusions were criticized by CRUICKSHANK [28], however, who was unable to reduce the titers by means of appropriate absorptions. Nor was he able to elute an autoantibody from glomeruli taken from fatal cases. FREEDMAN and MARKOWITZ [46] also failed to elute an anti-kidney antibody from diseased kidneys.

The observation that patients with acute glomerulonephritis had their own gamma globulin and complement attached to glomerular tissue indicated that an antigen-antibody reaction of some sort had occurred and that complement was bound to the antigen-antibody complexes. It thus seemed reasonable to search for streptococcal components as antigens attached to the glomerulus in such cases. The findings have been controversial [94, 117, 124, 160].

This situation was further explored by LANGE and his co-workers [93, 183, 184], who took kidney biopsies from a number of patients with acute glomerulonephritis and examined them by means of fluorescein-labeled antibodies to IgG and to complement. After suitable preparation and conjugation, the IgG fractions stained the glomerular basement membrane in the biopsy sections obtained from the same patients and also in those obtained from all other patients with early acute glomerulonephritis. These fractions did not stain normal renal tissue or tissue from patients with subacute or chronic glomerulonephritis or other kidney diseases. It was presumed that a circulating antibody against some factor present only in the kidney tissue from patients with this acute disease was present in their serum, and absorption with various bacterial products was attempted to explore the nature of this factor. Several strains of nephritogenic β-hemolytic streptococci and various other bacterial organisms were used. When the bacteria were used as absorbing agents in their intact form, no loss of staining activity resulted in the absorbed serum. When a freeze-thawed preparation of nephritogenic streptococci was used, the staining was markedly reduced or even completely eliminated in the resulting absorbed serum; in contrast, no loss of staining capacity was obtained after attempted absorption with freeze-thawed preparations of the various other bacteria. It seemed that an antigen capable of absorbing the specific antibody was liberated from the nephritogenic β-hemolytic streptococci. These bacteria were then fractionated into preparations of bacterial wall, M protein, and plasma membrane. The plasma membrane was the only one which eliminated the staining ability of the serum preparations.

Antisera were then prepared against β-hemolytic streptococcal plasma membrane, and after fluorescein-labeling these rabbit antisera were found to stain the glomeruli from early acute glomerulonephritics in the same way as the globulin fractions from the corresponding human sera. The specific activity of the streptococcal organism and the plasma membrane constituents was verified quantitatively [162]. Plasma membrane was the only active component. Acrylamide gel electrophoresis revealed that this preparation contained at least 9 constituents. Some degree of fractionation has been accomplished, and two or three fractions of special interest for further study have been prepared. Two antigens were isolated, one of which was soluble in buffer solution and the other insoluble. The soluble component was judged to be a lipoprotein with a molecular weight of approximately 120000.

Thus streptococcal components are present in the glomeruli of patients with acute poststreptococcal glomerulonephritis. These components are specifically derived from the plasma membrane, the structure under the cell wall that provides an osmotic barrier and regulates the transport of substances in and out of the cell. In general terms, the two major constituents of plasma membranes are lipids and proteins, which are present in approximately equal proportions. Part of the protein group can be found in patients' glomeruli. However, they can only be detected during the early phase of the disease, before all antigenic sites are fully saturated and when smaller amounts of antibody are available. It seems unlikely that antigen is removed after the initial damage, as antibody and complement bound in the original process are still demonstrable after antigen can no longer be stained. The constituent in the IgG fraction is directed against a specific component of β-hemolytic streptococci, as suggested by the absorption studies discussed above. All the patients with acute glomerulonephritis examined so far have seemed to share the same antibody, and many normal subjects have also shared it. The presence of the antibody in "normal" subjects may be due to previous contact with the specific streptococcus, resulting in a long-lasting antibody level [93, 183]. The chronic form of glomerulonephritis may involve quite different mechanisms. In this condition, the long duration of deposition of γ-globulin and complement over several decades made LANGE *et al.* [94] suggest a persistent autoimmune process as a probable mechanism. This concept can be combined with the ideas of LERNER *et al.* [102], who found anti-GBM antibodies in some cases of glomerulonephritis (but not acute cases), and suggested that there might well be some mechanism of autoimmunization in these situations.

The immunological findings in human glomerulonephritis suggest that no one experimental model can reproduce all features of the disease in animals. The data relating to the various experimental models, and experiments on the toxicity of antibody for renal cells in cell culture, as noted above, suggest that human glomerulonephritis is not a single entity. These experimental models include: 1. circulating antibody-nonglomerular antigen complexes, 2. glomerulonephritis induced by means of tubular antigen, 3. nephritis in NZB mice [14, 89, 122, 181], 4. glomerulonephritis caused by anti-glomerular (anti-GBM) antibodies, as shown by nephrotoxic sera or by direct immunization with GBM. It must be borne in mind that different mechanisms may operate in the different clinical forms, which include acute poststreptococcal, subacute, and chronic forms, and Goodpasture's syndrome.

Chapter 8

Mechanisms of Immunopathology

Autoimmune processes leading to tissue damage or malfunction are based on various mechanisms.

The cellular phenomenon in lesion formation generally involves an infiltration of certain white blood cells, although this is not always seen in autoimmune disease. In many of these diseases the typical tissue lesion involves an accumulation of mononuclear cells, as WAKSMAN has emphasized [23]. This is characteristic of experimental autoimmune thyroiditis, where there is extensive infiltration with lymphocytes and macrophages as the major cellular types. There are perivascular accumulations of cells in the brain tissue in allergic encephalomyelitis. Similar pictures are seen in other examples. We still know too little about the chemotactic influence that causes an invasion of these cells to offer any interpretation. Another mechanism is the attack that causes tissue cell death, as in experimental aspermatogenesis, where death of the epithelial cells of the tubule is observed rather than inflammatory responses. A similar effect is sometimes seen in thyroiditis, where desquamation of the epithelium is sometimes seen as well as cellular infiltration. Thus there are mechanisms that cause an invasion of cells and others that cause toxicity to local tissue cells or at least a loosening of their attachment to basement membrane.

The mechanisms can be grouped into two major categories. One category embraces the effects of circulating autoantibody acting as a tissue-specific antibody. Thus, the action of a cytotoxic antibody with an appropriate specificity for the target tissue may be aided by an interaction with complement, and may also be followed by a chemotactic attraction for certain lymphoid cells. The second category includes mechanisms based on cell mediated immune responses, which would involve delayed hypersensitivity directly attuned to the particular target tissue. In this situation, the prominent circulating autoantibody is simply a byproduct or a hallmark of the disease, rather than a pathogenic factor.

Although the data and interpretations have been considered for each of the autoimmune diseases already discussed, it would be simpler to use a single tissue to illustrate some general principles. We have chosen the thyroid gland and autoimmune thyroiditis as a model to examine the relationship between the tissue damage and the tissue-specific antigens.

Since the discovery of experimental autoimmune thyroiditis in 1956, many studies have been devoted to two problems central to the question of whether the circulating autoantibody is a causative agent in the formation of lesions. One of these problems is the relationship between the titer of circulating antibody and the degree of lesion damage. Many of the reports are ambiguous, but the general conclusion is that there is no convincing correlation between antibody titers and severity of lesions. The report by TERPLAN *et al.* [22] contains typical observations. ROSE *et al.* [16] have also stated that there is no significant correlation between the titer in passive hemagglutination and the degree of thyroiditis.

The second problem is the transfer of thyroiditis to normal animals by transfer of serum. Efforts to do this consistently failed in the early stages. The first report indicating that thyroiditis could be transferred by lymphoid cells appeared in 1961 [2]. This was a very brief preliminary report, but it prompted a chain of studies and reports indicating with increasing emphasis that a form of delayed hypersensitivity was more likely than the action of circulating autoantibody to be the causative agent in thyroiditis. This chain can be traced to bring us to our present state of knowledge.

MCMASTER *et al.* [10] claimed that there was some correlation in guinea pig studies between the development of experimental thyroiditis and that of delayed hypersensitivity, although the role of circulating antibody also had to be admitted. The passive hemagglutination test revealed no antibody in the first five days after isoimmunization of the guinea pigs, but there were signs of thyroiditis and also of mild delayed-type hypersensitivity reactions in skin tests with thyroglobulin. At seven weeks, delayed hypersensitivity reactions were seen in all the animals with thyroiditis, but there was also a good correlation with antibody titer. The authors concluded that there was a good correlation between experimental thyroiditis and delayed hypersensitivity. A group of guinea pigs immunized with thyroglobulin in incomplete Freund's adjuvant had low titers of circulating antibody, but neither tissue damage nor skin reactions.

ROSE *et al.* [1, 16] showed that the response of autoantibody formation could be dissociated from the response of tissue lesion development. They were able to stimulate a high titer of antibody production by immunizing rabbits with alum-precipitated antigen; in these conditions there was no development of thyroiditis. When the preparation was combined with complete Freund's adjuvant, however, the immunization resulted in the severe inflammatory thyroid changes characteristic of thyroiditis and also in the development of delayed skin hypersensitivity and circulating autoantibodies.

A very different approach was used by MIESCHER and his colleagues [12] in an effort to exert different effects on the antibody and the hypersensitivity responses. They showed a close relationship between the incidence of delayed hypersensitivity to thyroglobulin and the incidence of immune thyroiditis in guinea pigs immunized with a picrylated preparation of guinea pig thyroglobulin with complete Freund's adjuvant. This immunization technic led to a considerably reduced antibody response, but the delayed hypersensitivity response was largely unchanged. They did not establish any correlation between the titer of circulating antibodies and either tissue damage or delayed hypersensitivity, however; they found, for example, that approximately 60% of the immunized animals developed thyroiditis after an interval of 17 days following the initial injection. Of the same animals, approximately 70% developed delayed hypersensitivity to intradermal test injections of thyroglobulin, while circulating antibody against thyroglobulin, as measured by passive hemagglutination, was only elicited in either 5% or 30% of two groups of animals, depending on the dosage of thyroglobulin injected. There was no difference in the incidence of tissue reactions between the two groups. In a number of the animals they found that skin tests were positive, although thyroiditis was absent. They did not feel that this finding contradicted their thesis that delayed hypersensitivity to thyroglobulin was the pathogenic pathway for experimental thyroiditis, which was based on the feeling that the first stage in this mechanism would be the development of delayed hypersensitivity and that thyroiditis would appear at a later stage.

In a later study, SPIEGELBERG and MIESCHER [21] evaluated the possible mechanisms for the pathogenesis of thyroiditis by studying the different consequences of two alternative antimetabolites, 6-mercaptopurine and aminopterin, on the course of immunization. It had already been reported that both these drugs actively inhibit the development of delayed hypersensitivity in the guinea pig [6, 8] but that antibody formation in the guinea pig is only suppressed by aminopterin [6, 7], so that it appeared that the mechanism of action of these two compounds would be quite different with regard to the immune responses in guinea pigs. These workers therefore administered various dosage levels of each of these antimetabolites during different stages of the immunization phase in the experimental animals. They found that both compounds depressed the formation of delayed hypersensitivity and the development of immune thyroiditis. The formation of circulating antibody was strongly depressed by aminopterin but not significantly affected by 6-mercaptopurine. Furthermore, it was possible to induce thyroiditis in animals that had been treated with aminopterin and in which antibody formation was therefore not demonstrable. They again showed that there was generally a good correlation between a positive skin test and the appearance of thyroiditis, as indicated in earlier studies.

A group of papers by FLAX and his co-workers have illustrated some histological features of the condition they refer to as *experimental allergic thyroiditis* [3, 4, 5]. They reported a good correlation between the intensity of the delayed hypersensitivity and the severity of thyroiditis in various individual members of the immunized groups of guinea pigs but were not able to show any correlation between the titers of circulating antibody to thyroglobulin and the degree of thyroid pathogenicity. It was concluded that a mechanism of delayed hypersensitivity to thyroid antigen was of importance in the pathogenesis of thyroiditis. In some studies, the sequential development of the thyroid lesions after immunization with homologous thyroid material was examined in some detail. The lesions were described histologically with reference to the various types of cells that invade the tissues as the inflammatory response evolves. In the later study [4] correlations were attempted between the morphological changes in the development of experimental thyroiditis and certain functional aspects of the thyroid follicles manifested by the uptake of iodine. The reduced ability to take up iodine evolved at about the same rate as the infiltration with mononuclear cells, suggesting that cellular infiltration might very well be a causative factor in the damage to the thyroid tissue; no specific mechanism for the production of damage could be proposed, but it was stressed that a process of delayed-type hypersensitivity was inherent in the alterations.

WASSERMAN and PACKALÉN [24] also emphasized the importance of delayed hypersensitivity in the formation of experimental thyroiditis in guinea pigs. They confirmed the correlation found by others between skin sensitivity and experimental thyroiditis. They also showed that the eventual regression of the thyroiditis was accompanied by a decrease in the skin reactivity, and that there was no correlation between delayed hypersensitivity and the circulating antibodies. They then attempted to use cell migration as an alternative indicator of delayed hypersensitivity, testing for leukocyte migration in the presence or absence of thyroglobulin or other antigen preparations. They found, however, that the delayed hypersensitivity demonstrated by skin reactivity to thyroglobulin did not show any connection with the inhibitory effect of thyroglobulin on the migration of the leukocytes. They felt this was a technical problem and that a better correlation might well have been obtained with the use of macrophage and monocyte cells in place of leukocytes. However, the titers of serum antibody correlated with the degree of leukocyte sensitivity, which suggested to them that the possible role of humoral antibody in cellular hypersensitivity *in vitro* should be re-examined. More recently, these authors have confirmed the observation that antibody, and more precisely, γ_2-globulin antibody, will inhibit the migration of leukocytes in the presence of its antigen in a different model system [14].

As we have seen from the above discussion, many indications accumulated in the published reports to suggest that delayed hypersensitivity was the causative mechanism in thyroiditis and in the manifestation of the typical lesion. The evidence that the humoral autoantibody was only some indication of the disease, a kind of by-product, and not a causative agent became increasingly convincing; therefore, there was no close correlation between its concentration and the severity of the disease. Other data, however, supported the other side of the argument, suggesting that the autoantibody itself was a causative factor in the formation of the lesions.

Some of the data in the literature have suggested serum antibodies as a possible trigger factor in the development of experimental thyroiditis. ROITT *et al.* [15], for example, reported that rats injected with rabbit anti-rat thyroid serum following pretreatment with Freund's adjuvant did develop thyroiditis. However, this process could not be repeated with autoantibody, and there was some doubt as to whether interpretations of the mechanism of autoimmune thyroiditis were admissible on the basis of experiments with heteroantibodies. Serum from humans with thyroiditis is cytotoxic to thyroid cells in culture. It was suggested that cytotoxic antibody produces injury in the thyroid gland as a second step, after the action of sensitized cells that produce initial cell-surface damage.

In more recent studies, MCMASTER and his colleagues [11] indicated the importance of two additional factors in the mechanism of production of experimental thyroiditis. These factors are the immunizing dose and the genetic constitution of the experimental animal. Although it had been appreciated in other work that the dose of antigen and also the dose of mycobacteria affected the frequency and severity of autoimmune disease in experimental animals, this study emphasized certain aspects of this relationship peculiar to autoimmune thyroiditis. Both the dose of thyroid antigen and the dose of tubercle bacilli in the immunizing emulsion were found to be important, and large amounts of both were necessary to produce severe disease. If the dose of either is decreased, the severity of the lesions, and ultimately the incidence of disease, is decreased. They also emphasized the importance of the genetic constitution of the experimental animal. They compared the results in two strains of animals, namely, Hartley strain and strain 13 guinea pigs. Thyroiditis was more frequent and more severe in Hartley strain than in the strain 13 animals in response to higher doses [11].

The same study also cast some doubt on the concept that had been developing for a number of years that delayed hypersensitivity was the mechanism to be correlated with the appearance of thyroiditis. The experiments showed that delayed hypersensitivity developed in animals given immunizing doses too small to produce disease. The authors also pointed out that in certain earlier studies, delayed hypersensitivity in a group of experimental animals gradually diminished until it was undetectable one year after immunization, even though the disease itself persisted throughout a second year [11]. Thus it is possible that an association between delayed hypersensitivity and thyroiditis is only found if the tissue damage results from more than one type of immune response factor.

In very recent studies the significance of circulating autoantibody has once more been emphasized after many years of neglect. NAKAMURA and WEIGLE [13, 25] have described the possible damage or changes produced in the thyroglobulin molecule by mixing it with the Freund's adjuvant components, and they have also studied the successful transfer of thyroiditis development achieved by serum transfer in some detail. In the former study, they concluded that the thyroglobulin antigen was not modified by emulsification with the tubercle bacilli or the mineral oil. They believed that some change was induced in the molecule more rapidly after injection, because of the attraction of certain enzyme-liberating cells which also lowered the pH. They felt that this acid environment promoted swifter modification of the thyroglobulin antigen [25].

The following five points summarize the major arguments against autoantibody as a causative agent that prevailed at least until 1969.

1. There is no significant correlation between the antibody titers and the severity of the lesions.

2. Passive transfer of serum from an animal with thyroiditis to a normal animal has consistently failed to produce lesions in the recipient.

3. The formation of autoantibody can be dissociated from the induction of tissue lesions. This has been done in the thyroiditis studies by the use of both alum adjuvants and Freund's complete adjuvant. It has also been accomplished in some cases by the use of incomplete Freund's adjuvant, as against complete Freund's adjuvant.

4. A close correlation has often been reported by the severity of lesions and the results of skin tests, *i.e.*, the phenomenon of delayed hypersensitivity.

5. Passive transfer of the disease has been produced by transfer of lymphoid cells. For example, MCMASTER and LERNER [9] transferred lymph node cells in histocompatible guinea pigs (strain 13) and succeeded in producing thyroiditis in 28% of the recipient animals.

Evidence in support of the opinion that the basic and important mechanism of tissue damage in thyroiditis and in most other autoimmune diseases was related to a phenomenon of delayed hypersensitivity continued to accumulate until very recently. However, even though all the above arguments appear to indicate strongly that serum antibodies are not the causative agent and that lymphoid cells and a mechanism of delayed hypersensitivity are the causative factors in the tissue damage, objections to each must be considered.

1. The antibody titer is a total of many classes and subclasses of immunoglobulins and these have different, possibly opposed, functions. Some of them may be protective, while others in the same antiserum are cytotoxic.
2. Perhaps the failure to transfer the disease by the transfer of serum in all previous studies has been due to faulty technics.
3. Autoantibodies can be formed without resultant lesions, but this does not nullify the possibility that they may still be involved in the formation of lesions.
4. Some of the studies reported indicate that the correlation between delayed hypersensitivity and lesion severity is no better than that between antibody titer and lesion severity.
5. Even though lymphoid cells have produced passive transfer of the disease, a higher success rate would be more convincing; 28% is not high.

NAKAMURA and WEIGLE [13] found that it was possible to transfer serum from immunized animals in such a way as to induce thyroiditis in approximately 50% of the recipient normal animals. Success proved to be dependent on three factors. It was necessary to use a group of serum samples taken in a sequence of bleedings and to transfer these to recipient animals with the same time schedules. Secondly, the donor animals had to have been thyroidectomized before immunization. The thyroidectomy presumably prevents the soaking-up of the significant autoantibody and consequent removal of it from the circulation. Thirdly, it was necessary to use early bleedings and not late bleedings. The most effective samples were those taken during the first two weeks after the first injection while those taken approximately two months after the injection had no effect.

GHAYASUDDIN and colleagues [20] described the sequence of formation of 19 S and 7 S autoantibodies to thyroglobulin in immunized rabbits in 1968. Very early bleedings taken from rabbits 7–14 days after the first injection contained 19 S antibody, although in low titer, along with a higher level of 7 S antibody. Late bleedings taken from rabbits about 53 to 75 days after the first injection also contained both 19 S and 7 S antibody, but the content of the 19 S form was extremely low in comparison to the other, implying that it was disappearing from the circulation. It was impossible to say definitively which class appeared first. They may well be produced at the same time but in variable proportions. Other functional aspects of these two classes of autoantibody need further exploration; the work of NAKAMURA and WEIGLE [13] suggests that these different immunoglobulin classes cause cell injury by completely different actions.

Very probably both mechanisms—autoantibody and delayed hypersensitivity—are involved in the induction of experimental thyroiditis. The studies on experimental aspermatogenesis discussed in Chapter 5 have already led to the conclusion that both are involved. RUDDLE and WAKSMAN [17–19] have investigated the mechanisms of production of tissue damage by delayed hypersensitivity.

A final point must be made on the significance of the autoantigenic determinant groups in the antigenic molecule. As has already been discussed in Chapter 2, only two, three, or four antigenic groups of the thyroglobulin molecule are autoantigenic, while there may be forty or fifty groups that are heteroantigenic. We must therefore extend our knowledge of the particular antigenic stimulus produced by these few groups before we can explain the mechanisms of autoimmune damage in any more detail.

References

Chapter 1. Concepts of Specificity

1. Abramoff, P., La Via, M. F.: Biology of the Immune Response. New York: McGraw-Hill 1970.
2. Arbesman, C. E., Langlois, C., Bronson, P., Shulman, S.: The allergic response to stinging insects. VII. Fractionation of whole body and venom sac extracts of yellow jacket. J. Allergy **38**, 1—8 (1966).
3. Arbesman, C. E., Langlois, C., Shulman, S.: The allergic response to stinging insects. IV. Cross-reactions between bee, wasp, and yellow jacket. J. Allergy **36**, 147—157 (1965).
4. Arquilla, E. R., Finn, J.: Insulin antibody variations in rabbits and guinea pigs and multiple antigenic determinants on insulin. J. Exp. Med. **118**, 55—71 (1963).
5. Arquilla, E. R., Finn, J.: Genetic differences in antibody production to determinant groups on insulin. Science **142**, 400—401 (1963).
6. Arquilla, E. R., Ooms, H., Mercola, K.: Immunological and biological properties of iodo-insulin labeled with one or less atoms of iodine per molecule. J. Clin. Invest. **47**, 474—487 (1968).
7. Beutner, E. H., Witebsky, E., Ricken, D., Adler, R. H.: Studies on autoantibodies in myasthenia gravis. J. Am. Med. Assoc. **182**, 46—58 (1962).
8. Bordet, J.: Sur l'agglutination et la dissolution des globules rouges par le sérum d'animaux injectés de sang défibriné. Ann. Inst. Pasteur **12**, 688—695 (1898).
9. Bordet, J.: Mécanisme de l'agglutination. Ann. Inst. Pasteur **13**, 225—250 (1899).
10. Boyd, W. C.: Fundamentals of Immunology, 4th ed. New York: John Wiley 1966.
11. Chance, R. E., Ellis, R. M., Bromer, W. W.: Porcine proinsulin: Characterization and amino acid sequence. Science **161**, 165—167 (1968).
12. Colombani, J., Milgrom, F.: Studies on leukocyte-specific antigens. Vox Sanguinis **10**, 429—438 (1965).
13. Coombs, R. R. A.: The mixed agglutination reactions in the study of normal and malignant cells. Cancer Res. **21**, 1198—1202 (1961).
14. Dameshek, W., Witebsky, E., Milgrom, F. (Eds.): Autoimmunity-Experimental and Clinical Aspects. Ann. N. Y. Acad. Sci. **124**, 1965.
15. Deckert, T.: Autoimmunological aspects of diabetes mellitus. Acta Med. Scand. Suppl. **476**, 20—41 (1967).
16. Djanian, A. Y., Beutner, E. H., Witebsky, E.: Tanned-cell hemagglutination test for detection of antibodies in sera of patients with myasthenia gravis. J. Lab. Clin. Med. **63**, 60—70 (1964).
17. Doerr, R.: Die Immunitätsforschung. Ergebnisse und Probleme in Einzeldarstellungen. Volume III: Die Antigene, p. 197—212. Wien: Springer 1948.
18. Fagraeus, A., Espmark, A.: Use of a 'mixed haemadsorption' method in virus-infected tissue cultures. Nature **190**, 370—371 (1961).
19. Fisch, C.: Studies on lactoserum and on other cell-sera. St. Louis Courier of Medicine **22**, 90—102 (1900).
20. Fleisher, M. S.: Relationship of various anti-organ sera. J. Immunol. **7**, 51—67 (1922).
21. Fleisher, M. S., Arnstein, N.: Specificity of anti-organ sera. J. Immunol. **6**, 223—234 (1921).
22. Fleisher, M. S., Hall, T. G., Arnstein, N.: Serological relationships of liver and kidney. J. Immunol. **5**, 437—453 (1920).
23. Glynn, L. E., Holborow, J.: Autoimmunity and Disease. Philadelphia: F. A. Davis 1965.

24. Goldstein, G., Hofman, W. W.: Electrophysiological changes similar to those of myasthenia gravis in rats with experimental autoimmune thymitis. J. Neurol. Neurosurg. Psychiat. **31**, 453—459 (1968).

25. Goldstein, G., Strauss, A. J. L., Pickeral, S.: Antigens in thymus and muscle effective in inducing experimental autoimmune thymitis and the release of thymin. Clin. Exp. Immunol. **4**, 3—16 (1969).

26. Goldstein, G., Whittingham, S.: Experimental autoimmune thymitis: An animal model of human myasthenia gravis. Lancet **1966 II**, 315—318.

27. Goldstein, G., Whittingham, S.: Histological and serological features of experimental autoimmune thymitis in guinea-pigs. Clin. Exp. Immunol. **2**, 257—268 (1967).

28. Halbert, S. P., Manski, W.: Organ specificity with special reference to the lens. Progr. Allergy **7**, 107—186 (1963).

29. Hale, W. L., Beutner, E. H.: Studies of the serological relation of myosin and actomyosin to antigens reactive with muscle antibodies in the sera of maystehnia gravis patients. Federation Proc. **24**, 693 (1965).

30. Hektoen, L., Fox, H., Schulhof, K.: Specificness in the precipitin reaction of thyroglobulin. J. Infect. Diseases **40**, 641—646 (1927).

31. Hektoen, L., Schulhof, K.: The precipitin reaction of thyroglobulin. Proc. Nat. Acad. Sci. **11**, 481—484 (1925).

32. Intorp, H. W., Milgrom, F.: Thermostable kidney antigen and its excretion into urine. J. Immunol. **100**, 1195—1203 (1968).

33. Irvine, W. J., Scarth, L., Clarke, B. F., Cullen, D. R., Duncan, L. J. P.: Thyroid and gastric autoimmunity in patients with diabetes mellitus. Lancet **1970 II**, 163—168.

34. Kalden, J. R., Williamson, W. G., Johnston, R. J., Irvine, W. J.: Studies on experimental autoimmune thymitis in guinea pigs. Clin. Exp. Immunol. **5**, 319—340 (1969).

35. Kerp, L., Kasemir, H., Kieling, F., Steinhilber, S.: Localization of antibody-binding sites on insulin molecules. Intern. Arch. Allergy Appl. Immunol. **36**, 143—151 (1969).

36. Landsteiner, K.: The Specificity of Serological Reactions p. 13—75. Cambridge/Mass.: Harvard University Press 1946.

37. Landsteiner, K., van der Scheer, J.: On the antigens of red blood corpuscles. II. Flocculation reactions with alcoholic extracts of erythrocytes. J. Exp. Med. **42**, 123—142 (1925).

38. Lang, R., Shulman, S.: Precipitation analysis of muscle antibodies in human serum. Federation Proc. **23**, 342 (1964).

39. Lang, R., Shulman, S., Beutner, E., Witebsky, E.: Precipitation of muscle extracts by myasthenia gravis serum. Ann. N. Y. Acad. Sci. **135**, 601—605 (1966).

40. Langlois, C., Shulman, S., Arbesman, C. E.: The allergic response to stinging insects. II. Immunologic studies of human sera from allergic individuals. J. Allergy **36**, 12—22 (1965).

41. Langlois, C., Shulman, S., Arbesman, C. E.: The allergic response to stinging insects. III. The specificity of venom sac antigens. J. Allergy **36**, 109—120 (1965).

42. Langlois, C., Shulman, S., Kozmycz, S., Arbesman, C. E.: The allergic response to stinging insects. VI. Fractionation of whole body and venom sac extracts of wasp. J. Allergy **37**, 359—365 (1966).

43. Manski, W., Halbert, S. P., Auerbach-Pascal, T., Javier, P.: On the use of antigenic relationships among species for the study of molecular evolution. I. The lens proteins of the agnatha and chondrichthyes. Intern. Arch. Allergy Appl. Immunol. **31**, 38—56 (1967).

44. Manski, W., Halbert, S. P., Javier, P.: On the use of antigenic relationships among species for the study of molecular evolution. II. The lens proteins of the choanichthyes and early actinopterygii. Intern. Arch. Allergy Appl. Immunol. **31**, 475—489 (1967).

45. Manski, W., Halbert, S. P., Javier, P., Auerbach-Pascal, T.: On the use of antigenic relationships among species for the study of molecular evolution. III. The lens proteins of the late actinopterygii. Intern. Arch. Allergy Appl. Immunol. **31**, 529—545 (1967).

46. Margoliash, E., Nisonoff, A., Reichlin, M.: Immunological activity of cytochrome c. I. Precipitating antibodies to monomeric vertebrate cytochromes c. J. Biol. Chem. **245**, 931—939 (1970).

47. Maurer, P. H.: The cross reactions between albumins of different species and gamma globulins of different species. J. Immunol. **72**, 119—122 (1954).

48. MELCHER, L. R., MASOUREDIS, S. P., REED, R.: The immunological relationship between human and bovine serum albumin. J. Immunol. **70**, 125—128 (1953).
49. METZGAR, R. S.: Human pancreas-specific isoantigens. Nature **203**, 660—661 (1964).
50. METZGAR, R. S.: Immunologic studies of pancreas-specific isoantigens. J. Immunol. **93**, 176—182 (1964).
51. MIESCHER, P. A., MÜLLER-EBERHARD, H. J. (Eds.): Textbook of Immunopathology. New York/London: Grune and Stratton; Vol. I, 1968; Vol. II, 1969.
52. MILGROM, F.: Autoimmunity in relation to transplantation. In: RAPAPORT, F. T., DAUSSET, J. (Eds.): p. 587—600. Human Transplantation, New York/London: Grune and Stratton 1968.
53. MILGROM, F.: Tissue specificity. In: ROSE, N. R., MILGROM, F. (Eds.): p. 270—278. International Convocation on Immunology, Buffalo, N. Y. 1968, Basel/New York: S. Karger 1969.
54. MILGROM, F., INTORP, H. W., WITEBSKY, E.: Studies on antigenic structure of bovine aortic intima. J. Immunol. **99**, 164—170 (1967).
55. MILGROM, F., KANO, K., BARRON, A. L., WITEBSKY, E.: Mixed agglutination in tissue culture. J. Immunol. **92**, 8—16 (1964).
56. MILGROM, F., TUGGAC, M., CAMPBELL, W. A., WITEBSKY, E.: Thermostable ethanol-insoluble antigens of brain. J. Immunol. **92**, 82—90 (1964).
57. MILGROM, F., TUGGAC, M., WITEBSKY, E.: Immunological studies on adrenal glands. III. Interspecies relations of thermostable adrenal-specific antigens. Immunology **6**, 105—118 (1963).
58. MILGROM, F., TUGGAC, Z. M., WITEBSKY, E.: Studies on species specificity. J. Immunol. **93**, 902—909 (1964).
59. MILGROM, F., TUGGAC, Z. M., WITEBSKY, E.: Organ-specific antigens of liver, testicle and pituitary. J. Immunol. **94**, 157—163 (1965).
60. MILGROM, F., WITEBSKY, E.: Immunological studies on adrenal glands. I. Immunization with adrenals of foreign species. Immunology **5**, 46—66 (1962).
61. MILGROM, F., WITEBSKY, E.: Autoantibodies and autoimmune diseases. J. Am. Med. Assoc. **181**, 706—716 (1962).
62. NAMBA, T., GROB, D.: Autoantibodies and myasthenia gravis, with special reference to muscle ribonucleoprotein, Ann. N. Y. Acad. Sci. **135**, 606—630 (1965).
63. NASTUK, W. L., PLESCIA, O. J., OSSERMAN, K. E.: Changes in serum complement activity in patients with myasthenia gravis. Proc. Soc. Exp. Biol. Med. **105**, 177—184 (1960).
64. NISONOFF, A., REICHLIN, M., MARGOLIASH, E.: Immunological activity of cytochrome c. II. Localization of a major antigenic determinant of human cytochrome c. J. Biol. Chem. **245**, 940—946 (1970).
65. NUTTALL, G. H. F.: Blood Immunity and Blood Relationship. Cambridge: The University Press 1904.
66. OPPENHEIM, T. J., GOLDSTEIN, G.: Enhanced thymic lymphocyte response to phytohemagglutinin in experimental autoimmune thymitis. Nature **222**, 192—193 (1969).
67. POPE, C. G.: The immunology of insulin. Advan. Immunol. **5**, 209—244 (1966).
68. RIFÉ, U.: Localization of thermostable, adrenal-specific antigen in subcellular fractions. Intern. Arch. Allergy Appl. Immunol. **32**, 366—372 (1967).
69. ROSE, N. R., METZGAR, R. S., WITEBSKY, E.: Studies on organ specificity. XI. Isoantigens of rabbit pancreas. J. Immunol. **85**, 575—587 (1960).
70. ROSE, N. R., WITEBSKY, E.: Studies on organ specificity. II. Serological interrelationships among thyroid extracts of various species. J. Immunol. **75**, 282—290 (1955).
71. SHULMAN, S.: Allergic responses to insects. Ann. Rev. Entomol. **12**, 323—346 (1967).
72. SHULMAN, S.: Insect allergy: Biochemical and immunological analyses of the allergens. Progr. Allergy **12**, 246—317 (1968).
73. SHULMAN, S., BIGELSEN, F., LANG, R., ARBESMAN, C.: The allergic response to stinging insects: Biochemical and immunologic studies on bee venom and other bee body preparations. J. Immunol. **96**, 29—38 (1966).
74. SHULMAN, S., LANG, R., BEUTNER, E., WITEBSKY, E.: Precipitation of autoantibody in serum from patients with myasthenia gravis. Immunology **10**, 289—303 (1966)
75. SHULMAN, S., LANGLOIS, C., ARBESMAN, C. E.: The allergic response to stinging insects. I. Preparation of extracts and their biochemical characterization. J. Allergy **35**, 446—463 (1964).

76. SHULMAN, S., LANGLOIS, C., MILLER, J. B., ARBESMAN, C. E.: The allergic response to stinging insects. V. Fractionation of whole body and venom sac extracts of bee. J. Allergy **37**, 350—358 (1966).

77. SHULMAN, S., MILGROM, F., WITEBSKY, E.: Immunological studies on adrenal glands. IV. Chemical studies on the bovine thermostable adrenal-specific antigen. Immunology **7**, 605—615 (1964).

78. SIMPSON, J. A.: Myasthenia gravis: a new hypothesis. Scot. Med. J. **5**, 419—486 (1960).

79. SNELL, F., SHULMAN, S., SPENCER, R. P., MOOS, C.: Biophysical Principles of Structure and Function. Reading, Mass.: Addison-Wesley 1965.

79a. SPRINGER, G. F.: Blood-group and Forssman antigenic determinants shared between microbes and mammalian cells. Progr. Allergy **15**, 9—77 (1971).

80. STRAUSS, A. J. L., SEEGAL, B. C., HSU, J. C. BURKHOLDER, P. M., NASTUK, W. L., OSSERMAN, K. E.: Immunofluorescence demonstration of a muscle binding, complement-fixing serum globulin fraction in myasthenia gravis. Proc. Soc. Exp. Biol. Med. **105**, 184—191 (1960).

81. STRAUSS, A. J. L., VAN DER GELD, H. W. R., SMITH, C. W., MCFARLIN, D. E., BARLOW, M.: 'Autoimmune' reactivities in serums of patients with thymomas unassociated with myasthenia gravis. Federation Proc. **24**, 693 (1965).

82. SURMACZYNSKA, B., METZ, R.: Hormonal and immunological properties of insulin fragments: I. The individual peptide chains. Endocrinology **85**, 368—372 (1969).

83. SURMACZYNSKA, B., METZ, R., BARRETT, R., LUCENA, G.: Hormonal and immunological properties of insulin fragments: II. Products obtained by enzymatic hydrolysis. Endocrinology **85**, 577—581 (1969).

84. UHLENHUTH, P.: Zur Lehre von der Unterscheidung verschiedener Eiweißarten mit Hilfe spezifischer Sera. In: Festschrift zum Sechzigsten Geburtstag von Robert Koch, pp. 49—74. Jena: Gustav Fischer 1903.

85. UHLENHUTH, P.: Ein Verfahren zur biologischen Unterscheidung von Blut verwandter Tiere. Deut. Med. Wochschr. **31**, 1673—1676 (1905).

86. UHLENHUTH, P., SEIFFERT, W.: Die biologische Eiweißdifferenzierung mittels der Präcipitation mit besonderer Berücksichtigung der Technik. In: Handbuch der pathogenen Mikroorganismen, pp. 365—468. Berlin/Wien: Urban and Schwarzenberg 1930.

87. VAN DER GELD, H., OOSTERHUIS, H. J. G. H.: Muscle and thymus antibodies in myasthenia gravis. Vox Sanguinis **8**, 196—204 (1963).

88. VARANDANI, P. T.: Studies on the nature of antigenicity of A- and B-chains of bovine insulin. Biochemistry **6**, 100—104 (1967).

89. WASSERMANN, A., SCHÜTZE, A.: Über eine neue forensische Methode zur Unterscheidung von Menschen- und Thierblut. Berl. Klin. Wochschr. **38**, 187—190 (1901).

90. WEIL, A. J., WILSON, L., FINKLER, A. E.: Immunological test for semen on female genitalia as evidence of intercourse. J. Forensic Sci. **4**, 372—377 (1959).

91. WHITE, R. G., MARSHALL, A. H. E.: The autoimmune response in myasthenia gravis. Lancet **1962 I**, 120—123.

92. WHITTINGHAM, S., MATHEWS, J. D., MACKAY, I. R., STOCKS, A. E., UNGAR, B., MARTIN, F. I. R.: Diabetes mellitus, autoimmunity and ageing. Lancet **1971 I**, 763—767.

93. WIENER, A. S., GORDON, E. B.: Examination of blood stains in forensic medicine. J. Forensic Sci. **3**, 89—102 (1956).

94. WITEBSKY, E.: Die serologische Analyse von Zellen und Geweben. Naturwissenschaften **17**, 771—776 (1929).

95. WITEBSKY, E., BEHRENS, H. O.: Die serologische Differenzierung zwischen Vorderlappen und Hinterlappen der Hypophyse. Z. Immunitätsforsch. **73**, 415—428 (1932).

96. WITEBSKY, E., KLINKE, J.: Die serologische Spezifität des Nebennierenmarks. Z. Immunitätsforsch. **78**, 509—523 (1933).

97. WITEBSKY, E., KOMIYA, K.: Über Leukozyten-Antikörper. Z. Immunitätsforsch. **67**, 480—496 (1930).

98. WITEBSKY, E., MILGROM, F.: Immunological studies on adrenal glands. II. Immunization with adrenals of the same species. Immunology **5**, 67—78 (1962).

99. WITEBSKY, E., ROSE, N. R., NADEL, H.: Studies on organ specificity. X. The serologic specificity of pancreas extracts. J. Immunol. **85**, 568—574 (1960).

100. WITEBSKY, E., ROSE, N. R., SHULMAN, S.: Studies of normal and malignant tissue antigens. Cancer Res. **16**, 831—841 (1956).
101. WITEBSKY, E. STEINFELD, J.: Untersuchungen über spezifische Antigenfunktionen von Organen. I. Mitteilung. Z. Immunitätsforsch. **58**, 271—296 (1928).
102. WITEBSKY, E., ZEISSIG, A.: Zur serologischen Analyse der Schleimhaut des Intestinaltraktus. Z. Immunitätsforsch. **76**, 266—284 (1932).
103. WOLSTENHOLME, G. E. W., CAMERON, M. P. (Eds.): Immunoassay of Hormones. Ciba Foundation Colloquia on Endocrinology, Vol. XIV. Boston: Little, Brown 1962.
104. YAGI, Y., MAIER, P., PRESSMAN, D.: Antibodies against the component polypeptide chains of bovine insulin. Science **147**, 617—619 (1965).

Chapter 2. The Thyroid Gland

1. ADANT, M., SPEHL, P.: La spécificité immunologique des thyroglobulines. Compt. Rend. Soc. Biol. **117**, 230—233 (1934).
2. ALOJ, S., SALVATORE, G., ROCHE, J.: Isolation and properties of a native subunit of lamprey thyroglobulin. J. Biol. Chem. **242**, 3810—3814 (1967).
3. ANDRADA, J. A., ROSE, N. R., KITE, J. H., jr.: Experimental thyroiditis in the rhesus monkey. IV. The role of thyroglobulin and cellular antigens. Clin. Exp. Immunol. **3**, 133—151 (1968).
4. ASSEM, E. S. K., TROTTER, W. R., BELYAVIN, G.: The heterogeneity of human thyroglobulin. Biochim. Biophys. Acta **100**, 163—178 (1965).
5. BALFOUR, B. M., DONIACH, D., ROITT, I. M., COUCHMAN, K. G.: Fluorescent antibody studies in human thyroiditis: Autoantibodies to an antigen of the thyroid colloid distinct from thyroglobulin. Brit. J. Exp. Pathol. **42**, 307—316 (1961).
6. BECKERS, C., DE VISSCHER, M.: Thyroid proteins in endemic goiter. Metabolism **10**, 695—706 (1961).
7. BECKERS, C., DE VISSCHER, M.: Thyroid proteins in sporadic non-toxic goiter. J. Clin Endocrinol. Metab **23**, 149—155 (1963).
8. BEUTNER, E. H., WITEBSKY, E.: Studies on organ specificity. XIV. Immunofluorescent studies of thyroid reactive autoantibodies in human sera. J. Immunol. **88**, 462—475 (1963).
9. BLOTH, B., BERGQUIST, R.: The ultrastructure of human thyroglobulin. J. Exp. Med. **128**, 1129—1136 (1968).
10. BOUCHILLOUX, S., ROLLAND, M., TORRESANI, J., ROQUES, M., LISSITZKY, S.: Microhétérogénéité de la thyroglobuline. Purification par chromatographie sur diéthylaminoéthyl cellulose et interprétation. Biochim. Biophys. Acta **93**, 15—30 (1964).
11. CHEFTEL, C., BOUCHILLOUX, S., LISSITZKY, S.: Glyco-peptides issus de la thyroglobuline. Compt. Rend. Acad. Sci. Paris **259**, 1458—1460 (1964).
12. CHENG, H. F., PETERSON, R. E., EVANS, T. C.: Preparation of highly purified human thyroglobulin, Biochim. Biophys. Acta **168**, 161—164 (1968).
13. COLE, R. K., KITE, J. H., jr., WITEBSKY, E.: Hereditary autoimmune thyroiditis in the fowl. Science **160**, 1357—1358 (1968).
14. DE CROMBRUGGHE, B., EDELHOCH, H.: The properties of thyroglobulin. XIV. The structure of reoxidized thyroglobulin. Biochemistry **5**, 2238—2245 (1966).
15. DE CROMBRUGGHE, B., PITT-RIVERS, R., EDELHOCH, H.: The properties of thyroglobulin. XI. The reduction of the disulfide bonds. J. Biol. Chem. **241**, 2766—2773 (1966).
16. DEGROOT, L. J., CARVALHO, E.: Studies on proteins of normal and diseased thyroid glands. J. Clin. Endocrinol. Metab. **20**, 21—34 (1960).
17. DEGROOT, L. J., CARVALHO, E.: Iodide binding in thyroid cellular fractions. J. Biol. Chem. **235**, 1390—1397 (1960).
18. DEGROOT, L. J., STANBURY, J. B.: The syndrome of congenital goiter with butanol-insoluble serum iodine. Am. J. Med. **27**, 586—595 (1959).
19. DERRIEN, Y., MICHEL, R., PEDERSEN, K. O., ROCHE, J.: Recherches sur la préparation et sur les propriétés de la thyroglobuline pure. II. Biochim. Biophys. Acta **3**, 436—441 (1949).
20. DERRIEN, Y., MICHEL, R., ROCHE, J.: Recherches sur la préparation et les propriétés de la thyroglobuline pure. I. Biochim. Biophys. Acta **2**, 454—470 (1948).

21. DOEBBLER, T. K., ROSE, N. R.: Experimental thyroiditis in the rhesus monkey. II. Precipitating, haemagglutinating and anaphylactogenic antibodies. Clin. Exp. Immunol. **1**, 159—169 (1966).
22. DOWLING, T. J., INGBAR, S. H., FREINKEL, N.: Abnormal iodoproteins in the blood of eumetabolic goitrous adults. J. Clin. Endocrinol. Metab. **21**, 1390—1401 (1961).
23. EDELHOCH, H.: The properties of thyroglobulin. I. The effects of alkali. J. Biol. Chem. **235**, 1326—1334 (1960).
24. EDELHOCH, H.: I. Recent advances in thyroid chemistry and physiology. The structure of thyroglobulin and its role in iodination. In: Recent Progress in Hormone Research, Vol. 21 (PINCUS, G., Ed.), p. 1—31. New York: Academic Press 1965.
25. EDELHOCH, H., CARLOMAGNO, M. S., SALVATORE, G.: Iodine and the structure of thyroglobulin. Arch. Biochem. Biophys. **134**, 264—265 (1969).
26. EDELHOCH, H., DE CROMBRUGGHE, B.: The properties of thyroglobulin. XIII. The structure of reduced alkylated thyroglobulin. J. Biol. Chem. **241**, 4357—4365 (1966).
27. EDELHOCH, H., METZGER, H.: The properties of thyroglobulin. V. The properties of denatured thyroglobulin. J. Am. Chem. Soc. **83**, 1428—1435 (1961).
28. EDELHOCH, H., RALL, J. E.: The proteins and enzymes of the thyroid. In: The Thyroid Gland, Vol. 1 (PITT-RIVERS, R., TROTTER, W. R., Eds.), p. 113—130. London: Butterworths 1964.
29. EDELHOCH, H., STEINER, R. F.: Properties of thyroglobulin. XII. Comparison of the configurational states of reduced and unreduced thyroglobulin. Biopolymers **4**, 999—1014 (1966).
30. FALCONER, I. R., ROITT, I. M., SEAMARK, R. F., TORRIGIANI, G.: Studies of the congenitally goitrous sheep. Iodoproteins of the goitre. Biochem. J. **117**, 417—424 (1970).
31. FLANAGAN, T. D., BARRON, A. L., BEUTNER, E. H., WITEBSKY, E.: Retention of histologic characteristics and antigens in organ cultures of rhesus thyroid. J. Immunol. **97**, 539—545 (1966).
32. FURTH, E. D., AGRAWAL, R. B., PROPP, R. P.: Secretion of iodoalbumin and iodoprealbumin by a congenital goiter containing thyroglobulin and the iodoalbumins. J. Clin. Endocrinol. Metab. **31**, 60—69 (1970).
33. GHAYASUDDIN, M., SHULMAN, S.: Immunochemical studies on fragments of thyroglobulin. Abstracts, Seventh International Congress of Biochemistry, Tokyo 1967, p. 1024.
34. GHAYASUDDIN, M., SHULMAN, S.: Molecular forms of immunologlobulins in experimental autoimmune thyroiditis in rabbits. Federation Proc. **26**, 340 (1967).
35. GHAYASUDDIN, M., SHULMAN, S.: Antigenic fragments of rabbit thyroglobulin. Federation Proc. **27**, 275 (1968).
36. GHAYASUDDIN, M., SHULMAN, S.: Studies on thyroid proteins. VII. Immunochemical properties of some enzymatic fragments of rabbit thyroglobulin. Immunology **19**, 225—237 (1970).
37. GOODMAN, H. C., EXUM, D. E., ROBBINS, J.: Radioimmunoelectrophoresis of thyroid antigens and anti-thyroglobulin antibodies in clinical and experimental thyroiditis. J. Immunol. **92**, 843—853 (1964).
38. GOURLAY, F.: The proteids of the thyroid and the spleen. J. Physiol. (London) **16**, 23—33 (1894).
39. HEIDELBERGER, M., PALMER, W. W.: The preparation and properties of thyroglobulin. J. Biol. Chem. **101**, 433—439 (1933).
40. HEIDELBERGER, M., PEDERSEN, K. O.: The molecular weight and isoelectric point of thyroglobulin. J. Gen. Physiol. **19**, 95—108 (1935).
41. HEKTOEN, L., FOX, H., SCHULHOF, K.: Specificness in the precipitin reaction of thyroglobulin. J. Infect. Diseases **40**, 641—646 (1927).
42. HEKTOEN, L., SCHULHOF, K.: The precipitin reaction of thyroglobulin. J. Am. Med. Assoc. **80**, 386—387 (1923).
43. HJORT, T.: The occurrence of antibody against 'second colloid antigen' (CA-2 antibody) in patients with and without thyroid disease. Acta Med. Scand. **174**, 147—154 (1963).
44. HOLBOROW, E. J., BROWN, P. C., ROITT, I. M., DONIACH, D.: Cytoplasmic localization of complement-fixation autoantigens in human thyroid epithelium. Brit. J. Exp. Pathol. **40**, 583—588 (1959).
45. HUTCHISON, R.: The chemistry of the thyroid gland and the nature of its active constituent. J. Physiol. (London) **20**, 474—496 (1896).
46. INGBAR, S. H., ASKONAS, B. A., WORK, T. S.: Observations concerning the heterogeneity of bovine thyroglobulin. Endocrinology **64**, 110—122 (1959).

47. IRVINE, W. J.: Thyroid auto-immunity as a disorder of immunological tolerance. Quart. J. Exp. Physiol. **49**, 324—337 (1964).
48. IRVINE, W. J.: Automated determinations of thyroid and gastric complement-fixing antibody; comparison with the fluorescent antibody and manual complement-fixation methods. Clin. Exp. Immunol. **1**, 341—354 (1966).
49. JAKOBY, W. B., LABAW, L., EDELHOCH, H., PASTAN, I., RALL, J. E.: Thyroglobulin: Evidence for crystallization and association. Science **153**, 1671—1672 (1966).
50. JONCKHEER, M. H.: Présence d'une albumine comme constituant normal des protéines thyroïdiennes. Ann. Endocrinol. **24**, 756—760 (1963).
51. JONCKHEER, M. H., HAELST, L. V., OTTEN, J.: Studies on thyralbumin. Excerpta Medica No. 157, Third International Congress of Endocrinology (1968).
52. JONCKHEER, M. H., KARCHER, D. M.: Thyroid albumin. I. Isolation and characterization. J. Clin. Endocrinol. Metab. **32**, 7—17 (1971).
53. KITE, J. H., jr., ARGUE, H., ROSE, N. R.: Experimental thyroiditis in the rhesus monkey. I. Cytotoxic, mixed-agglutinating and complement-fixing antibodies. Clin. Exp. Immunol. **1**, 139—157 (1966).
54. KIVIKANGAS, V., LAMBERG, B. A. MÄENPÄÄ, J.: Thyroidal iodine and proteins in autoimmune thyroiditis. Scand. J. Clin. Lab. Invest. **25**, 263—268 (1970).
55. KOFFLER, D., FRIEDMAN, A. H.: Localization of immunoglobulins in chronic thyroiditis. Lab. Invest. **13**, 239—245 (1964).
56. KOFFLER, D., PARONETTO, F.: Complement-fixing antibody to colloid and epithelium in monkey thyroiditis. Nature **207**, 773—774 (1965).
57. KOFFLER, D., PARONETTO, F.: Serologic and immunofluorescent studies of humoral antibody and γ-globulin localization in experimental autoimmune thyroiditis. J. Immunol. **94**, 329—336 (1965).
58. KORNGOLD, L., VAN LEEUWEN, G., BRENER, J. L.: The determination of the molecular weight of different autoprecipitins in Hashimoto's disease by a new immunologic method. J. Lab. Clin. Med. **53**, 517—524 (1959).
59. LISSITZKY, S., BISMUTH, J., CODACCIONI, J.-L., CARTOUZOU, G.: Congenital goiter with iodoalbumin replacing thyroglobulin and defect of deiodination of iodotyrosines. Serum origin of the thyroid iodoalbumin. J. Clin. Endocrinol. Metab. **28**, 1797—1806 (1968).
60. LISSITZKY, S., CODACCIONI, J.-L., BISMUTH, J., DEPIEDS, R.: Congenital goiter with hypothyroidism and iodo-serum albumin replacing thyroglobulin. J. Clin. Endocrinol. Metab. **27**, 185—196 (1967).
61. LISSITZKY, S., CODACCIONI, J.-L., CARTOUZOU, G., MANTE, S.: Eumetabolic goitrous adult with iodoprealbumin in thyroid tissue and blood. J. Clin. Endocrinol. Metab. **24**, 305—312 (1964).
62. LISSITZKY, S., ROLLAND, M., BERGOT, J.: Données sur la structure de la thyroglobuline de mouton. Biochim. Biophys. Acta **111**, 543—546 (1965).
63. LISSITZKY, S., ROLLAND, M., REYNAUD, J., SAVARY, J., LASRY, S.: Structure sous-unitaire de la thyroglobuline de mouton. European J. Biochem. **4**, 464—471 (1968).
64. LOBO, L. C. G., FRIDMAN, J., REBELLO, M. A., HARGREAVES, F., FIGUEREDO, J. G.: Studies on the thyroidal proteins. Metabolism **15**, 330—337 (1966).
65. LUNDGREN, H. P., WILLIAMS, J. W.: Ultracentrifugal analysis and stability in protein systems. J. Phys. Chem. **43**, 989—1002 (1939).
65a. MANGKORNKANOK, M., MARKOWITZ, A. S., BATTIFORA, H. A.: Chronic thyroiditis in the rabbit induced with homologous thyroid microsomes. Science **178**, 316—318 (1972).
66. MATES, G. P., SHULMAN, S.: Studies on thyroid proteins. III. Precipitating activity of autoimmune and heteroimmune antisera with human thyroglobulin. Immunochemistry **4**, 319—330 (1967).
67. MATES, G. P., SHULMAN, S.: Studies on thyroid proteins. IV. Hemagglutinating activity of molecular fragments of human thyroid proteins. Immunology **14**, 89—98 (1967).
68. MATES, G. P., SHULMAN, S.: Studies on thyroid proteins. V. Immunochemical heterogeneity of human thyroglobulin. Immunochemistry **4**, 475—483 (1967).
69. MATES, G. P., SHULMAN, S.: Studies on thyroid proteins. VI. Immunochemical studies on the 4S and 7S tissue-specific thyroid proteins. Immunochemistry **6**, 35—42 (1969).
70. MCMASTER, P. R. B.: Auto-antibodies and autosensitivity. N. Y. State J. Med. **58**, 2980—2986 (1958).

71. McQuillan, M. T., Trikojus, V. M.: Thyroglobulin. In: Glycoproteins (Gottschalk, A., Ed.), p. 516—531. Amsterdam: Elsevier Publ. 1966.

72. Metzger, H., Sharp, C. C., Edelhoch, H.: The properties of thyroglobulin. VII. The immunologic activity of thyroglobulin fragments. Biochemistry **1**, 205—214 (1962).

73. Miescher, P., Gorstein, F., Benacerraf, B., Gell, P. G.: Studies on the pathogenesis of experimental immune thyroiditis. Proc. Soc. Exp. Biol. Med. **107**, 12—16 (1961).

74. Mouriz, J., Stanbury, J. B.: Purification of human 19S thyroglobulin by gel filtration. Can. J. Biochem. Physiol. **46**, 51—54 (1967).

75. Nakamura, R. M., Weigle, W. O.: In vivo behavior of homologous and heterologous thyroglobulin and induction of immunologic unresponsiveness to heterologous thyroglobulin. J. Immunol. **98**, 653—662 (1967).

76. Narasimha Murthy, P. V., Raghupathy, E., Abraham, S., Chaikoff, I. L.: Isolation and characterization of a glycopeptide from sheep thyroglobulin. Biochem. Biophys. Res. Commun. **14**, 514—522 (1964).

77. Narasimha Murthy, P. V., Raghupathy, E., Chaikoff, I. L.: Studies on thyroid proteins. I. Isolation and properties of a glycopeptide from sheep thyroglobulin. Biochemistry **4**, 611—618 (1965).

78. Nissley, P., Cittanova, N., Edelhoch, E.: The properties of thyroglobulin. XVIII. Isolation of thyroglobulin subunits. Biochemistry **8**, 443—448 (1969).

79. Nunez, J., Mauchamp, J., Pommier, J., Cirković, T., Roche, J.: Relationship between iodination and conformation of thyroglobulin. Biochem. Biophys. Res. Commun. **23**, 761—768 (1966).

80. O'Donnell, I. J., Baldwin, R. L., Williams, J. W.: Correlation of the N$\rightleftharpoons\alpha$ reaction of thyroglobulin with the type of breakdown produced by papain. Biochim. Biophys. Acta **28**, 295—308 (1958).

81. Oswald, A.: Die Eiweißkörper der Schilddrüse. Hoppe-Seylers Z. Physiol. Chem. **27**, 14—49 (1899).

82. Otten, J., Jonckheer, M., Dumont, J. E.: Thyroid albumin. II. In vitro synthesis of a thyroid albumin by normal human thyroid tissue. J. Clin. Endocrinol. Metab. **32**, 18—26 (1971).

83. Owen, C. A., jr.: A review of 'auto-immunization' in Hashimoto's disease. J. Clin. Endocrinol. Metab. **18**, 1015—1023 (1958).

84. Owen, S. G., Smart, G. A.: Thyroid antibodies in myxoedema. Lancet **1958 II**, 1034—1036.

85. Paseyro, P., Negrin, E., Morató-Manaro, J., Grosso, O. F.: Antithyroid antibodies: Their utilization in the investigation of antigenic thyroid substances in material obtained by cytologic aspiration. J. Clin. Endocrinol. Metab. **23**, 387—390 (1962).

86. Perelmutter, L., Devlin, W., Stephenson, N. R.: The purification of beef thyroglobulin with the use of gel filtration. Can. J. Biochem. Physiol. **41**, 2493—2500 (1963).

87. Perelmutter, L., Stephenson, N. R.: Immunochemical properties of thyroid proteins. Can. J. Biochem. Physiol. **42**, 1169—1176 (1964).

88. Pierce, J. G., Rawitch, A. B., Brown, D. M., Stanley, P. G.: Human thyroglobulin: Studies on the native and S-carboxymethylated protein. Biochim. Biophys. Acta **111**, 247—257 (1965).

89. Pinchera, A., Liberti, P., Martino, E., Fenzi, G. F., Grasso, L., Rovis, L., Baschieri, L., Doria, G.: Effects of antithyroid therapy on the long-acting thyroid stimulator and the antithyroglobulin antibodies. J. Clin. Endocrinol. Metab. **29**, 231—238 (1969).

90. Pitt-Rivers, R.: Heterogeneity of rat thyroglobulin labelled with ^{131}I in vivo. Biochem. J. **87**, 340—343 (1963).

91. Pitt-Rivers, R., Schwartz, H. L.: The thiol groups of thyroglobulin. Biochem. J. **105**, 28c—29c (1967).

92. Porter, D. D., Fennell, R. H., jr.: Serologic and immunohistochemical study of human and experimental thyroiditis. New Engl. J. Med. **265**, 830—834 (1961).

93. Pressman, D., James, A. W., Yagi, Y., Hiramoto, R., Woernley, D., Maxwell, W. T.: Rapidly sedimenting properties of specifically precipitating component of a Hashimoto's disease serum. Proc. Soc. Exp. Biol. Med. **96**, 773—777 (1957).

94. Ramagopal, E., Spiro, M. J., Stanbury, J. B.: Some properties of the soluble iodoproteins from normal and certain abnormal thyroid glands. J. Clin. Endocrinol. Metab. **25**, 742—752 (1965).

95. Rawstron, J. R., Farthing, C. P.: A comparison of tests for thyroglobulin antibody. J. Clin. Pathol. **15**, 153—155 (1962).

96. Robbins, J.: Thyroglobulin fractionation on diethylaminoethyl-cellulose columns. J. Biol. Chem. **238**, 182—188 (1963).

97. Robbins, J., Salvatore, G., Vecchio, G., Ui, N.: Thyroglobulin and 27-S iodoprotein. Iodination and ultracentrifugal heterogeneity. Biochim. Biophys. Acta **127**, 101—111 (1966).

98. Robbins, J., Rall, J. E.: Proteins associated with the thyroid hormones. Physiol. Rev. **40**, 415—489 (1962).

99. Robbins, J., Van Zyl, A., Van Der Walt, K.: Abnormal thyroglobulin in congenital goiter of cattle. Endocrinology **78**, 1213—1223 (1966).

100. Robbins, J., Wolff, J., Rall, J. E.: Iodoproteins in thyroid tissue and blood of rats with a transplantable thyroid tumor. Endocrinology **64**, 12—36 (1959).

101. Robbins, J., Wolff, J., Rall, J. E.: Iodoproteins in normal and abnormal human thyroid tissue and in normal sheep thyroid. Endocrinology **64**, 37—52 (1959).

102. Roche, J., Nunez, J., Gruson, M.: Sur l'hétérogénéité de la thyroglobuline. Compt. Rend. Soc. Biol. **154**, 2194—2201 (1960).

103. Roche, J., Salvatore, G., Sena, L., Aloj, S., Covelli, I.: Thyroid iodoproteins in vertebrates: Ultracentrifugal pattern and iodination rate. Comp. Biochem. Physiol. **27**, 67—82 (1968).

104. Roitt, I. M., Campbell, P. N., Doniach, D.: The nature of the thyroid auto-antibodies present in patients with Hashimoto's thyroiditis (lymphadenoid goitre). Biochem. J. **69**, 248—256 (1958).

105. Roitt, I. M., Doniach, D.: Human auto-immune thyroiditis: Serological studies. Lancet **1958 II**, 1027—1033.

106. Roitt, I. M., Doniach, D.: Thyroid auto-immunity. Brit. Med. Bull. **16**, 152—158 (1960).

107. Roitt, I. M., Doniach, D., Campbell, P. N., Hudson, R. V.: Autoantibodies in Hashimoto's disease (lymphadenoid goitre). Lancet **1956 II**, 820—821.

108. Roitt, I. M., Doniach, D., Wilson, E. G., Couchman, K.: Biochemical studies of thyroid auto-antigens. Bull. Soc. Chim. Biol. **42**, 1165—1170 (1960).

109. Roitt, I. M., Jones, H. E. H., Mills, G. L.: The activity of different fractions of homologous thyroid extract in the production of allergic thyroiditis in the rat. Immunology **9**, 281—286 (1965).

110. Roitt, I. M., Torrigiani, G., Doniach, D.: Immunochemical studies on the thyroglobulin autoantibody system in human thyroiditis. Immunology **15**, 681—696 (1968).

111. Rolland, M., Bismuth, J., Fondarai, J., Lissitzky, S.: Composition en acides aminés de la thyroglobuline de differentes espèces animales. Acta Endocrinol. **53**, 286—296 (1966).

112. Rolland, M., Lissitzky, S.: Succinylation of thyroglobulin. Relation between dissociation into subunit and iodine content. Biochim. Biophys. Acta **214**, 282—289 (1970).

113. Rose, N. R., Metzgar, R. S., Isaacs, E.: Studies on organ specificity. VIII. Serologic interrelationships among thyroid extracts of various species revealed by gel-diffusion precipitation techniques. J. Immunol. **84**, 649—658 (1960).

114. Rose, N. R., Shulman, S., Witebsky, E.: Studies on organ specificity. XIII. Immunological analysis of thyroglobulin and thyralbumin. J. Immunol. **88**, 229—239 (1962).

115. Rose, N. R., Skelton, F. R., Kite, J. H., jr., Witebsky, E.: Experimental thyroiditis in the rhesus monkey. III. Course of the disease. Clin. Exp. Immunol. **1**, 171—188 (1966).

116. Rose, N. R., Stylos, W. A.: Splitting of human thyroglobulin. I. Reduction and alkylation. Clin. Exp. Immunol. **5**, 129—140 (1969).

117. Rose, N. R., Witebsky, E.: Studies on organ specificity. II. Serological interrelationships among thyroid extracts of various species. J. Immunol. **75**, 282—290 (1955).

118. Rose, N. R., Witebsky, E.: Experimental autoimmune thyroiditis. In: Textbook of Immunopathology. Vol. I (Mischer, P. A., Müller-Eberhard, H. J., Eds.), p. 150—163. New York/London: Grune and Stratton 1968.

119. Rose, N. R., Witebsky, E., Beierwaltes, W. H.: Thyroiditis, In: Immunological Diseases (Samter, M., Alexander, H. L., Eds.), p. 821—842. Boston: Little, Brown 1965.

119a. Salabè, G. B., Davoli, C., Fontana, S.: The immunoreaction of auto and heteroantisera with modified human thyroglobulin. Intern. Arch. Allergy Appl. Immunol. **44**, 181—196 (1973).

119b. SALABÈ, G. B., FONTANA, S., ANDREOLI, M.: Radioimmunoassay for human antithyroglobulin antibodies. I. The relationship between tanned cell haemagglutination and a double antibody technique. Hormones **3**, 1—13 (1972).

120. SALVATORE, G., ALOJ, S., SALVATORE, M., EDELHOCH, H.: Hybridization of half molecules of guinea pig thyroglobulin. J. Biol. Chem. **242**, 5002—5007 (1967).

121. SALVATORE, G., SALVATORE, M., CAHNMANN, H. J., ROBBINS, J.: Separation of thyroidal iodoproteins and purification of thyroglobulin by gel filtration and density gradient centrifugation, J. Biol. Chem. **239**, 3267—3274 (1964).

122. SALVATORE, G., VECCHIO, G., SALVATORE, M., CAHNMANN, H. J., ROBBINS, J.: 27S thyroid iodoproteins. J. Biol. Chem. **240**, 2935—2943 (1965).

123. SHULMAN, S.: Preparation of hog thyroglobulin. Federation Proc. **15**, 613 (1956).

124. SHULMAN, S.: The Modeling of Biomolecular Structures. Cambridge, Massachusetts: The Ealing Press 1963.

125. SHULMAN, S.: Immunochemical and biochemical studies on thyroglobulin and other thyroid proteins. Gunma Symposia on Endocrinology **5**, 117—134 (1968).

126. SHULMAN, S.: Tissue specificity and autosensitization: The thyroid model. In: International Convocation on Immunology, Buffalo, N. Y. 1968 (ROSE, N. R., MILGROM, F., Eds.), p. 313—322. Basel: S. Karger 1969.

127. SHULMAN, S.: The thyralbumins: A 4S, iodinated, thyroid protein fraction. In preparation.

128. SHULMAN, S.: Thyroid antigens and autoimmunity. In: Advances in Immunology, Vol. 14 (DIXON, F. J., KUNKEL, H. G., Eds.), p. 85—185. New York: Academic Press 1971.

129. SHULMAN, S., ARMENIA, J. P.: Studies on thyroid proteins. I. The components of hog thyroid tissue, and the preparation of purified thyroglobulin, by column chromatography. J. Biol. Chem. **238**, 2723—2731 (1963).

130. SHULMAN, S., GHAYASUDDIN, M., WITEBSKY, E.: Studies on organ specificity. XX. Molecular forms in the antibody response to isoimmunization with thyroid proteins. J. Immunol. **101**, 1059—1067 (1968).

131. SHULMAN, S., MATES, G., BRONSON, P.: Studies on thyroid proteins. II. Purification of human thyroid proteins by gel filtration. Biochim. Biophys. Acta **147**, 208—221 (1967).

132. SHULMAN, S., ROSE, N. R., WITEBSKY, E.: Studies on organ specificity. III. Ultracentrifugal and elektrophoretic examinations of thyroid extracts. J. Immunol. **75**, 291— 300 (1955).

133. SHULMAN, S., ROSE, N. R., WITEBSKY, E.: Thyralbumin-a new antigen from thyroid tissue. Federation Proc. **16**, 433 (1957).

134. SHULMAN, S., STANLEY, P.: Preparation of pure proteins from hog thyroid glands by column chromatography. Australian J. Biol. Sci. **14**, 475—484 (1961).

135. SHULMAN, S., WITEBSKY, E.: Studies on organ specificity. IX. Biophysical and immunochemical studies on human thyroid autoantibody. J. Immunol. **85**, 559—567 (1960).

136. SHULMAN, S., WITEBSKY, E.: The thyroid gland as source and target in autosensitization. Ann. N. Y. Acad. Sci. **86**, 400—416 (1960).

137. SHULMAN, S., WITEBSKY, E.: Studies on organ specificity. XII. Fractionation of hog thyroid, preparation of thyroglobulin and thyralbumin, J. Immunol. **88**, 221—228 (1962)

138. SMITH, D. J., Biochemical and immunological studies on human thyroglobulin and 27 S thyroidiodoprotein. Ph. D. Thesis, New York Medical College 1972.

139. SMITH, D. J., SHULMAN, S.: Succinylation of normal and goitrous human thyroglobulin. Federation Proc. **30**, 1320 (1971).

140. SNELL, F. M. SHULMAN, S., SPENCER, R. P., MOOS, C.: Biophysical Principles of Structure and Function. Reading, Massachusetts: Addison-Wesley 1965.

141. SPIRO, R. G.: Glycoproteins: Structure, metabolism and biology. New Engl. J. Med. **269**, 566—573 (1963).

142. SPIRO, R. G.: The carbohydrate units of thyroglobulin. J. Biol. Chem. **240**, 1603—1610 (1965).

143. SPIRO, M. J.: Studies on the protein portion of thyroglobulin. Amino acid compositions and terminal amino acids of several thyroglobulins. J. Biol. Chem. **245**, 5820—5837 (1970).

144. SPIRO, R. G., SPIRO, M. J.: The carbohydrate of thyroglobulin. Federation Proc. **22**, 538 (1963).

145. SPIRO, R. G., SPIRO, M. J.: The carbohydrate composition of the thyroglobulins from several species. J. Biol. Chem. **240**, 997—1001 (1965).

146. STANLEY, P. G.: Proteins of normal and pathological human thyroid tissue. Acta Endocrinol. **45**, 161—170 (1964).

147. STANLEY, P. G.: Proteins of normal and pathological human thyroid tissue. 2. Nature of iodoproteins in two glands containing discrete malignant nodules. Acta Endocrinol. **46**, 675—678 (1964).
148. STEINER, R. F., EDELHOCH, H.: The properties of thyroglobulin. VI. The internal rigidity of native and denatured thyroglobulin. J. Am. Chem. Soc. **83**, 1435—1444 (1961).
149. STOKINGER, H. E., HEIDELBERGER, M.: A quantitative theory of the precipitin reaction. VI. The reaction between mammalian thyroglobulins and antibodies to homologous and heterologous preparations. J. Exp. Med. **66**, 251—272 (1937).
150. STYLOS, W. A., ROSE, N. R.: Splitting of human thyroglobulin. II. Enzymatic digestion. Clin. Exp. Immunol. **5**, 285—297 (1969).
151. TARUTANI, O., SHULMAN, S.: Sialic acid and the structural heterogeneity of thyroglobulin. Federation Proc. **29**, 645 (1970).
152. TARUTANI, O., SHULMAN, S.: Properties of carbohydrate-stripped thyroglobulin. I. Preparation and physicochemical properties of desialized thyroglobulin. Biochim. Biophys. Acta **229**, 642—648 (1971).
153. TARUTANI, O., SHULMAN, S.: Properties of carbohydrate-stripped thyroglobulin. II. Heterogeneity in sialic acid content in thyroglobulin subfractions. Biochim. Biophys. Acta **236**, 384—390 (1971).
154. TARUTANI, O., SHULMAN, S.: Properties of carbohydrate-stripped thyroglobulin. III. The role of sialic acid in the solubility properties of thyroglobulin. In preparation.
155. TARUTANI, O., SMITH, D. J., SHULMAN, S.: Properties of carbohydrate-stripped thyroglobulin. IV. Susceptibility of galactose units of desialized thyroglobulin to β-galactosidase and properties of desialodegalacto-thyroglobulin. In preparation.
156. TARUTANI, O., KONDO, T., SMITH, D. J., SHULMAN, S.: The subunit structure of thyroidal 27-S protein. In preparation.
157. TARUTANI, O., UI, N.: Accumulation of non-iodinated thyroglobulin in the thyroid of goitrogen-treated hogs. Biochem. Biophys. Res. Commun. **33**, 733—738 (1968).
158. TARUTANI, O., UI, N.: Subunit structure of hog thyroglobulin: Dissociation by treatment with sodium dodecyl sulfate. Biochim. Biophys. Acta **181**, 116—135 (1969).
159. TARUTANI, O., UI, N.: Subunit structure of hog thyroglobulin: Dissociation of noniodinated and highly iodinated preparations. Biochim. Biophys. Acta **181**, 136—145 (1969).
160. TATA, J. R., RALL, J. E., RAWSON, R. W.: Studies on an iodinated protein in the serum of subjects with cancer of the thyroid. J. Clin. Endocrinol. Metab. **16**, 1554—1569 (1956).
161. THEMANN, H., ANDRADA, J. A., ROSE, N. R., ANDRADA, E. C., WITEBSKY, E.: Experimental thyroiditis in the rhesus monkey. V. Electron microscopic investigations. Clin. Exp. Immunol. **3**, 491—508 (1968).
162. THOMSON, J. A., BISSETT, J. M.: Ultracentrifugal patterns of the thyroid proteins from human pathological thyroid glands. Acta Endocrinol. **62**, 577—586 (1969).
163. THOMSON, J. A., MCGIRR, E. M.: Defective deiodinase activity and abnormal thyroidal iodoproteins. J. Clin. Endocrinol. Metab. **29**, 1259—1260 (1969).
164. TORO-GOYCO, E., MATOS, M.: Abnormal iodoproteins in serum: Separation by gel filtration. J. Clin. Endocrinol. Metab. **25**, 916—922 (1965).
165. TORRIGIANI, G., ROITT, I. M.: Sedimentation characteristics of human thyroid auto-antibodies. Immunology **6**, 73—80 (1963).
166. TORRIGIANI, G., ROITT, I. M., DONIACH, D.: Quantitative distribution of human thyroglobulin autoantibodies in different immunoglobulin classes. Clin. Exp. Immunol. **3**, 621—630 (1968).
167. TROTTER, W. R., BELYAVIN, G., WADDAMS, A.: Precipitating and complement-fixing antibodies in Hashimoto's disease. Proc. Roy. Soc. Med. **50**, 961—962 (1957).
168. UI, N., TARUTANI, O.: Purification of hog thyroglobulin. J. Biochem. **50**, 508—518 (1961).
169. UI, N., TARUTANI, O., KONDO, Y., TAMURA, H.: Chromatographic fractionation of hog thyroglobulin. Nature **191**, 1199—1201 (1961).
170. UJEJSKI, L., GLEGG, R. E.: Carbohydrates in thyroglobulin and the lens capsule. Can. J. Biochem. Physiol. **33**, 199—201 (1955).
171. VALENTA, L., KYNCL, F., NIEDERLE, B., JIROUSEK , L.: Soluble proteins in thyroid neoplasia. J. Clin. Endocrinol. Metab. **28**, 442—450 (1968).
172. VALENTA, L., LISSITZKY, S., AQUARON, R.: Thyroglobulin-iodine in thyroid tumors. J. Clin. Endocrinol. Metab. **28**, 437—441 (1968).

173. VAN ZYL, A., THERON, C. N., VAN DER WALT, B.: The use of agarose for the preparation of pure 19-S thyroglobulin. Biochim. Biophys. Acta **171**, 337—339 (1969).
174. VAN JAARSVELD, P., VAN DER WALT, B., THERON, C. N.: Afrikander cattle congenital goiter: Purification and partial identification of the complex iodoprotein pattern. Endocrinology **91**, 470—482 (1972).
175. VECCHIO, G., EDELHOCH, H., ROBBINS, J., WEATHERS, B.: Studies on the structure of the 27S thyroid iodoproteins. Biochemistry **5**, 2617—2623 (1966).
176. WEIGLE, W. O.: The induction of autoimmunity in rabbits following injection of heterologous or altered homologous thyroglobulin. J. Exp. Med. **121**, 289—308 (1965).
177. WEIGLE, W. O.: The production of thyroiditis and antibody following injection of unaltered thyroglobulin without adjuvant into rabbits previously stimulated with altered thyroglobulin. J. Exp. Med. **122**, 1049—1062 (1965).
178. WEIGLE, W. O.: Inhibition of the production of autoimmune thyroiditis in the rabbit. Immunology **13**, 241—248 (1967).
179. WEIGLE, W. O., HIGH, G. L.: The behavior of autologous thyroglobulin in the circulation of rabbits immunized with either heterologous or altered homologous thyroglobulin. J. Immunol. **98**, 1105—1114 (1967).
180. WEIGLE, W. O., HIGH, G. L.: The effect of antigenic competition on antibody production to heterologous proteins, termination of immunologic unresponsiveness and induction of autoimmunity. J. Immunol. **99**, 392—398 (1967).
181. WEIGLE, W. O., NAKAMURA, R. M.: The development of autoimmune thyroiditis in rabbits following injection of aqueous preparations of heterologous thyroglobulins. J. Immunol. **99**, 223—231 (1967).
182. WEIGLE, W. O., NAKAMURA, R. M.: Perpetuation of autoimmune thyroiditis and production of secondary renal lesions following periodic injections of aqueous preparations of altered thyroglobulin. Clin. Exp. Immunol. **4**, 645—657 (1969).
183. WHITE, R. G.: An immunological investigation of Hashimoto's disease. Proc. Roy. Soc. Med. **50**, 953—954 (1957).
184. WITEBSKY, E.: Die serologische Analyse von Zellen und Geweben. Naturwissenschaften **40**, 771—776 (1929).
185. WITEBSKY, E.: Experimental thyroiditis. In: The Thyroid (HAZARD, J. B., SMITH, D. E., Eds.), p. 143—151. Baltimore: Williams & Wilkins 1964.
186. WITEBSKY, E., KITE, J. H., jr., WICK, G., COLE, R. K.: Spontaneous thyroiditis in the obese strain of chickens. I. Demonstration of circulating autoantibodies. J. Immunol. **103**, 708—715 (1969).
187. WITEBSKY, E., ROSE, N. R.: Studies on organ specificity. IV. Production of rabbit thyroid antibodies in the rabbit. J. Immunol. **76**, 408—416 (1956).
188. WITEBSKY, E., ROSE, N. R., SHULMAN, S.: Studies on organ specificity. I. The serological specificity of thyroid extracts. J. Immunol. **75**, 269—281 (1955).
189. WITEBSKY, E., ROSE, N. R., SHULMAN, S.: Studies of normal and malignant tissue antigens. Cancer Res. **16**, 831—841 (1956).
190. WITEBSKY, E., ROSE, N. R., SHULMAN, S.: The auto-antibody nature of the thyroiditis antibody and the role of thyroglobulin in the reaction. Lancet **1958 I**, 808—810.
191. WITEBSKY, E., ROSE, N. R., TERPLAN, K., PAINE, J. R., EGAN, R. W.: Chronic thyroiditis and autoimmunization. J. Am. Med. Assoc. **164**, 1439—1447 (1957).
192. WOLFF, J., ROBBINS, J., RALL, J. E.: Iodine trapping without organification in a transplantable rat thyroid tumor. Endocrinology **64**, 1—11 (1959).
193. WOLLMAN, S. H., WARREN, L.: Effects of thyrotropin and thiouracil on the sialic acid concentration in the thyroid gland. Biochim. Biophys. Acta **47**, 251—256 (1961).

Chapter 3. The Adrenal Gland

1. ANDERSON, J. R., GOUDIE, R. B., GRAY, K., STUART-SMITH, D. A.: Immunological features of idiopathic Addison's disease: An antibody to cells producing steroid hormones. Clin. Exp. Immunol. **3**, 107—117 (1968).

2. ANDERSON, J. R., GOUDIE, R. B., GRAY, K. G., TIMBURY, G. C.: Auto-antibodies in Addison's disease. Lancet **1957 I**, 1123—1124.
3. ANDRADA, J. A., SKELTON, F. R., ANDRADA, E. C., MILGROM, F., WITEBSKY, E.: Experimental autoimmune adrenalitis in rats. Lab. Invest. **19**, 460—465 (1968).
4. BARNETT, E. V., DUMONDE, D. C., GLYNN, L. E.: Induction of autoimmunity to adrenal gland. Immunology **6**, 382—402 (1963).
5. BEISER, S. M., ERLANGER, B. F., AGATE, F. J., LIEBERMAN, S.: Antigenicity of steroid-protein conjugates. Science **129**, 564—565 (1959).
6. BIGAZZI, P. L., ANDRADA, J. A., ANDRADA, E. C., BEUTNER, E. H., WITEBSKY, E.: Immunofluorescence studies on Addison's disease. Intern. Arch. Allergy Appl. Immunol. **34**, 455—469 (1968).
7. BLIZZARD, R. M., CHEE, D., DAVIS, W.: The incidence of parathyroid and other antibodies in the sera of patients with idiopathic hypoparathyroidism. Clin. Exp. Immunol. **1**, 119—128 (1966).
8. BLIZZARD, R. M., CHEE, D., DAVIS, W.: The incidence of adrenal and other antibodies in the sera of patients with idiopathic adrenal insufficiency (Addison's disease). Clin. Exp. Immunol. **1**, 19—30 (1967).
9. BLIZZARD, R. M., KYLE, M. A.: Studies of the adrenal antigens and antibodies in Addison's disease. J. Clin. Invest. **42**, 1653—1660 (1963).
10. BLIZZARD, R. M., KYLE, M. A., CHANDLER, R. W., HUNG, W.: Adrenal antibodies in Addison's disease. Lancet **1962 II**, 901—903.
11. BLIZZARD, R. M., TOMASI, T. B., CHRISTY, N. P.: Autoantibodies against thyroid and adrenal tissue in a patient with multiple, primary endocrine deficiencies, J. Clin. Endocrinol. Metab. **23**, 1179—1180 (1963).
12. CARTER, A. C., KAPLAN, S. A., DEMAYO, A. P., ROSENBLUM, D. J.: An unusual case of idiopathic hypoparathyroidism, adrenal insufficiency, hypothyroidism and metastatic calcification. J. Clin. Endocrinol. Metab. **19**, 1633—1641 (1959).
13. CENTENO, E.: Chemical studies on the adrenal auto-antigen. Federation Proc. **21**, 42 (1962).
14. CENTENO, E. R., SHULMAN, S.: Isolation and characterization of a rabbit adrenal autoantigen. Immunology **24**, 901—910 (1973).
15. CENTENO, E., SHULMAN, S., MILGROM, F., WITEBSKY, E.: Immunological studies on adrenal glands. VI. The multiple nature of the rabbit adrenal autoantigens. Immunology **8**, 160—169 (1965).
16. CHRISTY, N. P., HOLUB, D. A., TOMASI, T. B.: Primary ovarian, thyroidal and adrenocortical deficiencies simulating pituitary insufficiency, associated with diabetes mellitus. J. Clin. Endocrinol. Metab. **22**, 155—160 (1962).
17. COLOVER, J., GLYNN, L. E.: Experimental iso-immune adrenalitis. Immunology **1**, 172—178 (1958).
18. COPE, C. L.: Adrenal Steroids and Disease, p. 338 and 426. Philadelphia: Lippincott 1964.
19. D'AMELIO, V., PERLMANN, P.: The distribution of soluble antigens in cellular structures of rat liver. Exp. Cell. Res. **19**, 383—398 (1960).
20. GOUDIE, R. B., ANDERSON, J. R., GRAY, K. G., WHITE, W. G.: Autoantibodies in Addison's disease. Lancet **1966 I**, 1173—1176.
21. GOUDIE, R. B., MCDONALD, E., ANDERSON, J. R., GRAY, K.: Immunological features of idiopathic Addison's disease: Characterization of the adrenocortical antigens. Clin. Exp. Immunol. **3**, 119—131 (1968).
22. GOUDIE, R. B., STUART-SMITH, D. A., BOYLE, I. T., FERGUSON, A.: Serological diagnosis of idiopathic Addison's disease in patients on prolonged prednisolone therapy for steatorrhoea. Lancet **1969 I**, 186—188.
23. GUARINI, G., MACALUSO, M.: Steatorrhea in Addison's disease. Lancet **1963 I**, 955—966.
24. HELLE, K. B.: Comparative studies on the soluble protein fractions of bovine, equine, porcine and ovine adrenal chromaffin granules. J. Biochem. **100**, 6c—7c (1966).
25. HELLE, K.: Antibody formation against soluble protein from bovine adrenal chromaffin granules. Biochim. Biophys. Acta **117**, 107—110 (1966).
26. HOENIG, E. M., HIRANO, A., LEVINE, S., GHATAK, N. R.: The early development and fine structure of allergic adrenalitis, Lab. Invest. **22**, 198—205 (1970).
27. HUNG, W., MIGEON, C. J., PARROTT, R. H.: A possible autoimmune basis for Addison's disease in three siblings, one with idiopathic hypoparathyroidism, pernicious anemia and superficial moniliasis. New Engl. J. Med. **269**, 658—663 (1963).

28. IRINO, T., GROLLMAN, A.: Induction of adrenal insufficiency in the rat by sensitization with homologous tissue. Metabolism **17**, 717—724 (1968).
29. IRINO, T., GROLLMAN, A.: Ultrastructure of the adrenal cortical insufficiency induced in rats by immunization with adrenal antigen. Texas Rep. Biol. Med. **27**, 81—91 (1969).
30. IRVINE, W. J.: A clinical and immunological study of adrenal insufficiency. J. Endocrinol. **26**, 32—33 (1963).
31. IRVINE, W. J.: Adrenal disease and auto-immunity. Proc. 9th Int. Cong. Int. Med., Excerpta Medica Intern. Cong. Series No. 137, p. 93—98 (1966).
32. IRVINE, W. J.: Clinical and immunological associations in adrenal disorders. Proc. Roy. Soc. Med. **61**, 271—275 (1968).
33. IRVINE, W. J., CHAN, M. M. W., SCARTH, L.: The further characterization of autoantibodies reactive with extra-adrenal steroid-producing cells in patients with adrenal disorders. Clin. Exp. Immunol. **4**, 489—503 (1969).
34. IRVINE, W. J., CHAN, M. M. W., SCARTH, L., KOLB, F. O., HARTOG, M., BAYLISS, R. I. S., DRURY, M. I.: Immunological aspects of premature ovarian failure associated with iodiopathic Addison's disease. Lancet **1968 II**, 883—887.
35. IRVINE, W. J., STEWART, A. G., SCARTH, L.: A clinical and immunologic study of adrenocortical insufficiency (Addison's disease). Clin. Exp. Immunol. **2**, 31—70 (1967).
36. KRACHT, J., FISCHER, K., MOEBIUS, G.: Durch Autoaggression hervorgerufene Veränderungen der Nebenniere. Verhandl. Deut. Ges. Pathol. **46**, 152—157 (1962).
37. KUNIN, A. S., MACKAY, B. R., BURNS, S. L., HALBERSTAM, M. J.: The syndrome of hypoparathyroidism and adrenocortical insufficiency, a possible sequal of hepatitis. Am. J. Med. **34**, 856—866 (1963).
38. LEVINE, S.: Allergic adrenalitis and adenohypophysitis: Further observations on production and passive transfer. Endocrinology **84**, 469—475 (1969).
39. LEVINE, S., HOENIG, E. M.: Induced localization of allergic adrenalitis and encephalomyelitis at sites of thermal injury. J. Immunol. **100**, 1310—1318 (1968).
40. LEVINE, S., SOWINSKI, R.: Passive transfer of allergic adrenalitis and encephalomyelitis with whole blood. Proc. Soc. Exp. Biol. Med. **129**, 221—222 (1968).
41. LEVINE, S., SOWINSKI, R.: Allergic adrenalitis and encephalomyelitis produced by injection into lymph nodes. Clin. Exp. Immunol. **4**, 177—178 (1969).
42. LEVINE, S., SOWINSKI, R.: Allergic adrenalitis and adrenal isografts. Transplantation **10**, 92—99 (1970).
43. LEVINE, S., WENK, E. J.: The production and passive transfer of allergic adrenalitis. Am. J. Pathol. **52**, 41—53 (1968).
44. MCBRIEN, D. J., VAUGHAN JONES, R., CREAMER, B.: Steatorrhea in Addison's disease. Lancet **1963 I**, 25—26.
45. MEAD, R. K.: Autoimmune Addison's disease. New Engl. J. Med. **266**, 583—586 (1961).
46. MILCOU, M., POP, A., LUPULESCOU, A., TAGA, M.: L'autoimmunization expérimentale de la surrénale chez le lapin. Ann. Endocrinol. (Paris) **20**, 799—804 (1959).
47. MILGROM, F., CAMPBELL, W. A., WITEBSKY, E.: Studies on immunization with organ-specific haptens. Proc. Soc. Exp. Biol. Med. **115**, 165—169 (1964).
48. MILGROM, F., TUGGAC, M., WITEBSKY, E.: Immunological studies on adrenal glands. III. Interspecies relations of thermostable adrenal-specific antigens. Immunology **6**, 105—118 (1963).
49. MILGROM, F., WITEBSKY, E.: Immunological studies on adrenal glands. I. Immunization with adrenals of foreign species. Immunology **5**, 46—78 (1962).
50. NERUP, J., ANDERSEN, V., BENDIXEN, G.: Anti-adrenal, cellular hypersensitivity in Addison's disease. Clin. Exp. Immunol. **4**, 355—363 (1969).
50a. NERUP, J., ANDERSEN, V., BENDIXEN, G.: Anti-adrenal cellular hypersensitivity in Addison's disease. IV. In vivo and in vitro investigations on the mitochondrial fraction. Clin. Exp. Immunol. **6**, 733—739 (1970).
51. NERUP, J., BENDIXEN, G.: Anti-adrenal cellular hypersensitivity in Addison's disease. II. Correlation with clinical and serological findings. Clin. Exp. Immunol. **5**, 341—353 (1969).
52. NERUP, J., BENDIXEN, G.: Anti-adrenal cellular hypersensitivity in Addison's disease. III. Species specificity and subcellular localization of the antigen. Clin. Exp. Immunol. **5**, 355—364 (1969).
53. OKADA, T. S.: Tissue-specificity in the soluble antigens in kidney microsomes. Nature **194**, 306—307 (1962).

54. PATON, E., MURRAY, E. S., WATSON, W. C.: Intestinal disaccharidase activity in rosacea. Brit. Med. J. **1966 I**, 459—460.
55. PERLMANN, P., MORGAN, W. S.: Immunological studies of microsomal structure and function. In: Biological Structure and Function (GOODWIN, T. W., LINDBERG, O., Eds.), p. 209—219. New York: Academic Press 1961.
56. RIFÉ, U.: Localization of thermostable, adrenal-specific antigen in subcellular fractions. Intern. Arch. Allergy Appl. Immunol. **32**, 366—372 (1967).
57. SANERKIN, N. G., EL-SHABOURY, A. H.: Chronic adrenalitis with bronchial asthma. Lancet **1965 II**, 468—470.
58. SHULMAN, S., CENTENO, E. R.: Isolation and characterization of a rabbit non-tissue-specific autoantigen which is shared by kidney, heart, adrenal and liver, Immunology **24**, 925—937 (1973).
59. SHULMAN, S., CENTENO, E., MILGROM, F., WITEBSKY, E.: Immunological studies on adrenal glands. V. Chemical studies on the rabbit adrenal-specific autoantigen. Immunology **8**, 531—538 (1965).
60. SHULMAN, S., MILGROM, F., WITEBSKY, E.: Immunological studies on adrenal glands. IV. Chemical studies on the bovine thermostable adrenal-specific antigen. Immunology **7**, 605—615 (1964).
61. SLOPER, J. C.: A pathology of the thyroid in Addison's disease. J. Pathol. Bacteriol. **66**, 53—61 (1953).
62. SPINNER, M. W., BLIZZARD, R. M., CHILDS, B.: Clinical and genetic heterogeneity in idiopathic Addison's disease and hypoparathyroidism. J. Clin. Endocrinol. Metab. **28**, 795—804 (1968).
63. STEINER, J. W., LANGER, B., SCHATZ, D. L., VOLPE, R.: Experimental immunologic adrenal injury. A response to injections of autologous and homologous adrenal antigens in adjuvant. J. Exp. Med. **112**, 187—202 (1960).
64. TERPLAN, K., WITEBSKY, E., MILGROM, F.: Histopathology of adrenals in animals immunized with tissue antigens. Arch. Pathol. **76**, 333—338 (1963).
65. VOGT, P. K.: The immunology of liver microsomes. I. The properties of the quantitative precipitin system. Z. Naturforsch. **15B**, 221 (1960).
66. WELLS, H. G.: Addison's disease with selective destruction of the suprarenal cortex. Arch. Pathol. **10**, 499ff. (1930).
67. WERDELIN, O., BOEHME, D. H.: Immunization of BSVS mice with heterologous and homologous adrenal gland. Immunology **16**, 205—215 (1969).
68. WERDELIN, O., MCCLUSKEY, R. T., WITEBSKY, E.: In situ labeling of popliteal lymph node cells with tritiated thymidine in rats with allergic adrenalitis. Lab. Invest. **23**, 144—149 (1970).
69. WERDELIN, O., WITEBSKY, E.: Experimental allergic rat adrenalitis. A study on its elicitation and lymphokinetics. Lab. Invest. **23**, 136—143 (1970).
70. WHITAKER, J., LANDING, B. H., ESSELBORN, V. M., WILLIAMS, R. R.: The syndrome of familial juvenile hypoadrenocorticism, hypoparathyroidism and superficial moniliasis. J. Clin. Endocrinol. Metab. **16**, 1374—1387 (1956).
71. WINKLER, H., HÖRTNAGL, H., HÖRTNAGL, H., SMITH, A. D.: Membranes of the adrenal medulla. Behavior of insoluble proteins of chromaffin granules on gel electrophoresis. Biochem. J. **118**, 303—310 (1970).
72. WITEBSKY, E., KLINKE, J.: Die serologische Spezifität des Nebennierenmarks. Z. Immunitätsforsch. **78**, 509—523 (1933).
73. WITEBSKY, E., MILGROM, F.: Immunological studies on adrenal glands. II. Immunization with adrenals of the same species. Immunology **5**, 67—78 (1962).

Chapter 4. The Brain

1. ABDULLA, Y. H., MCFARLANE, E.: Evidence for the presence of complement in human myelin. Biochem. Biophys. Res. Commun. **46**, 1072—1073 (1972).
2. ALVORD, E. C., jr.: Distribution and nature of the 'antigen' responsible for experimental meningoencephalomyelitis in the guinea pig. Proc. Soc. Exp. Biol. Med. **67**, 459—461 (1948).
3. ALVORD, E. C., jr.: Brain antigens and antibodies: The possible relationship between carcinomatous and experimental allergic neuroencephalomyelitides. In: The Remote Effects of Cancer on the Nervous System (BRAIN, LORD, NORRIS, F. H., jr., Eds.), p. 188—203. New York: Grune and Stratton 1965.

4. ALVORD, E. C., jr.: The relationship of hypersensitivity to infection, inflammation and immunity. J. Neuropathol. Exp. Neurol. **25**, 1—17 (1966).
5. ALVORD, E. C., jr.: Hypersensitivity states affecting the nervous system. In: The Biological Basis of Pediatric Practice (COOKE, R. E., Ed.), p. 1251—1266. New York: McGraw-Hill 1968.
6. ALVORD, E. C., jr.: The etiology and pathogenesis of experimental allergic encephalomyelitis. In: The Central Nervous System (BAILEY, O. T., SMITH, D. E., Eds.), p. 52—70. Baltimore: Williams & Wilkins 1968.
7. ALVORD, E. C., jr., HRUBY, S., AUGUST, C. S., KIES, M. W.: Multiplicity of organ-specific antigens in encephalitogenic basic proteins. Federation Proc. **25**, 355 (1966).
8. ALVORD, E. C., jr., HRUBY, S., SHAW, C. M., KIES, M. W.: Multiplicity of encephalitogenic myelin basic proteins. II. Antigenic determinants related to species of origin and relative molecular size. Add. ad Intern. Arch. Allergy Appl. Immunol. **36**, 276—292 (1969).
9. ALVORD, E. C., jr., SHAW, C.-M., FAHLBERG, W. J., KIES, M. W.: An analysis of various types of inhibition of experimental 'allergic' encephalomyelitis in the guinea pig. Z. Immunitätsforsch. **126**, 217—227 (1962).
10. ALVORD, E. C., jr., SHAW, C. M., HRUBY, S., KIES, M. W.: Encephalitogen-induced inhibition of experimental allergic encephalomyelitis: Prevention, suppression and therapy. Ann. N. Y. Acad. Sci. **122**, 333—345 (1965).
11. ALVORD, E. C., jr., SHAW, C. M., LISAK, R. P., FALK, G. A., KIES, M. W.: Relationships between antibodies and experimental allergic encephalomyelitis. V. Antibodies and delayed hypersensitivity in production and prevention of experimental allergic encephalomyelitis. Intern. Arch. Allergy Appl. Immunol. **38**, 403—412 (1970).
12. ALVORD, E. C., jr., SUDDUTH, W. H., HRUBY, S., HUGHES, K.: A search for brain antigens in canine distemper: A preliminary report. Neurology **18**, 112—116 (1968).
13. ARNASON, B. G., RICHMAN, D. P.: Effect of oral contraceptives on experimental demyelinating disease. Arch. Neurol. **21**, 103—108 (1969).
14. AUGUST, C. S., KIES, M. W., ALVORD, E. C., jr.: Delayed-type skin sensitivity to human encephalitogen in experimental allergic encephalomyelitis. Nature **214**, 1021—1022 (1967).
15. AUGUST, C. S., KIES, M. W., HRUBY, S., SHAW, C. M.: Separation of organ and species specific antigens in brain proteins. Federation Proc. **25**, 356 (1966).
16. BEHAN, P. O., GESCHWIND, N., LAMARCHE, J. B., LISAK, R. P., KIES, M. W.: Delayed hypersensitivity to encephalitogenic protein in disseminated encephalomyelitis. Lancet **1968 II**, 1009—1012.
17. BENDA, P., LIGHTBODY, J., SATO, G., LEVINE, L., SWEET, W.: Differentiated rat glial cell strain in tissue culture. Science **161**, 370—371 (1968).
18. BENNETT, G. S., EDELMAN, G. M.: Isolation of an acidic protein from rat brain. J. Biol. Chem. **243**, 6234—6241 (1968).
19. BEUTNER, E. H., WITEBSKY, E., ROSE, N. R., GERBASI, J. R.: Localization of thyroid and spinal cord autoantibodies by fluorescent antibody technic. Proc. Soc. Exp. Biol. Med. **97**, 712—716 (1958).
20. BOGDANOVE, L. H., CLARK, G.: The induction of exacerbations of allergic meningoencephalomyelitis. J. Neuropathol. Exp. Neurol. **16**, 57—60 (1957).
21. BRANDRISS, M. W., SMITH, J. W., FRIEDMAN, R. M.: Suppression of experimental allergic encephalomyelitis by anti-metabolites. Ann. N. Y. Acad. Sci. **122**, 356—368 (1965).
22. BRANDT, R., GUTH, H., MÜLLER, R.: Zur Frage der Organ-spezifität von Lipoidantikörpern. Klin. Wochschr. **5**, 655 (1926).
23. BROCKMAN, J. A., STIFFEY, A. V., TESAR, W. C.: An in vitro assay for encephalitogenic components of central nervous tissue. J. Immunol. **100**, 1230—1236 (1968).
24. BROSTOFF, S., BURNETT, P., LAMPERT, P., EYLAR, E. H.: Isolation and characterization of a protein from sciatic nerve myelin responsible for experimental allergic neuritis. Nature **235**, 210—212 (1972).
25. BROSTOFF, S., EYLAR, E. H.: Localization of methylated arginine in the Al protein from myelin. Proc. Nat. Acad. Sci. **68**, 765—769 (1971).
26. BURNETT, P. R., EYLAR, E. H.: Allergic encephylomyelitis. Oxidation and cleavage of the single tryptophan residue of the Al protein from bovine and human myelin. J. Biol. Chem. **246**, 3425—3430 (1971).

27. CALISSANO, P., BANGHAM, A. D.: Effect of two brain specific proteins (S 100 and 14.3.2) on cation diffusion across artificial lipid membranes. Biochem. Biophys. Res. Commun. **43**, 504—509 (1971).
28. CALISSANO, P., MOORE, B. W., FRIESEN, A.: Effect of calcium ion on S-100, a protein of the nervous system. Biochemistry **8**, 4318—4326 (1969).
29. CARNEGIE, P. R.: Autoimmune encephalomyelitis: Isolation, structure and properties of the main antigenic determinant from the basic protein of human brain. Hoppe-Seylers Z. Physiol. Chem. **352**, 23—24 (1971).
30. CARNEGIE, P. R., BENCINA, B., LAMOUREUX, G.: Experimental allergic encephalomyelitis; isolation of basic proteins and polypeptides from central nervous tissue. Biochem. J. **105**, 559—568 (1967).
31. CARNEGIE, P. R., LUMSDEN, C. E.: Encephalitogenic peptides from spinal cord. Nature **209**, 1354—1355 (1966).
32. CARNEGIE, P. R., MCPHERSON, T. A., ROBSON, G. S. M.: Experimental autoimmune encephalomyelitis. Digestion of basic protein of human myelin with cyanogen bromide and trypsin. Immunology **19**, 55—63 (1970).
33. CASPARY, E. A., FIELD, E. J.: An encephalitogenic protein of human origin; some chemical and biological properties. Ann. N. Y. Acad. Sci. **122**, 182—198 (1965).
34. CASPARY, E. A., FIELD, E. J.: Stability of radioiodinated encephalitogenic factor in vivo. Clin. Exp. Immunol. **3**, 747—749 (1968).
35. CASPARY, E. A., HUGHES, D., FIELD, E. J.: On the mode of action of antilymphocytic serum: Experiments on electrophoretic mobility of macrophages in experimental allergic encephalomyelitis. Clin. Exp. Immunol. **7**, 395—400 (1970).
36. CHAO, L.-P., EINSTEIN, E. R.: Isolation and characterization of an active fragment from enzymatic degradation of encephalitogenic protein. J. Biol. Chem. **243**, 6050—6055 (1968).
37. CHAO, L.-P., EINSTEIN, E. R.: Estimation of the molecular weight of flexible disordered proteins by exclusion chromatography. J. Chromatog. **42**, 485—492 (1969).
38. CHAO, L.-P., EINSTEIN, E. R.: Physical properties of the bovine encephalitogenic protein. Molecular weight and conformation. J. Neurochem. **17**, 1121—1132 (1970).
39. CHAO, L.-P., EINSTEIN, E. R.: Localization of the active site through chemical modification of the encephalitogenic protein. J. Biol. Chem. **245**, 6397—6403 (1970).
40. CICERO, T. J., MOORE, B. W.: Turnover of the brain specific protein, S-100. Science **169**, 1333—1334 (1970).
41. COLOVER, J.: Experimental allergic encephalomyelitis induced with combined 'purified' spinal cord and bacillary fractions. Nature **182**, 105—106 (1958).
42. DANNIES, P. S., LEVINE, L.: Demonstration of subunits in beef brain acidic protein (S-100). Biochem. Biophys. Res. Commun. **37**, 587—592 (1969).
43. DANNIES, P. S., LEVINE, L.: Demonstration of subunits in beef brain acidic protein (S-100). Biochem. Biophys. Res. Commun. **37**, 587—592 (1969).
44. DANNIES, P. S., LEVINE, L.: Structural properties of bovine brain S-100 protein. J. Biol. Chem. **246**, 6276—6283 (1971).
45. DANNIES, P. S., LEVINE, L.: The role of sulfhydryl groups in serological properties of bovine brain S-100 protein. J. Biol. Chem. **246**, 6284—6287 (1971).
46. DAS, B. R., DAS, S.: An immunochemical study of monkey (Macaca mulatta) brain cortex grey matter soluble proteins. Immunochemistry **6**, 189—198 (1969).
47. DAU, P. C., PETERSON, R. D. A.: Transformation of rodent lymphoid cells by an encephalitogen of human origin. Intern. Arch. Allergy Appl. Immunol. **35**, 353—368 (1969).
48. DAVID, J. R., PATERSON, P. Y.: In vitro demonstration of cellular sensitivity in allergic encephalomyelitis. J. Exp. Med. **122**, 1161—1171 (1965).
49. DAY, E. D., LASSITER, S.: The in vitro absorption of anti-brain radioantibodies with brain sediments: Some unusual properties and a quantitative method. J. Immunol. **98**, 56—61 (1967).
50. DAY, E. D., RIGSBEE, L., WILKINS, R., MAHALEY, jr., M. S.: Localization of anti-brain radioantibodies in rat brain. J. Immunol. **98**, 62—66 (1967).
51. DEIBLER, G. E., MARTENSON, R. E., KIES, M. W.: Gel filtration of proteins at acid pH. Application to molecular weight estimation of myelin basic proteins. Biochim. Biophys. Acta **200**, 342—352 (1970).

52. DOWLING, P. C., KIM, S. U., MURRAY, M. R., COOK. S. D.: Serum 19 S and 7 S demyelinating antibodies in multiple sclerosis. J. Immunol. **101**, 1101—1104 (1968).
53. EDGINGTON, T. S., DALESSIO, D. J.: The assessment of immunofluorescence methods of humoral antimyelin antibodies in man. J. Immunol. **105**, 248—255 (1970).
54. EINSTEIN, E. R., CSEJTEY, J., DAVIS, W. J., LAJTHA, A., MARKS, N.: Enzymatic degradation of the encephalitogenic protein. In: Pathogenesis and Etiology of Demyelinating Diseases (KALLOS, P., Ed.), p. 363—375. Basel: S. Karger 1969.
55. EINSTEIN, E. R., CSEJTEY, J., DAVIS, W. J., RAUCH, H. C.: Protective action of the encephalitogen and other basic proteins in experimental allergic encephalomyelitis. Immunochemistry **5**, 567—575 (1968).
56. EINSTEIN, E. R., CSEJTEY, J., MARKS, N.: Degradation of encephalitogen by purified brain acid proteinase. FEBS Letters **1**, 191—195 (1968).
57. EINSTEIN, E. R., DALAL, K. B., CSEJTEY, J.: Increased protease activity and changes in basic proteins and lipids in multiple sclerosis plaques. J. Neurol. Sci. **11**, 109—121 (1970).
58. ENG, L. F., CHAO, F.-C., GERSTL, B., PRATT, D., TAVASTSTJERNA, M. G.: The maturation of human white matter myelin. Fractionation of the myelin membrane proteins. Biochemistry **7**, 4455—4465 (1968).
59. EYLAR, E. H.: Amino acid sequence of the basic protein of the myelin membrane. Proc. Nat. Acad. Sci. **67**, 1425—1431 (1970).
60. EYLAR, E. H.: Basic Al protein of myelin: Relationship to experimental allergic encephalomyelitis. In: Proc. Assoc. Res. Nerv. Ment. Dis., Vol. 49: Immunological Disorders of the Nervous System (ROWLAND, L. P.: Ed.), p. 50—75. Baltimore: Williams & Wilkins 1971.
61. EYLAR, E. H., BROSTOFF, S., HASHIM, G., CACCAM, J., BURNETT, P.: Basic Al protein of the myelin membrane. The complete amino acid sequence. J. Biol. Chem. **246**, 5770—5784 (1971).
62. EYLAR, E. H., CACCAM, J., JACKSON, J. J., WESTALL, F. C., ROBINSON, A. B.: Experimental allergic encephalomyelitis: Synthesis of disease inducing site of the basic protein. Science **168**, 1220—1223 (1970).
63. EYLAR, E. H., HASHIM, G. A.: Allergic encephalomyelitis: The structure of the encephalitogenic determinant. Proc. Nat. Acad. Sci. **61**, 644—650 (1968).
64. EYLAR, E. H., HASHIM, G. A.: Allergic encephalomyelitis: Cleavage of the C-tryptophyl bond in the encephalitogenic basic protein from bovine myelin. Arch. Biochem. Biophys. **131**, 215—222 (1969).
65. EYLAR, E. H., JACKSON, J., ROTHENBERG, B., BROSTOFF, S. W.: Suppression of the immune response: Reversal of the disease state with antigen in allergic encephalomyelitis. Nature **236**, 74—76 (1972).
66. EYLAR, E. H., SALK, J., BEVERIDGE, G. C., BROWN, L. V.: Experimental allergic encephalomyelitis: An encephalitogenic basic protein from bovine myelin. Arch. Biochem. Biophys. **132**, 34—48 (1969).
67. EYLAR, E. H., THOMPSON, M.: Allergic encephalomyelitis: The physico-chemical properties of the basic protein encephalitogen from bovine spinal cord. Arch. Biochem. Biophys. **129**, 468—479 (1969).
68. EYLAR, E. H., WESTALL, F. C., BROSTOFF, S.: Allergic encephalitogenic peptide derived from the basic protein myelin. J. Biol. Chem. **246**, 3418—3424 (1971).
69. FALK, G. A., HEINZE, R. G., KIES, M. W., ALVORD, E. C., jr.: Skin-fixing antibody in experimental allergic encephalomyelitis. J. Immunol. **100**, 321—328 (1968).
70. FALK, G. A., KIES, M. W.: Passive transfer of experimental allergic encephalomyelitis (EAE) and delayed hypersensitivity to myelin basic protein (BP). Federation Proc. **27**, 544 (1968).
71. FALK, G. A., KIES, M. W., ALVORD, E. C., jr.: Delayed hypersensitivity to myelin basic protein in the passive transfer of experimental allergic encephalomyelitis. J. Immunol. **101**, 638—644 (1968).
72. FALK, G. A., KIES, M. W., ALVORD, E. C.: Passive transfer of experimental allergic encephalomyelitis: Mechanisms of suppression. J. Immunol. **103**, 1248—1253 (1969).
73. FLAD, H. D., PATERSON, P. Y., MIESCHER, P. A.: In vitro effects. of phytohemagglutinin and brain antigen on cell transfer of experimental autoimmune encephalomyelitis in Lewis rats. J. Immunol. **100**, 647—653 (1968).
74. FOLCH, J., LEES, M.: Proteolipids, a new type of tissue lipoproteins. Their isolation from brain. J. Biol. Chem. **191**, 807—817 (1951).

75. FOLCH, J., WEBSTER, G. R., LEES, M.: The preparation of proteolipids. Federation Proc. **18**, 228 (1959).

76. FREUND, J., STERN, E. R., PIGANI, T. M.: Isoallergic encephalomyelitis and radiculitis in guinea pigs after one injection of brain and mycobacteria in water-in-oil emulsion. J. Immunol. **57**, 179—194 (1947).

77. FRIEDMAN, H. P., WENGER, B. S.: Identification of two distinct rabbit antibodies directed against different antigenic components of avian brain. Immunology **9**, 467—475 (1965).

78. GIBBS, N., HRUBY, S., ALVORD, E. C., jr., SHAW, C.-M.: Relationships between antibodies and experimental allergic encephalomyelitis. IV. Cytophilic antibodies. Intern. Arch. Allergy Appl. Immunol. **38**, 394—402 (1970).

79. GOLDSTEIN, N. P., KOLB, L. C., MASON, H. L., SAYRE, G. P., KARLSON, A. G.: Relationship of homologous brain proteolipid to allergic encephalomyelitis in guinea pigs. Neurology **3**, 609—614 (1953).

79a. GOMBOS, G., ZANETTA, J.-P., MANDEL, P., VINCENDON, G.: Étude de la fraction protéique neurospécifique S-100: I. Présence in vivo des composants rapide et lent de la fraction protéique S-100. Biochimie **5**, 635—643 (1971).

79b. GOMBOS, G., ZANETTA, J.-P., MANDEL, P., VINCENDON, G.: Étude de la fraction protéique neurospécifique S-100: II. Hétérogénéité moléculaire de la fraction protéique S 100. Biochimie **5**, 645—655 (1971).

80. HAGOPIAN, A., EYLAR, E. H.: Glycoprotein biosynthesis: The basic protein encephalitogen from bovine spinal cord, a receptor for the polypeptidyl: N-acetylgalactosaminyl transferase from bovine submaxillary glands. Arch. Biochem. Biophys. **126**, 785—794 (1968).

81. HAGOPIAN, A., WESTALL, F. C., WHITEHEAD, J. S., EYLAR, E. H.: Glycosylation of the Al protein from myelin by a polypeptide N-acetylgalactosaminyltransferase. J. Biol. Chem. **246**, 2519—2523 (1971).

82. HARWIN, S. M., PATERSON, P. Y.: Antibrain antibodies of the 19 S γ-globulin type in rats with allergic encephalomyelitis. Nature **194**, 391—392 (1962).

83. HASHIM, G. A., EYLAR, E. H.: Allergic encephalomyelitis: Enzymatic degradation of the encephalitogenic basic protein from bovine spinal cord. Arch. Biochem. Biophys. **129**, 635—644 (1969).

84. HASHIM, G. A., EYLAR, E. H.: Allergic encephalomyelitis: Isolation and characterization of encephalitogenic peptides from the baic protein of bovine spinal cord. Arch. Biochem. Biophys. **129**, 645—654 (1969).

85. HASHIM, G. A., EYLAR, E. H.: The structure of the terminal regions of the encephalitogenic Al protein. Biochem. Biophys. Res. Commun. **34**, 770—776 (1969).

86. HATCHER, V. B., MACPHERSON, C. F. C.: Studies on brain antigens. II. Water soluble antigenic proteins of bovine brain. J. Immunol. **102**, 877—883 (1969).

87. HATCHER, V. B., MACPHERSON, C. F. C.: Studies on brain antigens. III. Purification and characterization of water-soluble bovine antigen specific for nervous tissue (α-BASNT). J. Immunol. **104**, 633—640 (1970).

88. HENLE, W., CHAMBERS, L. A., GROUPÉ, V.: The serological specificity of particulate components derived from various normal mammalian organs. J. Exp. Med. **74**, 495—510 (1941).

88a. HERSCHMAN, H. R.: Synthesis and degradation of a brain-specific protein (S100 protein) by clonal cultured human glial cells. J. Biol. Chem. **246**, 7569—7571 (1971).

89. HOCHWALD, G. M., THORBECKE, G. J.: Trace proteins in cerebrospinal fluid and other biological fluids. I. Effect of various fractionation procedures on β-trace and γ-trace proteins and methods for isolation of both proteins. Arch. Biochem. Biophys. **101**, 325—334 (1963).

90. HONEGGER, C. C.: Studies on basic proteins from the central nervous system. Ann. N. Y. Acad. Sci. **122**, 199—208 (1965).

91. HOTTLE, G. A., NEDZEL, G. A., WRIGHT, J. T., BELL, J. R.: Allergic encephalitis following injection of dialysate of brain tissue, Proc. Soc. Exp. Biol. Med. **72**, 289—291 (1949).

92. HRUBY, S., ALVORD, E. C., jr., SHAW, C. M.: Relationships between antibodies and experimental allergic encephalomyelitis. I. Production of hemagglutinating and gel-precipitating antibodies in rabbits and guinea pigs. Intern. Arch. Allergy Appl. Immunol. **36**, 599—611 (1969).

93. HRUBY, S., SHAW, C. M., ALVORD, E. C., jr., AUGUST, C. S., KIES, M. W.: Relationships between antibodies and experimental allergic encephalomyelitis. II. Identification and separation of spe-

cies-specific non-encephalitogenic contaminants of encephalitogenic basic proteins. Intern. Arch. Allergy Appl. Immunol. **37**, 532—545 (1970).

94. Jankovic, B. D., Išvaneski, M.: Experimental allergic encephalomyelitis in thymectomized, bursectomized and normal chickens. Intern. Arch. Allergy Appl. Immunol. **23**, 188—206 (1963).
95. Joffe, S.: Isolation and some properties of a succinylated protein-lipid complex derived from calf brain myelin. Arch. Biochem. Biophys. **146**, 46—53 (1971).
96. Joffe, S., Rapport, M. M., Graf, L.: Identification of an organ specific lipid hapten in brain. Nature **197**, 60—62 (1963).
97. Kabat, E. A., Wolf, A., Bezer, A. E.: The rapid production of acute disseminated encephalomyelitis in rhesus monkeys by injection of heterologous and homologous brain tissue with adjuvants. J. Exp. Med. **85**, 117—130 (1947).
98. Kabat, E. A., Wolf, A., Bezer, A. E.: Studies on acute disseminated encephalomyelitis produced experimentally in rhesus monkeys. III. J. Exp. Med. **88**, 417—425 (1948).
99. Kessler, D., Levine, L., Fasman, G.: Some conformational and immunological properties of a bovine brain acidic protein. Biochemistry **7**, 758—764 (1968).
100. Khan, A., Hill, J. M., Adachi, M.: L-Asparaginase in experimental auto-immune disease: Inhibition of allergic encephalomyelitis. J. Immunol. **105**, 256—258 (1970).
101. Kibler, R. F., Barnes, A. E.: Antibody studies in rabbit encephalomyelitis induced by a water-soluble protein fraction of rabbit cord. J. Exp. Med. **116**, 807—825 (1962).
102. Kibler, R. F., Fox, R. H., Shapira, R.: Isolation of a highly purified encephalitogenic protein from bovine cord. Nature **204**, 1273—1275 (1964).
103. Kibler, R. F., Re, P. K., McKneally, S., Shapira, R., Keeling, M. E.: Biological activity of an encephalitogenic fragment in the monkey. J. Biol. Chem. **247**, 969—972 (1972).
104. Kibler, R. F., Shapira, R.: Isolation and properties of an encephalitogenic protein from bovine, rabbit, and human central nervous system tissue. J. Biol. Chem. **243**, 281—286 (1968).
105. Kibler, R. F., Shapira, R., McKbeally, S., Jenkins, J., Seldon, P., Chou, F.: Encephalitogenic protein: Structure. Science **164**, 577—580 (1969).
106. Kies, M. W.: Chemical studies on an encephalitogenic protein from guinea pig brain. Ann. N. Y. Acad. Sci. **122**, 161—170 (1965).
107. Kies, M. W.: Panel discussion on species variability and multiple antigens in EAE. Summary statement. Ann. N. Y. Acad. Sci. **122**, 242—244 (1965).
108. Kies, M. W., Alvord, E. C., jr.: Prevention of allergic encephalomyelitis by prior injection of adjuvants. Nature **182**, 1106 (1958).
109. Kies, M. W., Alvord, E. C., jr. (Eds.): "Allergic" Encephalomyelitis. Springfield, Ill.: Ch. C. Thomas 1959.
110. Kies, M. W., Alvord, E. C., jr.: Encephalitogenic activity in guinea pigs of water-soluble protein fractions of nervous tissue. In: "Allergic" Encephalomyelitis (Kies, M. W., Alvord, E. C. jr., Eds.), p. 293—299. Springfield, Ill.: Ch. C. Thomas 1959.
111. Kies, M. W., Alvord, E. C., jr.: Multiplicity of encephalitogenic myelin basic proteins. I. Relative molecular sizes related to methods of preparation. Add. ad Intern Arch. Allergy Appl. Immunol. **36**, 182—202 (1969).
112. Kies, M. W., Alvord, E. C., jr., Martenson, R. E., Le Baron, F. N., Encephalitogenic activity of bovine basic proteins. Science **151**, 821—822 (1966).
113. Kies, M. W., Alvord, E. C., jr., Roboz, E.: The allergic encephalomyelitic activity of a collagen-like compound from bovine spinal cord—II. J. Neurochem. **2**, 261—264 (1958).
114. Kies, M. W., Alvord, E. C., jr., Roboz, E.: Production of experimental allergic encephalomyelitis in guinea pigs with fractions isolated from bovine spinal cord and killed tubercle bacilli. Nature **182**, 104—105 (1958).
115. Kies, M. W., Gordon, S., Laatsch, R. H., Alvord, E. C., jr.: Cellular localization of allergic encephalomyelitic activity in guinea pig brain. In: IV. International Congress for Neuropathology, Vol. 1 — Histochemistry and Biochemistry (Jacob, H., Ed.), p. 20—29. Stuttgart: G. Thieme 1962.
116. Kies, M. W., Laatsch, R. H., Silva, O. L., Alvord, E. C., jr.: Chemical and immunological studies on myelin from guinea pig brain. Z. Immunitätsforsch. **126**, 25—32 (1962).
117. Kies, M. W., Mueller, S., Alvord, E. C., jr.: Influence of ascorbic acid deficiency on immunologic mechanisms. Z. Immunitätsforsch. **126**, 228—233 (1962).

118. KIES, M. W., MURPHY, J. B., ALVORD, E. C. jr.: Fractionation of guinea pig brain proteins with encephalitogenic activity. Federation Proc. **19**, 207 (1960).
119. KIES, M. W., MURPHY, J. B., ALVORD, E. C., jr.: Studies on the encephalitogenic factor in guinea pig central nervous tissue. In: Chemical Pathology of the Nervous System (FOLCH-PI, J., Ed.), p. 197—204. London: Pergamon Press 1961.
120. KIES, M. W., THOMPSON, E. B., ALVORD, E. C., jr.: The relationship of myelin proteins to experimental allergic encephalomyelitis. Ann. N. Y. Acad. Sci. **122**, 148—160 (1965).
121. KLENK, E., GIELEN, W.: Über ein zweites hexosaminhaltiges Gangliosid aus Menschengehirn. Hoppe-Seylers Z. Physiol. Chem. **330**, 218—226 (1963).
122. KOPROWSKI, H., JERVIS, G. A.: Further studies in experimental allergic encephalomyelitis, in the guinea pig. Proc. Soc. Exp. Biol. Med. **69**, 472—476 (1948).
123. KOSINSKI, E., GRABAR, P.: Immunochemical studies of rat brain. J. Neurochem. **14**, 273—281 (1967).
124. KUHN, R., WIEGANDT, H., EGGE, H.: Structure of gangliosides. Angew. Chem. **73**, 580—581 (1961).
125. KUHN, R., WIEGANDT, H.: Constitution of ganglio-N-tetraose and the ganglioside, G_I. Chem. Ber. **96**, 866—890 (1963).
126. KUHN, R., WIEGANDT, H.: The constitution of the gangliosides G_{II}, G_{III}, and G_{IV}. Z. Naturforsch. **18b**, 541—543 (1963).
127. LAATSCH, R. H., KIES, M. W., GORDON, S., ALVORD, E. C., jr.: The encephalomyelitic activity of myelin isolated by ultracentrifugation. J. Exp. Med. **115**, 777—788 (1962).
128. LAMOUREUX, G., BORDUAS, A. G.: Immune studies in multiple sclerosis. Clin. Exp. Immunol. **1**, 363—376 (1966).
129. LAMOUREUX, G., CARNEGIE, P. R., MCPHERSON, T. A., JOHNSTON, D.: Experimental allergic encephalomyelitis: Immunological properties of encephalitogenic polypeptides and proteins. Clin. Exp. Immunol. **2**, 601—609 (1967).
130. LAMOUREUX, G., CARNEGIE, P. R., MCPHERSON, T. A., MACKAY, I. R., BERNARD, C.: Mécanisme d'action d'un polypeptide encéphalitogène dans l'induction de l'encéphalite allergique expérimentale. Ann. Inst. Pasteur **118**, 562—574 (1970).
131. LAMOUREUX, G., MCPHERSON, T. A., CARNEGIE, P. R.: Attempts to transfer experimental allergic encephalomyelitis in guinea-pigs in lymph node fragments in millipore chambers. Clin. Exp. Immunol. **2**, 253—255 (1967).
132. LAMOUREUX, G., MCPHERSON, T. A., CARNEGIE, P. R., MACKAY, I. R.: Lymph node localization and whole body distribution of radioiodinated encephalitogenic polypeptide in guinea-pigs. Clin. Exp. Immunol. **3**, 25—35 (1968).
133. LATERRE, E. C., HEREMANS, J. F., CARBONARA, A.: Immunological comparison of some proteins found in cerebrospinal fluid, urine and extracts from brain and kidney. Clin. Chim. Acta **10**, 197—209 (1964).
134. LEES, M. B.: The solubility properties of proteolipids. Ann. N. Y. Acad. Sci. **122**, 116—128 (1965).
135. LEIBOWITZ, S., LESSOF, M. H., KENNEDY, L. A.: The effect of anti-lymphocyte serum on experimental allergic encephalomyelitis in the guinea-pig. Clin. Exp. Immunol. **3**, 753—760 (1968).
136. LENNON, V. A., WHITTINGHAM, S., CARNEGIE, P. R., MCPHERSON, T. A., MACKAY, I. R.: Detection of antibodies ot the basic protein of human myelin by radioimmunoassay and immunofluorescence. J. Immunol. **107**, 56—62 (1971).
137. LENNON, V. A., WILKS, A. V., CARNEGIE, P. R.: Immunologie properties of the main encephalitogenic peptide from the basic protein of human myelin. J. Immunol. **105**, 1223—1230 (1970).
138. LEVINE, S.: Allergic encephalomyelitis: Cellular transformation and vascular blockade. J. Neuropathol. Exp. Neurol. **29**, 6—20 (1970).
139. LEVINE, S.: Relationship of experimental allergic encephalomyelitis to human disease. In: Proc. Assoc. Res. Nerv. Ment. Dis., Vol. 49: Immunological Disorders of the Nervous System (ROWLAND, L. P., Ed.), p. 33—49. Baltimore: Williams & Wilkins 1971.
140. LEVINE, S., COCHRANE, C. G., CARPENTER, C. B., BEHAN, P. O.: Allergic encephalomyelitis: Effect of complement depletion with cobra venom. Proc. Soc. Exp. Biol. Med. **138**, 285—289 (1971).
141. LEVINE, S., HOENIG, E. M.: A new form of localized allergic encephalomyelitis featuring polymorphonuclear neutrophilic leukocytes. Am. J. Pathol. **64**, 13—30 (1971).

142. Levine, S., Hoenig, E. M., Kies, M. W.: Allergic encephalomyelitis: Prevention of cellular passive transfer by an encephalitogenic basic protein from myelin. Science **161**, 1155—1156 (1968).

143. Levine, S., Hoenig, E. M., Kies, M. W.: Allergic encephalomyelitis: Immunologically specific inhibition of cellular passive transfer by encephalitogenic basic proteins. Clin. Exp. Immunol. **6**, 503—517 (1970).

144. Levine, S., Hoenig, E. M., Wenk, E. J.: Altered distribution of lesions after repeated passive transfers of allergic encephalomyelitis. Proc. Soc. Exp. Biol. Med. **126**, 454—458 (1967).

145. Levine, S., Prineas, J., Scheinberg, L. C.: Allergic encephalomyelitis: Inhibition of cellular passive transfer by X-radiation. Proc. Soc. Exp. Biol. Med. **131**, 986—990 (1969).

146. Levine, S., Sowinski, R.: Reduction of allergic encephalomyelitis incubation period to five days. Am. J. Pathol. **56**, 97—109 (1969).

147. Levine, S., Sowinski, R.: Immunologic competence of the liver for production of allergic encephalomyelitis. Arch. Pathol. **87**, 223—227 (1969).

148. Levine, S., Sowinski, R.: Allergic encephalomyelitis: New form featuring polymorphonuclear leukocytes. Science **171**, 498—499 (1971).

149. Levine, S., Sowinski, R., Kies, M. W.: Treatment of experimental allergic encephalomyelitis with encephalitogenic basic proteins. Proc. Soc. Exp. Biol. Med. **139**, 506—510 (1972).

150. Levine, S., Sowinski, R., Hoenig, E. M., Gruenewald, R.: Allergic encephalomyelitis: Passive transfer across major histocompatibility barrier. Proc. Soc. Exp. Biol. Med. **135**, 596—572 (1970).

151. Levine, S., Strebel, R.: Allergic encephalomyelitis: Inhibition of cellular passive transfer by exogenous and endogenous steroids. Experientia **25**, 189—190 (1969).

152. Levine, S., Wenk, E. J.: Encephalitogenic potencies of nervous system tissues. Proc. Soc. Exp. Biol. Med. **114**, 220—222 (1963).

153. Levine, S., Wenk, E. J.: Allergic encephalomyelitis: Rapid induction without the use of adjuvants. Science **141**, 519—530 (1963).

154. Levine, S., Wenk, E. J.: Induction of experimental allergic encephalomyelitis in rats without the aid of adjuvant. Ann. N. Y. Acad. Sci. **122**, 209—226 (1965).

155. Levine, S., Wenk, E. J.: Rapid passive transfer of allergic encephalomyelitis. J. Immunol. **99**, 1277—1285 (1967).

156. Levine, S., Wenk, E. J., Devlin, H. B., Pieroni, R. E., Levine, L.: Hyperacute allergic encephalomyelitis: Adjuvant effect of pertussis vaccines and extracts. J. Immunol. **97**, 363—368 (1966).

157. Levine, S., Wenk, E. J., Harman, P. J., Hovde, C. A.: Encephalitogenicity of sicca cells. J. Amer. Med. Assoc. **203**, 155—156 (1968).

158. Levine, S., Wenk, E. J., Hoenig, E. M.: Passive transfer of allergic encephalomyelitis between inbred rat strains: Correlation with transplantation antigens. Transplantation **5**, 534—541 (1967).

159. Levine, S., Wenk, E. J., Kies, M. W., Alvord, E. C., jr.: Central nervous system tissue. Is it an immunologic adjuvant? Neurology **15**, 560—564 (1965).

160. Liakopoulu, A., MacPherson, C. F. C.: Purification of a species restricted rat brain organ antigen. Federation Proc. **26**, 753 (1967).

161. Liakopoulu, A., MacPherson, C. F. C.: Studies on brain antigens. IV. Isolation and partial characterization of a rat species-restricted antigen of nervous tissue (SRANT). J. Immunol. **105**, 512—520 (1970).

162. Lisak, R. P., Falk, G. A., Heinze, R. G., Kies, M. W.: Effect of methotrexate on specific prevention of experimental allergic encephalomyelitis (EAE). Federation Proc. **27**, 473 (1968).

163. Lisak, R. P., Heinze, R. G., Falk, G. A.,Kies,M. W.: Search for anti-encephalitogen antibody in human demyelinative diseases. Neurology **18**, 122—128 (1968).

164. Lisak, R. P., Heinze, R. G., Kies, M. W.: Relationships between antibodies and experimental allergic encephalomyelitis. III. Coprecipitation and radioautography of I-labeled antigen-antibody complexes for detection of antibodies to myelin basic protein. Intern. Arch. Allergy Appl. Immunol. **37**, 621—629 (1970).

165. Lisak, R. P., Heinze, R. G., Kies, M. W., Alvord, E. C., jr.: Antibodies to encephalitogenic basic protein in experimental allergic encephalomyelitis. Proc. Soc. Exp. Biol. **130**, 814—818 (1969).
166. Lumsden, C. E.: Experimental allergic encephalomyelitis. II. On the nature of the encephalitogenic agent. Brain **72**, 517—537 (1949).
167. MacPherson, C. F. C.: Changes in the concentrations of the γ_c-globulin and the γG-globulin of bovine cerebrospinal fluid with maturation. J. Immunol. **98**, 1039—1044 (1967).
168. MacPherson, C. F. C., Cosgrove, J. B. R.: Immunochemical evidence for a gamma globulin peculiar to a cerebrospinal fluid. Can. J. Biochem. Physiol. **39**, 1567—1574 (1961).
169. MacPherson, C. F. C., Liakopoulu, A.: Studies on brain antigens. I. Water soluble antigenic proteins of rat brain. J. Immunol. **97**, 450—457 (1966).
170. Martenson, R. E., Le Baron, F. N.: Studies on the acid-extractable proteins of bovine brain white matter. J. Neurochem. **13**, 1469—1480 (1966).
171. Martenson, R. E., Deibler, G. E., Kies, M. W.: Charge heterogeneity of highly basic proteins from brain. Federation Proc. **27**, 619 (1968).
172. McFarland, H. H.: Immunofluorescent study of circulating antibody in experimental allergic encephalomyelitis. Proc. Soc. Exp. Biol. Med. **133**, 1195—1200 (1970).
173. McPherson, T. A., Marchalonis, J. J., Lennon, V.: Binding of encephalitogenic basic protein by serum α-globulins. Immunology **19**, 929—932 (1970).
174. McPherson, T. A., Robson, G. S. M., Carnegie, P. R.: Is encephalitogenic basic protein in human cerebrospinal fluid? Intern. Arch. Allergy Appl. Immunol. **39**, 566—579 (1970).
175. Milgrom. F., Tuggac, M., Campbell, W. A., Witebsky, E.: Thermostable ethanol-insoluble antigens of brain. J. Immunol. **92**, 82—90 (1964).
176. Milgrom, F., Tuggac, Z. M., Campbell, W., Witebsky, E.: Thermostable brain-specific auto antigen. J. Immunol. **98**, 359—363 (1967).
177. Miller, H., Schapira, K.: Aetiological aspects of multiple sclerosis. Brit. Med. J. **1959 I**, 737—740.
178. Moore, B. W.: A soluble protein characteristic of the nervous system. Biochem. Biophys. Res. Commun. **19**, 729—744 (1965).
179. Moore, B. W., McGregor, D.: Chromatographic and electrophoretic fractionation of soluble protein of brain and liver. J. Biol. Chem. **240**, 1647—1653 (1965).
180. Morgan, I. M.: Allergic encephalomyelitis in monkeys in response to injection of normal monkey nervous tissue. J. Exp. Med. **85**, 131—140 (1947).
181. Mueller, P. S., Kies, M. W., Alvord, E. C., jr., Shaw, C. M.: Prevention of experimental allergic encephalomyelitis (EAE) by vitamin C deprivation. J. Exp. Med. **115**, 329—338 (1962).
182. Mueller, P., Kies, M. W., Alvord, E. C., jr., Yamamoto, R. S.: Effect of experimental allergic encephalomyelitis on guinea pig plasma lipid fractions. Proc. Soc. Exp. Biol. Med. **115**, 1095—1099 (1964).
183. Nakao, A., Davis, W. J., Einstein, E. R.: Basic proteins from the acidic extract of bovine spinal cord. I. Isolation and characterization. Biochim. Biophys. Acta **130**, 163—170 (1966).
184. Nakao, A., Davis, W. J., Einstein, E. R.: Basic proteins from the acidic extract of bovine spinal cord. II. Encephalitogenic, immunologic and structural interrelationships. Biochim. Biophys. Acta **130**, 171—179 (1966).
185. Nakao, A., Roboz-Einstein, E.: Chemical and immunochemical studies with a dialyzable encephalitogenic compound from bovine spinal cord. Ann. N. Y. Acad. Sci. **122**, 171—181 (1965).
186. Newbould, B. B.: Production of allergic encephalomyelitis in rats by injections of spinal cord adjuvant into the inguinal lymph nodes. Immunology **9**, 613—614 (1965).
187. Niedieck, B., Kuwert, E., Palacios, O., Drees, O.: Immunochemical and serological studies on the lipid hapten of myelin with relationship to experimental allergic encephalomyelitis (EAE). Ann. N. Y. Acad. Sci. **122**, 266—276 (1965).
188. Okada, S., O'Brien, J. S.: Tay-Sachs disease: Generalized absence of a beta-D-N-acetylhexosaminidase component. Science **165**, 698—700 (1969).
189. Olitsky, P. K., Tal, C.: Acute disseminated encephalomyelitis produced in mice by brain proteolipids. Proc. Soc. Exp. Biol. Med. **79**, 50—53 (1952).
190. Oshiro, Y., Eylar, E. H.: Allergic encephalomyelitis: Preparation of the encephalitogenic basic protein from bovine brain. Arch. Biochem. Biophys. **138**, 392—396 (1970).

191. PALMER, F. B., DAWSON, R. M. C.: The isolation and properties of experimental allergic encephalitogenic protein. Biochem. J. **111**, 629—636 (1969).

192. PASCAL, T. A., SAIFER, A.: Immunochemical studies of isolated human brain ganglioside components. J. Neurochem. **16**, 301—307 (1969).

193. PASCAL, T. A., SAIFER, A., GITLIN, J.: Immunochemical studies on normal and Tay-Sachs' brain gangliosides. Proc. Soc. Exp. Biol. Med. **121**, 739—743 (1966).

194. PASCAL, T. A., SAIFER, A., GITLIN, J.: Comparative studies of normal human and Tay-Sachs gangliosides — an immunochemical approach. In: Inborn Disorders of Sphingolipid Metabolism (ARONSON, S. M., VOLK, B. W., Eds.), p. 289—301. New York: Pergamon Press 1966.

195. PATERSON, P. Y.: Transfer of allergic encephalomyelitis in rats by means of lymph node cells. J. Exp. Med. **111**, 119—135 (1960).

196. PATERSON, P. Y.: Cells, antibodies and auto-immune disease. In: Cell-Bound Antibodies (AMOS, B., KOPROWSKI, H., Eds.), p. 101—105. Philadelphia: Wistar Institute Press 1963.

197. PATERSON, P. Y.: Experimental allergic encephalomyelitis and autoimmune disease. Advan. Immunol. **5**, 131—208 (1966).

198. PATERSON, P. Y.: Experimental autoimmune (allergic) encephalomyelitis. In: Textbook of Immunopathology, Vol. I (MIESCHER, P. A., MÜLLER-EBERHARD, H. J., Eds.), p. 132—149. New York: Grune and Stratton 1968.

199. PATERSON, P. Y.: Cyclophosphamide treatment of experimental allergic encephalomyelitis in Lewis rats. J. Immunol. **106**, 1473—1479 (1971).

200. PATERSON, P. Y., COIA, E. M., JACOBS, A. F.: Complement-fixing antibrain antibodies and allergic encephalomyelitis. I. Characterization of the antibodies. Ann. N. Y. Acad. Sci. **122**, 256—265 (1965).

201. PATERSON, P. Y., DROBISH, D. G.: Cyclophosphamide: Effect on experimental allergic encephalomyelitis in Lewis rats. Science **165**, 191—192 (1969).

202. PATERSON, P. Y., DROBISH, D. G., HANSON, M. A., JACOBS, A. F.: Induction of experimental allergic encephalomyelitis in Lewis rats. Intern. Arch. Allergy Appl. Immunol. **37**, 26—40 (1970).

203. PATERSON, P. Y., HANSON, M. A.: Studies of cyclophosphamide suppression of experimental allergic encephalomyelitis in Wistar rats. J. Immunol. **103** 795—803 (1969).

204. PATERSON, P. Y., HANSON, M. A.: Cyclophosphamide inhibition of experimental allergic encephalomyelitis and cellular transfer of the disease in Lewis rats. J. Immunol. **103**, 1311—1316 (1969).

205. PATERSON, P. Y., HANSON, M. A., GERNER, E. W.: Cyclophosphamide inhibition of experimental allergic encephalomyelitis in Wistar rats. Proc. Soc. Exp. Biol. Med. **124**, 928—932 (1967).

206. PATERSON, P. Y., HARWIN, S. M.: Suppression of allergic encephalomyelitis in rats by means of antibrain serum. J. Exp. Med. **117**, 755—774 (1963).

207. PATERSON, P. Y., STEELE, F. M.: Cerebrospinal fluid beta-glucuronidase activity in rabbits with experimental allergic encephalomyelitis. Clin. Exp. Immunol. **7**, 759—768 (1970).

208. POULIK, M. D.: Starch gel electrophoresis in a discontinuous system of buffers. Nature **180**, 1477—1479 (1957).

209. RAJAM, P. C., BOGOCH, S.: Brain antigens: Components of subfractions from human grey matter. Immunology **11**, 211—215 (1966).

210. RAJAM, P. C., GAUDREAU, C. J., GRADY, A., RUNDLETT, S. T.: Preparation, derivation and partial characterization of organ-specific antigens from human brain. Immunology **17**, 367—385 (1969).

211. RAJAM, P. C., GAUDREAU, C. J., GRADY, A., RUNDLETT, S. T.: Species distribution of ribonucleoprotein-derived brain antigens. Immunology **17**, 813—818 (1969).

212. RAPPORT, M. M., GRAF, G.: Immunological reactions of myelin in vitro. Ann. N. Y. Acad. Sci. **122**, 277—279 (1965).

213. RAUCH, H. C., EINSTEIN, E. R.: Immunogenicity of bovine encephalitogenic protein. Intern. Arch. Allergy Appl. Immunol. **36**, 376—386 (1969).

214. RAUCH, H. C., FERRARESI, R. W., RAFFEL, S., EINSTEIN, E. R.: Inhibition of in vitro cell migration in experimental allergic encephalomyelitis. J. Immunol. **102**, 1431—1436 (1969).

215. RICHARDSON, W. P., PATERSON, P. Y.: Temporal dissociation of experimental allergic encephalomyelitis transfer activity and γ-globulin staining of lymphoid cells from sensitized Lewis rats. J. Immunol. **105**, 1563—1564 (1970).

216. RICHARDSON, W. P., PATERSON, P. Y.: The effect of antisera against rat immunoglobulins on cellular transfer of experimental allergic encephalomyelitis in Lewis rats. Clin. Exp. Immunol. **6**, 337—354 (1970).

217. ROBERTSON, D. M., BLIGHT, R., LUMSDEN, C. E.: Dialyzable peptide as the causative factor in experimental 'allergic' encephalomyelitis. Nature **196**, 1005 (1962).

218. ROBOZ, E., HENDERSON, N.: Preparation and properties of water-soluble proteins from bovine cord with 'allergic' encephalomyelitic activity. In: "Allergic" Encephalomyelitis (KIES, M. W., ALVORD, E. C., jr., Eds.), p. 281—292. Springfield, Ill.: Ch. C. Thomas 1959.

219. ROBOZ, E., HENDERSON, N., KIES, M. W.: A collagen-like compound isolated from bovine spinal cord—I. J. Neurochem. **2**, 254—260 (1958).

220. ROBOZ-EINSTEIN, E., ROBERTSON, D. M., DICAPRIO, J. M., MOORE, W.: The isolation from bovine spinal cord of a homogeneous protein with encephalitogenic activity. J. Neurochem. **9**, 353—361 (1962).

221. SAIFER, A., GERSTENFELD, S.: Photometric determination of sialic acids in serum and cerebrospinal fluid with the thiobarbituric acid method. Clin. Chim. Acta **7**, 467—475 (1962).

222. SALVIN, S. B., LIAUW, H. L.: Immunologic unresponsiveness, immunity and enhancement in experimental allergic encephalomyelitis. J. Immunol. **101**, 33—42 (1968).

223. SCHWENTKER, F. F., RIVERS, T. M.: The antibody response of rabbits to injections of emulsions and extracts of homologous brain. J. Exp. Med. **60**, 559—574 (1934).

224. SEIL, F. J., FALK, G. A., KIES, M. W., ALVORD, E. C., jr.: The in vitro demyelinating activity of sera from guinea pig sensitized with whole CNS and with purified encephalitogen. Exp. Neurol. **22**, 545—555 (1968).

225. SHAPIRA, R., MCKNEALLY, S. S., CHOU, F., KIBLER, R. F.: Encephalitogenic fragment of myelin basic protein. Amino acid sequence of bovine, rabbit, guinea pig, monkey, and human fragment. J. Biol. Chem. **246**, 4630—4640 (1971).

226. SHAW, C.-M.: Facilitatory and inhibitory effects of phytohemagglutinin on experimental allergic encephalomyelitis in guinea pigs. J. Immunol. **102**, 63—68 (1969).

227. SHAW, C. M., ALVORD, E. C., jr., FAHLBERG, W. J., KIES, M. W.: Adjuvant-antigen relationships in the production of experimental 'allergic' encephalomyelitis in the guinea pig. J. Exp. Med. **115**, 169—179 (1962).

228. SHAW, C. M., ALVORD, E. C., jr., FAHLBERG, W. J., KIES, M. W.: Specificity of encephalitogen-induced inhibition of experimental 'allergic' encephalomyelitis in the guinea pig. J. Immunol. **89**, 54—61 (1962).

229. SHAW, C. M., ALVORD, E. C., jr., FAHLBERG, W. J., KIES, M. W.: Substitutes for the mycobacteria in Freund's adjuvants in the production of experimental 'allergic' encephalomyelitis in the guinea pig. J. Immunol. **92**, 28—40 (1964).

230. SHAW, C. M., ALVORD, E. C., jr., KAKU, J., KIES, M. W.: Correlation of experimental allergic encephalomyelitis with delayed-type skin sensitivity to specific homologous encephalitogen. Ann. N. Y. Acad. Sci. **122**, 318—331 (1965).

231. SHAW, C.-M., ALVORD, E. C., jr., KIES, M. W.: Straight chain hydrocarbons as substitutes for the oil in Freund's adjuvants in the production of experimental 'allergic' encephalomyelitis in the guinea pig. J. Immunol. **92**, 24—27 (1964).

232. SHAW, C.-M., FAHLBERG, W. J., KIES, M. W., ALVORD, E. C., jr.: Suppression of experimental 'allergic' encephalomyelitis in guinea pigs by encephalitogenic proteins extracted from homologous brain. J. Exp. Med. **111**, 171—180 (1960).

233. SHULMAN, S., MILGROM, F., SWANBORG, R. H.: Immunochemical studies of an organ-specific thermostable antigen of bovine brain. Immunology **16**, 25—33 (1969).

234. SMYTHIES, J. R., BENINGTON, F., MORIN, R. D.: Encephalitogenic protein: a β-pleated sheet conformation (102—120) yields a possible molecular form of a serotonin receptor. Experientia **28**, 24—24 (1972).

235. STEWART, J. A.: Subunit composition of the tissue specific bovine brain S-100 protein. Biochem. Biophys. Res. Commun. **46**, 1405—1410 (1972).

236. STONE, S. H.: Transfer of allergic encephalomyelitis by lymph node cells in inbred guinea pigs. Science **134**, 619—620 (1961).

237. STONE, S. H., LERNER, E. M., II: Chronic disseminated allergic encephalomyelitis in guinea pigs. Ann. N. Y. Acad. Sci. **122**, 227—241 (1964).

238. STONE, S. H., LERNER, E. M., II., Goode, J. H.: Adoptive autoimmune encephalomyelitis in inbred guinea pigs: Immunological and histological aspects. Science **159**, 995—997 (1968).
239. STONE, S. H., LERNER, E. M., II, GOODE, J. H., jr.: Acute and chronic autoimmune encephalomyelitis: Age, strain and sex dependency. The importance of the source of antigen. Proc. Soc. Exp. Biol. Med. **132**, 341—344 (1969).
240. STONE, S. H., LERNER, E. M., II, MYERS, R. E., NIEMANN, W. H.: Autoimmune encephalomyelitis and ocular lesions in monkeys sensitized during the neonatal period. Science **151**, 473—475 (1966).
241. SVENNERHOLM, L.: The chemical structure of normal human brain and Tay-Sachs gangliosides. Biochem. Biophys. Res. Commun. **9**, 436—441 (1962).
242. SVET-MOLDAVSKY, G. J., SVET-MOLDAVSKAYA, I. A., RAFFKINA, L. I.: Various types of acquired resistance to experimental allergic encephalomyelitis. Nature **184**, 1552—1553 (1959).
243. SWANBORG, R. H.: Immunologic response to altered encephalitogenic protein in guinea pigs. J. Immunol. **102**, 381—388 (1969).
244. SWANBORG, R. H.: The effect of selective modification of tryptophan, lysine and arginine residues of basic brain protein on encephalitogenic activity. J. Immunol. **105**, 865—871 (1970).
245. SWANBORG, R. H., AMESSE, L. S.: Experimental allergic encephalomyelitis: Species variability of the encephalitogenic determinant. J. Immunol. **107**, 281—283 (1971).
246. SWANBORG, R. H., RADZIALKOWSKI, C. B.: Enhanced immunogenicity of altered encephalitogenic protein. Infection and Immunity **2**, 676—678 (1970).
247. SWANBORG, R. H., SHULMAN, S.: Purification of an organ-specific thermostable antigen found in bovine brain. Immunology **19**, 31—39 (1970).
248. SWANBORG, R. H., SHULMAN, S., WITEBSKY, E.: Immunochemical studies of thermostable brain-specific antigen of brain. Federation Proc. **24**, 176 (1965).
249. THOMAS, L., PATERSON, P. Y., SMITHWICK, B.: Acute disseminated encephalomyelitis following immunization with homologous brain extracts. J. Exp. Med. **92**, 133—152 (1950).
250. THOMPSON, E. B., KIES, M. W.: Kinetics of myelin dialysis. Federation Proc. **23**, 228 (1964).
251. THOMPSON, E. B., KIES, M. W.: Current studies on the lipids and proteins of myelin. Ann. N. Y. Acad. Sci. **122**, 129—147 (1965).
252. THOMPSON, E. B., KIES, M. W., ALVORD, E. C., jr.: Isolation of an encephalitogenic phospholipid-protein complex by dialysis of myelin in organic solvents. Biochem. Biophys. Res. Commun. **13**, 198—204 (1963).
253. TOMASI, L. G., KORNGUTH, S. E.: Purification and partial characterization of a basic protein from pig brain. J. Biol. Chem. **242**, 4933—4938 (1967).
254. UYEMURA, K., TOBARI, C., HIRANO, S.: Purifications and properties of basic proteins in pig spinal cord and peripheral nerve. Biochim. Biophys. Acta **214**, 190—197 (1970).
255. VOGEL, C. L., DeVITA, V. T., LISAK, R. P., KIES, M. W.: Suppression of experimental allergic encephalomyelitis by NSC 82196, a new imidazole carboxamide derivative. Cancer Res. **29**, 2249—2253 (1969).
256. WAKSMAN, B. H.: Allergic encephalomyelitis in rats and rabbits pretreated with nervous tissue. J. Neuropathol. Exp. Neurol. **18**, 397—417 (1959).
247. WAKSMAN, B. H.: Experimental allergic encephalomyelitis and the 'autoallergic' diseases. Intern. Arch. Allergy Appl. Immunol. (Suppl.) **14**, 1—87 (1959).
258. WAKSMAN, B. H., MORRISON, L. R.: Tuberculin type sensitivity to spinal cord antigen in rabbits with isoallergic encephalomyelitis. J. Immunol. **66**, 421—444 (1951).
259. WAKSMAN, B. H., PORTER, H., LEES, M. B., ADAMS, R. D., FOLCH, J.: A study of the chemical nature of components of bovine white matter effective in producing allergic encephalomyelitis in the rabbit. J. Exp. Med. **100**, 451—471 (1954).
260. WARECKA, K., BAUER, H.: Studies on 'brain-specific' proteins in aqueous extracts of brain tissue. J. Neurochem. **14**, 783—787 (1967).
261. WASSERMAN, E., LEVINE, L.: Quantitative micro-complement fixation and its use in the study of antigenic structure by specific antigen-antibody inhibition. J. Immunol. **87**, 290—295 (1961).
262. WENDER, M., ZGORZALEWICZ, B., WROBLEWSKI, T.: Activation of amino acids in the brain during experimental allergic encephalomyelitis. Acta Neurol. Scand. **47**, 52—58 (1971).
263. WESTALL, F. C., ROBINSON, A. B., CACCAM, J., JACKSON, J., EYLAR, E. H.: Essential chemical requirements for induction of allergic encephalomyelitis. Nature **229**, 22—24 (1971).

264. WITEBSKY, E., STEINFELD, J.: Untersuchungen über spezifische Antigenfunktionen von Organen. I. Mitteilung. Z. Immunitätsforsch. **58**, 271—296 (1928).
265. WITZ, I., YAGI, Y., PRESSMAN, D.: Brain localizing activity of hetero and isoimmune sera directed against lymphocytic cells. Proc. Soc. Exp. Biol. Med. **130**, 928—930 (1969).
266. WOLFGRAM, F.: Macromolecular constituents of myelin. Ann. N. Y. Acad. Sci. **122**, 104—115 (1965).
267. YOKOYAMA, M., ROBOZ-EINSTEIN, E.: Immunochemical analysis of cerebrospinal fluid. Ann. N. Y. Acad. Sci. **122**, 439—454 (1965).
268. YOKOYAMA, M., TRAMS, E. G., BRADY, R. O.: Immunochemical studies with gangliosides. J. Immunol. **90**, 372—380 (1963).

Chapter 5. The Reproductive System

1. ADLER, H.: Über Autospermotoxine. Z. Immunitätsforsch. **3**, 447—450 (1909).
2. AHMED, U., SHULMAN, S.: Fractionation of the antigens of canine prostatic fluid. J. Immunol. **108**, 432—445 (1972).
3. ALBERS, H. J., NEVES E CASTRO, M.: The protein components of rat uterine fluid. Fertility Sterility **12**, 142—150 (1961).
4. AMANO, Y., BEHRMAN, S. J.: Immunochemical studies on human seminal plasma. II. Isolation and characterization of major antigens. Intern. J. Fertility **13**, 61—70 (1968).
5. ANDRADA, J. A., ANDRADA, E. C., WITEBSKY, E.: Experimental autoallergic orchitis in rhesus monkeys. Proc. Soc. Exp. Biol. Med. **130**, 1106—1113 (1969).
6. ANSBACHER, R.: Sperm-agglutinating and sperm-immobilizing antibodies in vasectomized men. Fertility Sterility **22**, 629—632 (1971).
7. ASHITAKA, Y., ISOJIMA, S., UKITA, H.: Mechanism of experimental sterility induced in guinea pigs by injection of homologous testis and sperm. I. Relationship between sterility and anaphylactic reaction of the uterus. Fertility Sterility **15**, 206—212 (1964).
8. ASHITAKA, Y., ISOJIMA, S., UKITA, H.: Mechanism of experimental sterility induced in guinea pigs by injection of homologous testis and sperm. II. Relationship between sterility and a sperm-immobilizing antibody. Fertility Sterility **15**, 213—221 (1964).
9. BANDHAUER, K.: Zum Problem der Antigeneigenschaften des menschlichen Samenplasmas. Wien. Med. Wochschr. **116**, 318—321(1966).
10. BARKA, T.: Studies of acid phosphatase. I. Electrophoretic separation of acid phosphatases of rat liver on polyacrylamide gels. J. Histochem. Cytochem. **9**, 542—547 (1961).
11. BARKA, T.: Studies on acid phosphatases. II. Chromatographic separation of acid phosphatases of rat liver. J. Histochem. Cytochem. **9**, 564—571 (1961).
12. BARNES, G., SHULMAN, S., GONDER, M. J., SOANES, W. A.: Further studies of the immunological properties of human prostatic fluid. J. Lab. Clin. Med. **66**, 741—749 (1965).
13. BARNES, G., SOANES, W. A., MAMROD, L., GONDER, M. J., SHULMAN, S.: Immunologic properties of human prostatic fluid. J. Lab. Clin. Med. **61**, 578—591 (1963).
14. BEDFORD, J. M.: Morphological changes in rabbit spermatozoa during passage through the epididymis. J. Reprod. Fertility **5**, 169—177 (1963).
15. BEDFORD, J. M.: Fine structure of the sperm head in ejaculate and uterine spermatozoa of the rabbit. J. Reprod. Fertility **7**, 221—228 (1964).
16. BEER, A. E., BILLINGHAM, R. E.: Immunobiology of mammalian reproduction. In: Advances in Immunology, Vol. 14 (DIXON, F. J., KUNKEL, H. G., Eds.), p. 1—84. New York: Academic Press 1971.
17. BEHRMAN, S. J., AMANO, Y.: Immunochemical studies on human seminal plasma. I. Antigenicity of seminal protein. Intern. J. Fertility **12**, 291—298 (1967).
18. BEHRMAN, S. J., BUETTNER-JANUSCH, J., HEGLAR, R., GERSHOWITZ, H., TEW, W. L.: ABO(H) blood incompatibility as a cause of infertility: A new concept. Am. J. Obstet. Gynecol. **79**, 847—855 (1960).
19. BEHRMAN, S. J., NAKAYAMA, M.: Antitestis antibody: Its inhibition of pregnancy. Fertility Sterility **16**, 37—44 (1965).

20. Behrman, S. J., Otani, Y.: Transvaginal immunization of the guinea pig with homologous testis and epididymal sperm. Intern. J. Fertility **8**, 829—834 (1963).

21. Bennett, D., Goldberg, E., Dunn, L. C., Boyse, E. A.: Serological detection of a cell-surface antigen specified by the T (Brachyury) mutant gene in the house mouse. Prod. Nat. Acad. Sci. U.S. **69**, 2076—2080 (1972).

22. Billingham, R. E.: Transplantation immunity and the maternal-fetal relation. New Engl. J. Med. **270**, 667—672, 720—725 (1964).

23. Billington, W. D.: The invasiveness of transplanted mouse trophoblast and the influence of immunological factors. J. Reprod. Fertility **10**, 343—352 (1965).

24. Billington, W. D., Kirby, D. R. S., Owen, J. J. T., Ritter, M. A., Burtonshaw, M. D., Evans, E. P., Ford, C. E., Gauld, I. K., McLaren, A.: Placental barrier of maternal cells. Nature **224**, 704—766 (1969).

25. Bishop, D. W.: Aspermatogenesis induced by testicular antigen uncombined with adjuvant. Proc. Soc. Exp. Biol. Med. **107**, 115—120 (1961).

26. Bishop, D. W., Carlson, G. L.: Immunologically induced aspermatogenesis in guinea pigs. Ann. N. Y. Acad. Sci. **124**, 247—266 (1965).

27. Bishop, D. W., Narbaitz, R., Lessof, M.: Induced aspermatogenesis in adult guinea pigs injected with testicular antigen and adjuvant in neonatal stages. Develop. Biol. **3**, 444—485 (1961).

28. Boettcher, B.: Human ABO blood group antigens on spermatozoa from secretors and non-secretors. J. Reprod. Fertility **9**, 267—268 (1965).

29. Boettcher, B.: Blood group antigens in seminal plasma, and the nature of human sperm-coating antigen. In: Immunology and Reproduction (Edwards, R. G., Ed.), p. 148—154. London: International Planned Parenthood Federation 1969.

30. Boettcher, B., Hay, J. H.: An investigation of a proposed mechanism for infertility based on ABO blood group incompatibility. Am. J. Obstet. Gynecol. **100**, 437—441 (1968).

31. Boursnell, J. C., Johnson, P., Zamora, J.: An electrophoretic and ultracentrifugal study of boar seminal plasma. Biochim. Biophys. Acta **63**, 374—381 (1962).

32. Bratanov, K.: Antibodies in the reproductive process in the female. In: Immunology and Reproduction (Edwards, R. G., Ed.), p. 175—189. London: International Planned Parenthood Federation 1969.

33. Bratanov, K., Dikov, V.: Über den Einfluß einiger Immunfaktoren bei Fortpflanzungsstörungen der landwirtschaftlichen Nutztiere. Fortpfl. Haust. **3**, 153—159 (1967).

34. Bratanov, K., Dikov, V., Popova, Y.: On the formation of auto-spermoantibodies in brood animals. Compt. Rend. Acad. Bulgare Sci. **17**, 1117—1119 (1964).

35. Brown, P. C., Glynn, L. E., Holborow, E. J.: The pathogenesis of experimental allergic orchitis in guinea-pigs. J. Pathol. Bacteriol. **86**, 505—520 (1963).

36. Brown, P. C., Glynn, L. E., Holborow, E. J.: The dual necessity for delayed hypersensitivity and circulating antibody in the pathogenesis of experimental allergic orchitis in guinea-pigs. Immunology **13**, 307—314 (1967).

37. Brown, P. C., Holborow, E. J., Glynn, L. E.: The aspermatogenic antigen in experimental allergic orchitis in guinea-pigs. Immunology **9**, 255—260 (1965).

38. Camba, R.: Contributo all'interpretazione del diagramma elettroforetico dello sperma umano. Minerva Med. **77**, 43—45 (1957).

39. Charny, C. W., Meranze, D. R.: Testicular biopsy. Further studies in male infertility. Surg. Gynecol. Obstet. **74**, 836—842 (1942).

40. Coelingh, J. P., Rozijn, T. H., Montfort, C. H.: Isolation and partial characterization of a basic protein from bovine sperm heads. Biochim. Biophys. Acta **188**, 353—356 (1969).

41. Coombs, R. R. A., Rümke, P., Edwards, R. G.: Immunoglobulin classes reactive with spermatozoa in the serum and seminal plasma of vasectomised and infertile men. In: Second International Symposium on Immunology of Reproduction, Varna, Bulgaria 1971 (Bratanov, K., Ed.), p. 354—359. Sofia: Bulgarian Academy of Sciences Press 1973.

42. Davajan, V., Kunitake, G.: Fractional in vivo and in vitro examination of postcoital cervical mucus in the human. Fertility Sterility **20**, 197—210 (1969).

43. Davajan, V., Nakamura, R., Kharma, K.: Spermatozoan transport in cervical mucus. Obstet. Gynecol. Survey **25**, 1—43 (1970).

44. Davajan, V., Nakamura, R. M., Mishell, D. R., jr.: A simplified technique for evaluation of the biophysical properties of cervical mucus. Am. J. Obstet. Gynecol. **209**, 1042—1048 (1971).

45. DESJARDINS, C., KIRTON, K. T., HAFS, H. D.: Some chemical, immunochemical and electrophoretic properties of bovine follicular fluid. J. Reprod. Fertility **11**, 237—244 (1966).
46. DUFOUR, D., GAGNON, P. M., TREMBLAY, A., PROULX, J., LEMIEUX, S.: Charactérisation des relations antigéniques et enzymatiques entre la prostate et l'urine humaine. Laval Med. **36**, 643—645 (1965).
47. DUFOUR, D., LAFONTAINE, A., LILLE, S.: Polymorphisme d'une urophosphatase humaine. Rev. Immunol. **29**, 411—415 (1965).
48. DUFOUR, D., TREMBLAY, A., LEMIEUX, S.: Différence de spécificité immunologique entre la phosphatase urinaire humaine mâle et femelle. Rev. Fr. Etudes Clin. Biol. **11**, 89—92 (1966).
49. DUKES, C. D., FRANKLIN, R. R.: Sperm agglutinins and human infertility: Female. Fertility Sterility **19**, 263—267 (1968).
50. DZIEMBOR, E., GRYSZKIEWICZ, J., OSTROWSKI, W.: The role of neuraminic acid in the stability and enzymic activity of acid phosphatase of the human prostate gland. Experientia **26**, 947—948 (1970).
51. DZIEMBOR, E., GRYSZKIEWICZ, J., OSTROWSKI, W.: Properties of neuraminidase-treated acid phosphatase of prostate. Acta Biochim. Polon. **18**, 419—431 (1971).
52. EDWARDS, R. G.: Immunological control of fertility in female mice. Nature **203**, 50—53 (1964).
53. EDWARDS, R. G.: Transmission of antibodies across membranes of the reproductive tracts. In: Immunology and Reproduction (EDWARDS, R. G., Ed.), p. 28—48. London: International Planned Parenthood Federation 1969.
54. EKBOM, K., WETTERDAL, B.: Paper-electrophoretic studies on human semen with special interest in the distribution of administered Zn^{64}. Scand. J. Clin. Lab. Invest. **13**, 396—401 (1961).
55. EYQUEM, A., JOUANNE, C., LANDREIN, S.: Contribution a l'étude des constituants antigéniques du plasma séminal humain. Ann. Inst. Pasteur **110**, 89—94 (1966).
56. EYQUEM, A., KRIEG, H.: Experimental autosensitization of the testis. Ann. N. Y. Acad. Sci. **124**, 270—278 (1965).
57. FEIGELSON, M. KAY, E.: Protein patterns of rabbit oviductal fluid. Biol. Reprod. **6**, 244—252 (1972).
58. FELTKAMP, T. E. W., KRUYFF, K., LADIGES, N. C. J. J., RÜMKE, P.: Autospermagglutinins: Immunofluorescent studies. Ann. N. Y. Acad. Sci. **124**, 702—708 (1965).
59. FJÄLLBRANT, B.: Immunoagglutination of sperm in cases of sterility. Acta Obstet. Gynecol. Scand. **44**, 474—490 (1965).
60. FJÄLLBRANT, B.: Serological studies of seminal antigens. Acta Path. Microbiol. Scand. **66**, 280 (1966).
61. FJÄLLBRANT, B.: Sperm agglutinins in sterile and fertile men. Acta Obstet. Gynecol. Scand. **47**, 89—101 (1968).
62. FJÄLLBRANT, B.: Interrelation between high levels of sperm antibodies, reduced penetration of cervical mucus by spermatozoa, and sterility in men. Acta Obstet. Gynecol. Scand. **47**, 102—118 (1968).
63. FJÄLLBRANT, B., OBRANT, O.: Clinical and seminal findings in men with sperm antibodies. Acta Obstet. Gynecol. Scand. **47**, 451—468 (1968).
64. FLOCKS, R. H., BANDHAUR, K., PATEL, C., BEGLEY, B. J.: Studies on spermagglutinating antibodies in antihuman prostate sera. J. Urol. **87**, 475—478 (1962).
65. FLOCKS, R. H., URICH, V. C., PATEL, C. A., OPITZ, J. M.: Studies on the antigenic properties of prostatic tissue. I. J. Urol. **84**, 134—143 (1960).
66. FRANKLIN, R. R., DUKES, C. D.: Antispermatozoal antibody and unexplained infertility. Am. J. Obstet. Gynecol. **89**, 6—9 (1964).
67. FRANKLIN, R. R., DUKES, C. D.: Further studies on spermagglutinating antibody and unexplained infertility. J. Am. Med. Assoc. **190**, 682—683 (1964).
68. FREUND, J., LIPTON, M. M., THOMPSON, G. E.: Aspermatogenesis in the guinea pig induced by testicular tissue and adjuvants. J. Exp. Med. **97**, 711—725 (1953).
69. FREUND, J., LIPTON, M. M., THOMPSON, G. E.: Impairment of spermatogenesis in the rat after cutaneous injection of tesicular suspension with complete adjuvant. Proc. Soc. Exp. Biol. Med. **87**, 408—411 (1954).
70. FREUND, J., MCDERMOTT, K.: Sensitization to horse serum by means of adjuvants. Proc. Soc. Exp. Biol. Med. **49**, 548—553 (1942).

71. FREUND, J., THOMPSON, G. E., LIPTON, M. M.: Aspermatogenesis, anaphylaxis, and cutaneous sensitization induced in the guinea pig by homologous testicular extract. J. Exp. Med. **101**, 591—603 (1955).

72. FREUND, M.: Collection and liquefaction of guinea pig semen. Proc. Soc. Exp. Biol. Med. **98**, 538—540 (1958).

73. FREUND, M.: Interrelationship among the characteristics of guinea pig semen collected by electro-ejaculation. J. Reprod. Fertility **19**, 383—403 (1969).

74. GADDUM, P., BLANDAU, R. J.: Proteolytic reaction of mammalian spermatozoa on gelatin membranes. Science **170**, 749—751 (1970).

75. GARNER, D. L., SALISBURY, G. W., GRAVES, C. N.: Electrophoretic fractionation of bovine acrosomal proteins and proteinase. Biol. Reprod. **4**, 93—100 (1971).

76. GERSHOWITZ, H., BEHRMAN, S. J., NEEL, J. V.: Hemagglutinins in uterine secretions. Science **128**, 719—720 (1958).

77. GIBBONS, R. A.: Chemical properties of two mucoids from bovine cervical mucin. Biochem. J. **73**, 209—217 (1959).

78. GIBBONS, R. A., GLOVER, F. A.: The physico-chemical properties of two mucoids from bovine cervical mucin. Biochem. J. **73**, 217—225 (1959).

79. GIBBONS, R. A., MATTNER, P.: Some aspects of the chemistry of cervical mucus. Intern. J. Fertility **11**, 366—372 (1966).

80. GRAY, S., HUGGINS, C.: Electrophoretic analysis of human semen. Proc. Soc. Exp. Biol. Med. **50**, 351—353 (1942).

81. GUSDON, JR., J. J. P.: Immunologic studies of the fetal allograft. Obstet. Gynecol. **37**, 192—204 (1971).

82. GUYER, M. F.: Studies on cytolysins. III. Experiments with spermatoxins. J. Exp. Zool. **35**, 207—223 (1922).

83. HALPERN, B. N., KY, T., ROBERT, B.: Clinical and immunological study of an exceptional case of reaginic type sensitization to human seminal fluid. Immunology **12**, 247—258 (1967).

84. HAMNER, C. E., WILLIAMS, W. L.: Composition of rabbit oviduct secretions. Fertility Sterility **16**, 170—175 (1965).

85. HEGLAR, R.: Relationship between follicular fluid, ABO(H) system, and infertility. Intern. J. Fertility **7**, 321—325 (1962).

86. HEKMAN, A., RÜMKE, P.: The specificity of the antigens of human seminal plasma with special reference to lactoferrin as spermatozoa-coating antigen. In: Immunology of Spermatozoa and Fertilization (BRATANOV, K., Ed.), p. 107—110. Sofia: Bulgarian Academy of Sciences Press 1969.

87. HEKMAN, A., RÜMKE, P.: The antigens of human seminal plasma. Fertility Sterility **20**, 312—323 (1969).

87a. HEKMAN, A., RÜMKE, P.: Auto- and iso-immunity against spermatozoa. In: Textbook of Immunopathology, 2nd ed. (MIESCHER, P. A., MÜLLER-EBERHARD, H. J., Eds.) London/New York: Grune and Stratton 1974, in press.

88. HEKMAN, A., SHULMAN, S.: Antibodies to spermatozoa. III. Responses in rabbits and guinea pigs to immunization with guinea pig sperm cells. Clin. Exp. Immunol. **9**, 147—160 (1971).

89. HEKTOEN, L., MANLY, L. S.: Specific precipitin reaction of semen. J. Infect. Diseases **32**, 167—171 (1923).

90. HENLE, W.: The specificity of some mammalian spermatozoa. J. Immunol. **34**, 324—336 (1938).

91. HENLE, W., HENLE, G.: Spermatozoal antibodies and fertility. II. Attempt to induce temporary sterility in female guinea pigs by active immunization against spermatozoa. J. Immunol. **38**, 105—115 (1940).

92. HENLE, W., HENLE, G., CHAMBERS, L. A.: Studies on the antigenic structure of some mammalian spermatozoa. J. Exp. Med. **68**, 335—352 (1938).

93. HERMANN, G.: Le plasma seminal. In: Analyse Immuno-Électrophorétique (GRABAR, P., BURTIN, P., Eds.), p. 271—275. Paris: Masson 1960.

94. HERRMANN, W. P.: Immunologische Charakterisierung der Aminopeptidasen im menschlichen Spermaplasma. Arch. Klin. Exp. Dermatol. **233**, 269—276 (1968).

95. HERRMANN, W. P.: Immunologische Charakterisierung menschlicher Spermaplasmaproteine. Andrologie **1**, 11—18 (1969).

96. HERRMANN, W. P., HERMANN, G.: Immunoelectrophoretic and chromatographic demonstration of IgG, IgA, and fragments of γ-globulin in the human seminal fluid. Intern. J. Fertility **14**, 211—215 (1969).
97. HERRMANN, W. P. HERMANN, G.: Purification of the specific seminal fluid 3.72 S protein. Fertility Sterility **20**, 521—525 (1969).
98. HERRMANN, W. P., SCHIRREN, C.: Immunoelektrophoretische Untersuchungen des menschlichen Spermaplasma. Z. Haut-Geschlechtskrankh. **34**, 134—140 (1961).
99. HOMBURGER, F., BERNFELD, P., TREGIER, A., GROSSMAN, M. S., HARPEL, P.: Endometrial secretions. Ann. N. Y. Acad. Sci. **106**, 683—691 (1963).
100. HUGGINS, C., NEAL, W.: Coagulation and liquefaction of semen. Proteolytic enzymes and citrate in prostatic fluid. J. Exp. Med. **76**, 527—542 (1942).
101. HUGGINS, C. SOMMER, J. L.: Quantitative studies of prostatic secretion. III. Simultaneous measurement of size and secretion of the canine prostate and the interaction of androgenic and estrogenic substances thereon. J. Exp. Med. **97**, 663—680 (1953).
102. HUGGINS, E., TALALAY, P.: Sodium phenolphthalein phosphate as a substrate for phosphatase test. J. Biol. Chem. **159**, 399—410 (1945).
103. HULKA, J. F., OMRAN, K. F.: The uterine cervix as a potential local antibody secretor. Am. J. Obstet. Gynecol. **104**, 440—442 (1969).
104. ISOJIMA, S.: Relationship between antibodies to spermatozoa and sterility in females. In: Immunology and Reproduction (EDWARDS, R. G., Ed.), p. 267—279. London: International Parenthood Federation 1969.
105. ISOJIMA, S., GRAHAM, R. M., GRAHAM, J. B.: Sterility in female guinea pigs induced by injection with testis. Science **129**, 44 (1958).
106. ISOJIMA, S., LI, T. S.: Stepwise appearance of sperm-specific antigens in rats and their disappearance after fertilization. Fertility Sterility **19**, 999—1008 (1968).
107. ISOJIMA, S., LI, T. S., ASHITAKA, Y.: Immunologic analysis of sperm-immobilizing factor found in sera of women with unexplained sterility. Am. J. Obstet. Gynecol. **101**, 677—683 (1968).
108. ISOJIMA, S., STEPUS, S.: Antigenicity of guinea pig testis and ovary. Intern. Arch. Allergy Appl. Immunol. **15**, 350—359 (1959).
109. ISOJIMA, S., TSUZUKU, O.: Problem of ABO blood group incompatibility and sterility: The effect of blood group antibody on spermatozoa. Am. J. Obstet. Gynecol. **102**, 204—306 (1968).
110. JAGODZINSKI, R. V., YANTORNO, C., SHULMAN, S.: An experimental system for the production of antibodies in response to cryosurgical procedures. Cryobiology **3**, 456—463 (1967).
111. JOHNSON, M. W.: Changes in the blood-testis barrier in the guinea pig in relation to histological damage following iso-immunization with testis. J. Reprod. Fertility **33**, 119—127 (1970).
111a. JOHNSON, M. H., HEKMAN, A., RÜMKE, P.: The male and female genital tracts in allergic disease. In: Clinical Aspects of Immunology, 3rd ed (GELL, P. G. H., COOMBS, R. R. A., Eds.). Philadelphia: F. A. Davis 1973, in press.
112. JUNGE, J. M., BLANDAU, R. J.: Studies on the electrophoretic properties of the cornual fluids of rats in heat. Fertility Sterility **9**, 353—367 (1958).
113. KATSH, S.: The contribution of the bacterial components of adjuvant in the induction of aspermatogenesis and in the sensitization of the ilea of guinea pigs. Intern. Arch. Allergy Appl. Immunol. **15**, 172—188 (1959).
114. KATSH, S.: Immunology, fertility, and infertility: A historical survey. Am. J. Obstet. Gynecol. **77**, 946—956 (1959).
115. KATSH, S.: Infertility in female guinea pigs induced by injection of homologous sperm. Am. J. Obstet. Gynecol. **78**, 276—278 (1959).
116. KATSH, S.: Adjuvants and aspermatogenesis in the guinea pig. Intern. Arch. Allergy Appl. Immunol. **24**, 319—331 (1964).
117. KATSH, S.: Immunological control of reproduction in experimental animals: Implications regarding human fertility and infertility. Ann. Allergy **24**, 615—620 (1966).
118. KATSH, S., AGUIRRE, A.: Biochemical responses in organs of guinea pigs immunized with aspermatogenic antigen. Intern. Arch. Allergy Appl. Immunol. **33**, 141—150 (1968).
119. KATSH, S., AGUIRRE, A., KATSH, G. F.: Inactivation of sperm antigens by sera and tissues of the female reproductive tract. Fertility Sterility **19**, 740—747 (1968).

120. KATSH, S., BISHOP, D.: The effects of homologous testicular and brain and heterologous testicular homogenates combined with adjuvant upon the testes of guinea-pigs. J. Embryol. Exp. Morphol. **6**, 94—104 (1958).

212. KATSH, S., CROWLE, A. J., KATSH, G. F.: Non-mycobacterial adjuvant which mediates experimental aspermatogenesis. Nature **212**, 1486—1487 (1966).

122. KENNEDY, W. P.: The production of spermatoxins. Quart. J. Exp. Physiol. **14**, 279—283 (1924).

123. KIBRICK, S., BELDING, D. L., MERRILL, B.: Methods for the detection of antibodies against mammalian spermatozoa. I. A modified macroscopic agglutination test. Fertility Sterility **3**, 419—429 (1952).

124. KIBRICK, S., BELDING, D. L., MERRILL, B.: Methods for the detection of antibodies against mammalian spermatozoa. II. A gelatin agglutination test. Fertility Sterility **3**, 430—438 (1952).

125. KIDDY, C. A., STONE, W. H., TYLER, W. J., CASIDA, L. E.: Immunologic studies on fertility and sterility. III. Effect of isoimmunization with blood semen on fertility in cattle. J. Dairy Sci. **42**, 100—109 (1959).

126. KIRKPATRICK, C. H., KATSH, S.: Amino-acid content of antispermatogenic antigen. Nature **201**, 197—198 (1964).

127. KLOPSTOCK, A., HAAS, R., RIMON, A.: Immunoelectrophoretic analysis of seminal plasma. Fertility Sterility **14**, 530—534 (1963).

128. KRIEG, H.: Effects of blood group differences between parents on fertility and embryonic development. In: Immunology and Reproduction (EDWARDS, R. G., Ed.), p. 234—242. London: International Planned Parenthood Federation 1969.

129. KUNITAKE, G. M., NAKAMURA, R. M., WELLS, B. C., MOYER, D. L.: Studies on uterine fluid. I. Disc electrophoresis and disc-gel Ouchterlony analyses of rat uterine fluid. Fertility Sterility **16**, 120—124 (1965).

130. LANDSTEINER, K.: Zur Kenntnis der spezifisch auf Blutkörperchen wirkende Sera. Zentr. Bakteriol. Parasitenk. Abt. I (a) Ref. **25**, 546—549 (1899).

131. LANG, C. M.: A technique for the collection of semen from squirrel monkeys (Saimiri sciureus) by electro-ejaculation. Lab. Animal Care **17**, 218—221 (1967).

132. LARSON, B. L., GRAY, R. S., SALISBURY, G. W.: The proteins of bovine seminal plasma. II. Ultracentrifugal and immunological studies and comparison with blood and milk serum. J. Biol. Chem. **211**, 43—52 (1954).

133. LARSON, B. L., SALISBURY, G. W.: The proteins of bovine seminal plasma. I. Preliminary and electrophoretic studies. J. Biol. Chem. **206**, 741—749 (1954).

134. LAURENCE, K. A., CARPUK, O., PERLBACHS, M.: Transfer of testicular lesions by leukocytes from testes-immunized rats. Intern. J. Fertility **10**, 13—18 (1965).

135. LAURENCE, K. A., PERLBACHS, M.: Studies on the relationship of delayed hypersensitivity to experimental aspermatogenesis in rats. Bacteriol. Proc. **88**, 88 (1962).

136. LEVI, M.: Antigenicity of ovarian and cervical malignancies with a view toward possible immunodiagnosis. Am. J. Obstet. Gynecol. **109**, 689—698 (1971).

136a. LEVINE, B. B., SIRAGANIAN, R. P., SCHENKEIN, I.: Allergy to human seminal plasma. New Engl. J. Med. **288**, 894—896 (1973).

137. LEVINE, P.: Serological factors as possible causes in spontaneous abortions. J. Heredity **34**, 71—80 (1943).

138. LEVINE, P., CELANO, M. J.: The question of D (Rh_0) antigenic sites on human spermatozoa. Vox Sanguinis **6**, 720—723 (1961).

139. LEVINE, S., SOWINSKI, R.: Allergic inflammation, infarction and induced localization in the testis. Am. J. Pathol. **59**, 437—451 (1970).

140. LEWIS, J. H.: The antigenic relationship of the alcohol-soluble fractions of brain and testicle. J. Immunol. **27**, 473—478 (1934).

141. LI, T. S., BEHRMAN, S. J.: The sperm- and seminal plasma-specific antigens of human semen. Fertility Sterility **21**, 565—573 (1970).

142. LI, T. S., SHULMAN, S.: Immunoelectrophoretic analysis of human seminal plasma fractions after fractionation by various methods. Intern. J. Fertility **16**, 87—100 (1971).

143. LIPPES, J., ENDERS, R. G., PRAGAY, D., BARTHOLOMEW, W. R.: The collection and analysis of human fallopian tubal fluid. Contraception **5**, 85—103 (1972).

144. LIPPES, J., OGRA, S., TOMASI, T. B., JR., TOURVILLE, D. R.: Immunohistological localization of γG, γA, γM, secretory piece and lactoferrin in the human female genital tract. Contraception **1**, 163—183 (1970).
145. LIPPIELLO, L. A., EL-RUBAYE, F., WEIL, A. J.: Human spermatozoa-coating antigen. Studies on purification. Fertility Sterility **19**, 991—998 (1968).
146. LODGE, T. W., USHER, A.: Lewis blood group substances in seminal fluid. Vox Sanguinis **7**, 329—333 (1962).
147. LONDON, M., HUDSON, P. B.: Studies on the purification of acid prostatic phosphatase. Arch. Biochem. Biophys. **46**, 141—153 (1953).
148. LUNDQUIST, F.: Function of prostatic phosphatase. Nature **158**, 710—711 (1946).
149. MACALALAG, E. V., JR., PROUT, G. R., JR.: Anti-canine prostatic fluid serum and prostatic degeneration. Invest. Urol. **4**, 321—340 (1967).
150. MACALALAG, E. V., JR., PROUT, G. R., JR., DENIS, L. J.: Lactate dehydrogenase, its isozymes, and the canine prostate. Invest. Urol. **3**, 268—277 (1965).
151. MACKENZIE, A. R., HALL, T., LO, M-C., WHITMORE, W. F., JR.: Influence of castration and sex hormones on size, histology, and zinc content of canine prostate. J. Urol. **89**, 864—874 (1963).
152. MANARANG-PANGAN, S., MENGE, A. C.: Immunologic studies on human follicular fluid. Fertility Sterility **22**, 367—372 (1971).
153. MANCINI, R. E.: Cellular and subcellular aspects of allergic orchitis. In: Immunology and Reproduction (EDWARDS, R. G., Ed.), p. 49—54. London: International Planned Parenthood Federation 1969.
154. MANCINI, R. E., ANDRADA, J. A., SARACENI, D., BACHMANN, A. E., LAVIERI, J. C., NEMIROVSKY, M.: Immunological and testicular response in man sensitized with human testicular homogenate. J. Clin. Endocrinol. Metab. **25**, 859—875 (1965).
155. MANCINI, R. E., GUTIERREZ, O., FERNANDEZ-COLLAZO, E.: Immunohistochemical localization of antigens in human spermatozoa. Fertility Sterility **22**, 475—481 (1971).
156. MANCINI, R. E., MONASTIRSKY, R., FERNANDEZ-COLLAZO, E., SEIGUER, A. C., ALONSO, A.: Cytotoxic effect of antispermatic antibodies on guinea pig germinal cells in vitro. Fertility Sterility **20**, 779—798 (1969).
157. MANN, T.: The Biochemistry of Semen and of the Male Reproductive Tract. London: Metheun 1964.
158. MARUTA, H., MOYER, D. L.: Immunologic studies of the antigens of guinea pig semen. Fertility Sterility **18**, 649—658 (1967).
159. MASON, M. M., KEEFE, F., BORIA, T.: Specialized surgery of the canine bladder and prostate gland. J. Am. Vet. Med. Assoc. **139**, 1007—1014 (1961).
160. MASTROIANNI, L., JR., EHTESHAMZADEH, J.: Corona cell dispersing properties of rabbit tubal fluid. J. Reprod. Fertility **8**, 145—147 (1964).
161. MASTROIANNI, L., JR., MANSON, W. A., JR.: Collection of monkey semen by electroejaculation. Proc. Soc. Exp. Biol. Med. **112**, 1025—1027 (1963).
162. MASTROIANNI, L., JR., URZUA, M., STAMBAUGH, R.: Protein patterns in monkey oviductal fluid before and after ovulation. Fertility Sterility **21**, 817—820 (1970).
163. MATOUŠEK, J.: Effects on spermatogenesis in guinea-pigs, rabbits and sheep after their immunization with sexual organ fluids of bulls. J. Reprod. Fertility **19**, 63—72 (1969).
164. MATOUŠEK, J., SCHRÖFFEL, J.: Male sexual fraction in the sera of pigs and possible individual antigenic differences of some fluids of the genital tract in bulls. Folia Biol. (Prague) **10**, 30—35 (1964).
165. MATSUNAGA, E., ITOH, S.: Blood groups and fertility in a Japanese population, with special reference to intra-uterine selection due to maternal-foetal incompatibility. Ann. Hum. Genet. **22**, 111—131 (1958).
166. MATTILA, S.: Detection of two molecular forms of the human prostatic acid phosphatase. Invest. Urol. **6**, 337—344 (1969).
167. MATTILA, S.: Further studies on the prostatic tissue antigens; separation of two molecular forms of aminopeptidase. Invest. Urol. **7**, 1—9 (1969).
168. MCCARTNEY, J. L.: Further observations on the antigenic effects of semen. Mechanism of sterilization of female rat from injections of spermatozoa. Am. J. Physiol. **66**, 404—407 (1923).
169. MCCORMICK, J. N., FAULK, W. P., FOX, H., FUDENBERG, H. H.: Immunohistological and elution studies of the human placenta. J. Exp. Med. **133**, 1—18 (1971).

170. McLaren, A.: Immunological control of fertility in female mice. Nature **201**, 582—585 (1964).
171. McLaren, A.: Studies on the isoimmunization of mice with spermatozoa. Fertility Sterility **17**, 492—499 (1966).
172. Menge, A. C.: Induced infertility in cattle by isoimmunization with semen and testis. J. Reprod. Fertility **13**, 445—456 (1967).
173. Menge, A. C.: Fertilization, embryo and fetal survival rates in rabbits isoimmunized with semen, testis, and conceptus. Proc. Soc. Exp. Biol. Med. **127**, 1271—1275 (1968).
174. Menge, A. C.: Early embryo mortality in heifers isoimmunized with semen and conceptus. J. Reprod. Fertility **18**, 67—74 (1969).
175. Menge, A. C.: Immune reactions and infertility. J. Reprod. Fertility Suppl. **10**, 171—186 (1970).
176. Menge, A. C.: Survival of rabbit blastocysts after incubation with isoantisera against spermatozoa and seminal plasma. In: Immunology and Reproduction (Edwards, R. G., Ed.), p. 190—191. London: International Planned Parenthood Federation 1969.
177. Menge, A. C., Kiddy, C. A., Stone, W. H., Casida, L. E.: Immunological studies on fertility and sterility. V. Effect of antibodies against semen and erythrocytes on rabbit embryos. J. Reprod. Fertility **4**, 87—92 (1962).
178. Menge, A. C., Protzman, W. P.: Origin of the antigens in rabbit semen which induce antifertility antibodies. J. Reprod. Fertility **13**, 31—40 (1967).
179. Menge, A. C., Stone, W. H., Tyler, W. J., Casida, L. E.: Immunological studies on fertility and sterility. IV. Fertility of cattle and rabbits inseminated with semen treated with antibodies produced against semen, spermatozoa and erythrocytes. J. Reprod. Fertility **3**, 331—341 (1962).
180. Metalnikoff, S.: Études sur la spermotoxine. Ann. Inst. Pasteur **14**, 577—589 (1900).
181. Metchnikoff, E.: Études sur la résorption des cellules. Ann. Inst. Pasteur **13**, 737—770 (1899).
182. Milgrom, F., Tuggac, M., Witebsky, E.: Immunological studies on adrenal glands. III. Interspecies relations of thermostable adrenal-specific antigens. Immunology **6**, 105—118 (1963).
183. Milgrom, F., Tuggac, Z. M., Witebsky, E.: Thermostable organ specific antigens of bovine brain and testis. Federation Proc. **22**, 497 (1963).
184. Milgrom, F., Witebsky, E.: Immunological studies on adrenal glands. I. Immunization with adrenals of foreign species. Immunology **5**, 46—78 (1962).
185. Mischler, T. W., Reineke, E. P.: Some electrophoretic and immunological properties of human semen. J. Reprod. Fertility **12**, 125—129 (1966).
186. Moghissi, K. S.: Human fallopian tube fluid. I. Protein composition. Fertility Sterility **21**, 821—829 (1970).
187. Moghissi, K. A., Neuhaus, O. W.: Composition and properties of human cervical mucus. II. Immunoelectrophoretic studies of the proteins. Am. J. Obstet. Gynecol. **83**, 149—155 (1962).
188. Moghissi, K. A., Syner, F. N.: Studies on human cervical mucus: Mucoids and their relation to sperm penetration. Fertility Sterility **21**, 234—239 (1970).
189. Moghissi, K. A., Syner, F. N.: The effect of seminal protease on sperm migration through cervical mucus. Intern. J. Fertility **15**, 43—49 (1970).
190. Moncure, C. W., Prout, G. R., jr.: Antigenicity of human prostatic acid phosphatase. Cancer **25**, 463—467 (1970).
191. Moyer, D. L., Maruta, H.: Induced isoantibody to homologous seminal and spermatozoal antigens in female monkeys. Fertility Sterility **18**, 497—508 (1967).
192. Mudd, S.: A simple reaction for detecting the binding of agglutinins by difficultly agglutinable suspensions. J. Immunol. **13**, 113—121 (1927).
193. Mudd, S., Mudd, E. B. H.: The specificity of mammalian spermatozoa, with especial reference to electrophoresis as a means of serological differentiation. J. Immunol. **17**, 39—52 (1929).
194. Nakabayashi, N. T., Tyler, E. T., Tyler, A.: Immunologic aspects of human infertility. Fertility Sterility **12**, 544—550 (1961).
195. Odeblad, E.: Micro-NMR in high permanent magnetic fields: Theoretical and experimental investigations with an application to the secretions from single glandular units in the human uterine cervix. Acta Obstet. Gynecol. Scand. **45**, (Suppl. 2) 7—188 (1966).
196. Odeblad, E.: The functional structure of human cervical mucus. Acta Obstet. Gynecol. Scand. **47**, 57—79 (1968).
197. Odeblad, E.: Types of human cervical secretions. Acta Europ. Fertility **1**, 99—116 (1969).
198. Orsini, F., Shulman, S.: The antigens and autoantigens of the seminal vesicle. II. Immunochemical studies on rabbit vesicular fluid. In preparation.

199. OSSERMAN, E. F.: A modified technique of immunoelectrophoresis facilitating the identification of specific precipitin arcs. J. Immunol. **84**, 93—97 (1960).
200. OSTROWSKI, W., RYBARSKA, J.: Studies on human prostatic acid phosphomonoesterase. Further purification and molecular weight of the enzyme. Biochim. Biophys. Acta **105**, 196—198 (1965).
201. OSTROWSKI, W., WASYL, Z.: Stoke's radius and frictional ratio of human prostatic acid phosphatase. Biochim. Biophys. Acta **181**, 497—482 (1969).
202. OTANI, Y., BEHRMAN, S. J.: Immunization of the guinea pig with homologous testis and sperm. Fertility Sterility **14**, 456—467 (1963).
203. OTANI, Y., BEHRMAN, S. J., PORTER, C. W., NAKAYAMA, M.: Reduction of fertility in immunized guinea pigs. Intern. J. Fertility **8**, 835—837 (1963).
204. OTANI, Y., INO, H., KAGAMI, T.: Antigenicity of human semen, sperm and testis. Intern. J. Fertility **10**, 143—149 (1965).
205. OWNBY, C., SHIVERS, C. A.: Antigens of the hamster ovary and effects of anti-ovary serum on eggs. Biol. Reprod. **6**, 310—318 (1972).
206. PALM, J.: Maternal-fetal interactions and histocompatibility antigen polymorphisms. Transplantation Proc. **2**, 162—173 (1970).
207. PAOLELLA, A.: Electroforesi su carta di liquido seminale umano normale e patologico. Minerva Medicolegale **77**, 48—50 (1957).
208. PARISH, W. E., CARRON-BROWN, J. A., RICHARDS, C. B.: The detection of antibodies to spermatozoa and to blood group antigens in cervical mucus. J. Reprod. Fertility **13**, 469—483 (1967).
209. PAUFLER, S. K., FOOTE, R. H.: Sperm retention and resorption in sexually active rabbits with epididymal ligatures. Proc. Soc. Exp. Biol. Med. **131**, 1179—1183 (1969).
210. PEEL, S.: An immunologic study of dog prostate and the effects of injecting antidog prostate serum. Invest. Urol. **5**, 427—448 (1968).
211. PERNOT, E.: Recherches sur les constituants antigéniques des spermatozoides de cobayes. Bull. Soc. Chim. Biol. **38**, 1041—1054 (1956).
212. PERNOT, E., SZUMOWSKI, P.: Étude électrophorétique et immuno-électrophoretique des protéines du plasma séminal de taureau. Bull. Soc. Chim. Biol. **40**, 1423—1434 (1948).
213. PFEIFFER, L., ABLIN, R. J., GONDER, M. J., SOANES, W. A.: Antibodies to human prostatic acid phosphatase. Fertility Sterility **21**, 344—347 (1970).
214. PHADKE, A. M., PADUKONE, K.: Presence and significance of autoantibodies against spermatozoa in the blood of men with obstructed vas deferens. J. Reprod. Fertility **7**, 163—170 (1964).
215. PICADO, C., ROTTER, W.: Precipitines anti-testiculaires chez le pigeon male. Compt. Rend. Soc. Biol. **127**, 1096—1098 (1938).
216. POKORNÁ, Z.: Induction of autoimmune aspermatogenesis by non-cellular cytophilic material. Folia Biol. (Prague) **15**, 173—180 (1969).
217. POKORNÁ, Z.: Passive transfer of experimental autoimmune aspermatogenesis by noncellular cytophilic material in recipients treated with amethopterin. Folia Biol. (Prague) **16**, 222—224 (1970).
218. POKORNÁ, Z., VOJTÍŠKOVÁ, M., RYCHLÍKOVÁ, M., CHUTNÁ, J.: An isologous model of experimental autoimmune apsermatogenesis in mice. Folia Biol. (Prague) **9**, 203—209 (1963).
219. POPIVANOV, R., VULCHANOV, V. H.: Segretation of man's AB-group spermatozoa in A and B spermatozoa through agglutination with immune anti-A rabbit serum. Z. Immunitätsforsch. **124**, 206—210 (1962).
220. POPIVANOV, R., VULCHANOV, V. H.: Immunogenetics of human spermatozoa. In: Immunology and Reproduction (EDWARDS, R. G., Ed.), p. 155—167. London: International Planned Parenthood Federation 1969.
221. POPOVA, J.: Ultrastructural investigations of spermatozoa treated with desoxyribonuclease and ribonuclease. Compt. Rend. Acad. Bulgare Sci. **22**, 201—203 (1969).
222. QUINLIVAN, W. L. G.: Antigen-antibody reactions with human semen. Fertility Sterility **17**, 722—730 (1966).
223. QUINLIVAN, W. L. G.: The specific antigens of human seminal plasma. Fertility Sterility **20**, 58—66 (1969).
224. RABOCH, J.: Electrophoresis of seminal plasma proteins. Intern. J. Fertility **6**, 31—40 (1961).
225. RAITSINA, S. S., NILOVSKY, M. N.: Posttraumatic aspermatogenesis. Resemblance of pathogenesis of autoallergic and posttraumatic orchitis. Folia Biol. (Prague) **13**, 450—546 (1967).

226. RAO, S. S., SADRI, K. K.: Immunological studies with human semen and cervical mucus. In: Proceedings of the Sixth International Conference on Planned Parenthood, New Delhi 1959, p. 313—318. London: International Planned Parenthood Federation 1959.
227. RAO, S. S., SADRI, K. K.: The antigenic composition of buffalo semen. J. Comp. Pathol. Therap. **70**, 1—9 (1960).
228. RAO, S. S., SADRI, K. K., SHETH, A. R.: The antigenicity of human spermatozoa and its significance. In: The Proceedings of the Symposium on Proteins, August 1960, C.F.T.R.I., Mysore 1961, p. 1—8.
229. RAO, S. S. SHETH, A. R. SADRI, K. K.: Antigens of human spermatozoa. J. Reprod. Fertility **2**, 204 (1961).
230. RAPAPORT, F. T., SAMPATH, A., KANO, K., MCCLUSKEY, R. T., MILGROM, F.: Immunological effects of thermal injury. I. Inhibition of spermatogenesis in guinea pigs. J. Exp. Med. **130**, 1411—1425 (1969).
231. REID, B. L.: The behaviour of human sperm toward cultured fragments of human cervix uteri. Lancet **1964 I**, 21—23.
232. REINSTEIN, H., BENOTTI, N., MCBAY, A. J.: The demonstration of prostatic origin of seminal stain acid phosphatase. Am. J. Clin. Pathol. **39**, 583—585 (1963).
233. RIERA, C., YANTORNO, C., SHULMAN, S.: Antigenic specificity of seminal plasma and the formation of autoantibodies. Federation Proc. **26**, 532 (1967).
234. RINGLER, I.: Protein composition of rat uterine luminal fluid. Federation Proc. **15**, 152—153 (1956).
235. RINGLER, I.: The composition of rat uterine luminal fluid. Endocrinology **68**, 281—291 (1961).
236. ROBERTS, T. K., BOETTCHER, B.: Identification of human sperm-coating antigen. J. Reprod. Fertility **18**, 347—350 (1969).
237. ROSENKRANTZ, H., KIRDANI, E. S.: The proteolytic enzymes of canine prostatic fluid. Cancer Chemotherapy Rep. **15**, 9—16 (1961).
238. ROSENKRANTZ, H., LANGILLE, J.: A comparison of canine prostate and wheat germ acid phosphatase. Proc. Soc. Exp. Biol. Med. **108**, 417—419 (1961).
239. ROSENKRANTZ, H., LANGILLE, J., MASON, M. M.: The chemical analysis of normal canine prostatic fluid. Am. J. Vet. Res. **22**, 1057—1065 (1961).
240. ROSENKRANTZ, H., MASON, M. M.: The influence of hormones and pilocarpine on biochemical constituents of canine prostatic fluid. Cancer Chemotherapy Rep. **12**, 143—151 (1961).
241. ROSS, V.: Precipitin-reactions of human seminal plasma. J. Immunol. **52**, 87—96 (1946).
242. ROSS, V., MILLER, E. G., JR., MOORE, D. H., SIKORSKI, H.: Electrophoretic patterns of seminal plasma from some 'abnormal' human semens. Proc. Soc. Exp. Biol. Med. **54**, 179—181 (1943).
243. ROSS, V., MOORE, D. H., MILLER, E. G., JR.: Proteins of human seminal plasma. J. Biol. Chem. **144**, 667—677 (1942).
244. ROZIN, S., GRAFF, E., SHAFRIR, E.: Electrophoretic resolution and characterization of human seminal plasma proteins. Intern. J. Fertility **8**, 523—530 (1963).
245. RÜMKE, P.: The presence of sperm antibodies in the serum of two patients with oligozoospermia. Vox Sanguinis **4**, 135—140 (1954).
246. RÜMKE, P.: Auto-antibodies against spermatozoa in sterile men. In: Immunopathology First International Symposium, Basel/Seelisberg 1958, p. 145—153. Basel: Benno Schwabe 1959.
247. RÜMKE, P.: Autospermagglutinins: A cause of infertility in men. Ann. N.Y. Acad. Sci. **124**, 696—701 (1965).
248. RÜMKE, P.: Clinical aspects of autoimmunity to spermatozoa in men. In: Immunology and Reproduction (EDWARDS, R. G., Ed.), p. 251—266. London: International Planned Parenthood Federation 1969.
249. RÜMKE, P.: The spermatozoa and testes in allergic disease. In: Clinical Aspects of Immunology, 2nd ed. (GELL, P. G. H., COOMBS, R. R. A., Eds.), p. 1143—1159. Philadelphia: F. A. Davis 1968.
250. RÜMKE, P.: Sperm-agglutinating autoantibodies in relation to male infertility. Proc. Roy. Soc. Med. **61**, 275—278 (1968).
251. RÜMKE, P.: Sperm antibodies and their action upon human spermatozoa. Ann. Inst. Pasteur **118**, 525—528 (1970).
252. RÜMKE, P.: Autoantibodies against spermatozoa in men. Ann. Inst. Pasteur **117**, 877—878 (1969).
253. RÜMKE, P.: Autoantibodies to sperm in man. In: Immunology of Spermatozoa and Fertilization (BRATANOV, K., Ed.), p. 179—185. Sofia: Bulgarian Academy of Sciences Press 1969.

254. RÜMKE, P.: Autoantikörperbildung gegen Spermatozoen infolge Extravasation von Spermatozoen ins Interstitium der Epididymis älterer Männer. Schweiz. Med. Wochschr. **101**, 1439—1441 (1971).
255. RÜMKE, P., HELLINGA, G.: Autoantibodies against spermatozoa in sterile men. Am. J. Clin. Pathol. **32**, 357—363 (1959).
256. RÜMKE, P., TITUS, M.: Spermagglutinin formation in male rats by subcutaneously injected syngeneic epididymal spermatozoa and by vasoligation or vasectomy. J. Reprod. Fertility **21**, 69—79 (1970).
257. SCHNEIDER, W.: Neue Gesichtspunkte der Spermaelektrophorese. Symp. Deut. Ges. Endokrinol. **2**, 200—204 (1955).
258. SCHUMACHER, G. F. B.: Protein analysis of secretions of the female genital tract. J. Reprod. Med. **1**, 61—87 (1968).
259. SCHUMACHER, G. F. B., PEARL, M. J.: Cyclic changes of muramidase (lysozyme) in cervical mucus. J. Reprod. Med. **3**, 105—112 (1969).
260. SCHUMACHER, G. F. B., STRAUSS, E. K., WIED, G. L.: Serum proteins in cervical mucus. Am. J. Obstet. Gynecol. **91**, 1035—1049 (1965).
261. SCHWIMMER, W. B., USTAY, K. A., BEHRMAN, S. J.: An evaluation of immunologic factors of infertility. Fertility Sterility **18**, 167—180 (1967).
262. SEARCY, R. L., CRAIG, R. G., BERGQUIST, L. M.: Immunochemical properties of normal and pathological seminal plasma. Fertility Sterility **15**, 1—8 (1964).
263. SHIVERS, C. A., METZ, C. B., LUTWAK-MANN, C.: Some properties of pig follicular fluid. J. Reprod. Fertility **8**, 115—120 (1964).
264. SHULMAN, S.: Antibodies, autoantibodies, and the prostate gland. Bull. Millard Fillmore Hosp. **13**, 77 97 (1966).
265. SHULMAN, S.: Cryo-immunology and autoantibodies. J. St. Barnabas Med. Center **4**, 308—313 (1967).
266. SHULMAN, S.: Cryosurgery and cryo-immunology. Bull. Millard Fillmore Hosp. **14**, 87—95 (1967).
267. SHULMAN, S.: Cryo-immunology: The production of antibodies by the freezing of tissue. In: Cryosurgery (RAND, R. W., RINFRET, A. P., VON LEDEN, H., Eds.), p. 78—91. Springfield/Ill.: Ch. C. Thomas 1968.
268. SHULMAN, S.: Experimental cryosurgery and antibody response. J. Cryosurg. **2**, 90—96 (1969).
269. SHULMAN, S.: Antigenic analysis of the male tract. In: Immunology and Reproduction (EDWARDS, R. G., Ed.), p. 111—135. London: International Planned Parenthood Federation 1969.
270. SHULMAN, S.: Les autoantigènes de la vésicule séminale. Ann. Inst. Pasteur **118**, 529—538 (1970).
271. SHULMAN, S.: Antigenität und Autoimmunität bei der geschlechtlichen Fortpflanzung. Deut. Ärzteblatt **67**, 3342—3347 (1970).
272. SHULMAN, S.: Antigenicity and autoimmunity in sexual reproduction: A review. Clin. Exp. Immunol. **9**, 267—288 (1971).
273. SHULMAN, S.: Sperm antibodies as a cause of infertility. CRC Crit. Rev. Clin. Lab. Sci. **2**, 393—460 (1971).
274. SHULMAN, S.: Immunity and infertility: A review. Contraception **4**, 135—154 (1971).
275. SHULMAN, S.: Immunologic barriers to fertility. Obstet. Gynecol. Survey **27**, 553—606 (1972).
276. SHULMAN, S.: Agglutination of spermatozoa. In: Methods in Immunology and Immunochemistry, Vol. 4 (WILLIAMS, C. A., CHASE, M. W., Eds.). New York: Academic Press 1974.
276a. SHULMAN, S.: Sterilization, antibodies, and autoimmunity, In: Second International Conference on Sterilization (LUBELL, I., SCHIMA, M., Eds.). Amsterdam: Excerpta Medica 1974, in press.
276b. SHULMAN, S.: Antibodies to spermatozoa. IV. Human spermagglutinating activity in different tests with variation in semen source. Am. J. Obstet. Gynecol. **117**, 233—239 (1973).
276c. SHULMAN, S.: Sperm antibodies as a cause of problems in infertility and in vasectomy. In: First International Congress on Immunology in Obstetrics and Gynaecology (CENTARO, A., CARRETTI, N., ADDISON, G. M., Eds.). Amsterdam: Excerpta Medica 1974, in press.
276d. SHULMAN, S.: Sperm antibodies in the serum and cervical mucus of women. In: First International Congress on Immunology in Obstetrics and Gynaecology (CENTARO, A., CARRETTI, N., ADDISON, G. M., Eds.) .Amsterdam: Excerpta Medica 1974, in press.
277. SHULMAN, S., AHMED, U.: Prostate antigens and antibodies. Proc. Soc. Exp. Biol. Med. **137**, 97—100 (1971).

278. SHULMAN, S., BRANDT, E. J., YANTORNO, C.: Studies in cryo-immunology. II. Tissue specificity of the antibody response and comparison to isoimmunization. Immunology **14**, 149—158 (1968).

279. SHULMAN, S., BRONSON, P.: Immunochemical studies on human seminal plasma. I. Changes in composition during storage, as demonstrated by electrophoresis. Fertility Sterility **19**, 549—561 (1968).

280. SHULMAN, S., BRONSON, P.: Immunochemical studies on human seminal plasma. II. The major antigens and their fractionation. J. Reprod. Fertility **18**, 481—491 (1969).

281. SHULMAN, S., BRONSON, P., GONDER, M. J., SOANES, W. A.: Ultracentrifugal constituents of human and canine prostatic fluid. Nature **197**, 58—60 (1968).

282. SHULMAN, S., BRONSON, P., RIERA, C., BRANDT, E. J., YANTORNO, C.: Studies in cryo-immunology. III. The immunoglobulin nature of the antibody response. Immunology **14**, 541—551 (1968).

283. SHULMAN, S., FERBER, J.: Multiple forms of prostatic acid phosphatase. J. Reprod. Fertility **11**, 295—297 (1966).

283a. SHULMAN, S., FRIEDMAN, M. R.: Antibodies to spermatozoa. V. Antibody activity in human reproductive tissue. (in preparation).

284. SHULMAN, S., HEKMAN, A.: Antibodies to spermatozoa. I. A new macroscopic agglutination technic for their detection, using immotile sperm. Clin. Exp. Immunol. **9**, 137—146 (1971).

285. SHULMAN, S., HEKMAN, A., PANN, C.: Antibodies to spermatozoa. II. Spermagglutination technics for guinea pig and human cells. J. Reprod. Fertility **27**, 31—41 (1971).

286. SHULMAN, S., LEWIN, E., MYERS, S.: Sperm agglutinins in diverse patients with unexplained infertility. Federation Proc. **31**, 761 Abs. (1972).

287. SHULMAN, S., LI, T. S.: The analysis of the antigens of human seminal plasma. In: Second International Symposium on Immunology of Reproduction, Varna, Bulgaria, 1971 (BRATANOV, K., Ed.). p. 133—142. Sofia: Bulgarian Academy of Sciences Press 1973.

288. SHULMAN, S., MAMROD, L., GONDER, M. J., SOANES, W. A.: The detection of prostatic acid phosphatase by antibody reactions in gel diffusion. J. Immunol. **93**, 474—480 (1964).

289. SHULMAN, S., MAMROD, L., LANG, R., GONDER, M. J. SOANES, W. A.: Measurement of prostatic acid phosphatase by gel diffusion methods. J. Reprod. Fertility **10**, 55—60 (1965).

290. SHULMAN, S., MENNINGER, F., JR.: Electrophoretic analysis of human prostatic fluid by means of cellulose acetate membranes. I. The method and special problems. In preparation.

291. SHULMAN, S., MILGROM, F., WITEBSKY, E.: Immunological studies on adrenal glands. IV. Chemical studies on the bovine thermostable adrenal-specific antigen. Immunology **7**, 605—615 (1964).

292. SHULMAN, S., ORSINI, F.: The antigens of seminal vesicle and seminal plasma. Fertility Sterility **21**, 794—801 (1970).

293. SHULMAN, S., ORSINI, F.: The antigens and autoantigens of the seminal vesicle. I. Immunochemical studies on guinea pig vesicular fluid. J. Exp. Med. **134**, 120—140 (1971).

294. SHULMAN, S., RIERA, C., YANTORNO, C.: Studies on organ specificity. XIX. Antigenic specificity of seminal plasma and the formation of autoantibodies. J. Immunol. **100**, 682—688 (1968).

295. SHULMAN, S., SHULMAN, J. F.: Spermagglutinating activity in man and guinea pig. Fertility Sterility **22**, 633—638 (1971).

296. SHULMAN, S., SHULMAN, J. F., LEWIN, E.: Sperm antigens and human antibodies. In: Second International Symposium on Immunology of Reproduction, Varna, Bulgaria 1971 (BRATANOV, K., Ed.). p. 325—331. Sofia: Bulgarian Academy of Sciences Press 1973.

297. SHULMAN, S., YANTORNO, C., BARNES, G. W., GONDER, M. J., SOANES, W. A., WITEBSKY, E.: Studies on autosensitization to prostatic tissue and related tissues. Ann. N.Y. Acad. Sci. **124**, 279—291 (1965).

298. SHULMAN, S., YANTORNO, C., BRONSON, P.: Cryo-immunology: A method of immunization to autologous tissue. Proc. Soc. Exp. Biol. Med. **126**, 658—661 (1967).

299. SHULMAN, S., YANTORNO, C., SOANES, W. A., GONDER, M. J., WITEBSKY, E.: Studies on organ specificity. XVI. Urogenital tissues and autoantibodies. Immunology **10**, 99—113 (1966).

300. SHULMAN, S., ZAPPI, E., AHMED, U., DAVIS, J.: Immunologic consequences of vasectomy. Contraception **5**, 269—278 (1972).

301. SHULMAN, S., ZAPPI, E.: Cryo-immunology: An aspect of cyrobiology. In: Cryogenics in Surgery (VON LEDEN, H., CAHAN, W., Eds.), p. 42—79. Flushing, N. Y.: Medical Examination Publishing 1972.

302. SIMMONS, R. L., RUSSELL, P. S.: The antigenicity of mouse trophoblast. Ann. N.Y. Acad. Sci. **99**, 717—732 (1962).

303. SNELL, G. D.: Antigenic differences between the sperm of different inbred strains of mice. Science **100**, 272—273 (1944).
304. SOANES, W. A., SHULMAN, S., MAMROD, L., BARNES, G. W., GONDER, M. J.: Electrophoretic analysis of prostatic fluid. Classification according to agar gel electrophoresis. Invest. Urol. **1**, 269—278 (1963).
305. SOKOLOVSKAYA, I. I., RESHETNIKOVA, N. M.: Investigations of immunobiological factors in fertilization and early development. In: Immunology and Reproduction (EDWARDS, R. G., Ed.), p. 192—204. London: International Planned Parenthood Federation 1969.
306. SOLISH, G. I.: Distribution of ABO isohaemagglutinins among fertile and infertile women. J. Reprod. Fertility **18**, 459—474 (1969).
307. SOLISH, G. I., GERSHOWITZ, H., BEHRMAN, S. J.: Occurrence and titer of isohemagglutinins in secretions of the human uterine cervix. Proc. Soc. Exp. Biol. Med. **108**, 645—649 (1961).
308. STAMBAUGH, R., NORIEGA, C., MASTROIANNI, L., JR.: Bicarbonate ion: The corona cell dispersing factor of rabbit tubal fluid. J. Reprod. Fertility **18**, 51—58 (1969).
309. STEVENS, K. M., FOST, C. A.: Sperm and antibody production in rabbits following immunization with sperm and semen. Proc. Soc. Exp. Biol. Med. **117**, 125—127 (1964).
310. STEVENS, K. M., FOST, C. A., BALOWS, A.: Circulating antibodies to human seminal plasma in man. J. Reprod. Fertility **10**, 137—139 (1965).
311. STEVENS, K. R., HAFS, H. D., HUNTER, A. G.: Immunochemical and electrophoretic properties of oestrous rabbit uterine fluid proteins obtained by uterine ligation. J. Reprod. Fertility **8**, 319—324 (1964).
312. STRAUS, E. K.: Occurrence of antibody in human vaginal mucus. Proc. Soc. Exp. Biol. Med. **106**, 617—621 (1961).
313. SUTHERLAND, J. M., LANDING, B. H.: Failure to demonstrate antibody to sperm in serum of prostitutes. Lancet **1961 II**, 56.
314. TOAFF, R., AYALON, D., NELKEN, D.: Blood group antibody titres in homospecific and heterospecific pregnancies. J. Reprod. Fertility **12**, 81—89 (1966).
315. TOURVILLE, D. R., OGRA, S. S., LIPPES, J., TOMASI, T. B., JR.: The human female reproductive tract: Immunohistological localization of γA, γG, γM, secretory "piece", and lactoferrin. Am. J. Obstet. Gynecol. **108**, 1102—1108 (1970).
316. TUNG, K. S. K., UNANUE, E. R., DIXON, F. J.: The immunopathology of experimental allergic orchitis. Am. J. Pathol. **60**, 313—324 (1970).
317. TUNG, K. S. K., UNANUE, E. R., DIXON, F. J.: Pathogenesis of experimental allergic orchitis. I. Transfer with immune lymph node cells. J. Immunol. **106**, 1453—1462 (1971).
318. TUNG, K. S. K., UNANUE, E. R., DIXON, F. J.: Pathogenesis of experimental allergic orchitis. II. The role of antibody. J. Immunol. **106**, 1463—1472 (1971).
319. TYLER, A.: Conversion of agglutinins and precipitins into 'univalent' (non-agglutinating or non-precipitating) antibodies by photodynamic irradiation of rabbit antisera vs. pneumococci, sheep-red-cells and sea-urchin sperm. J. Immunol. **51**, 157—172 (1945).
320. TYLER, A., TYLER, E. T., DENNY, P. C.: Concepts and experiments in immunoreproduction. Fertility Sterility **18**, 153—166 (1967).
321. UPHOFF, D. E.: Maternal modification of antigenicity: An immunologic mechanism to ensure survival of mammalian fetuses. J. Nat. Cancer Inst. **45**, 1189—1196 (1970).
322. URBACH, G. I.: Fetal-maternal-placenta immunologic relationship. Fertility Sterility **21**, 356—360 (1970).
323. URZUA, M. A., STAMBAUGH, R., FLICKINGER, G., MASTROIANNI, L.: Uterine and oviduct fluid protein patterns in the rabbit before and after ovulation. Fertility Sterility **21**, 860—865 (1970).
324. VALLOTTON, M. B., FORBES, A. P.: Antibodies to cytoplasm of ova. Lancet **1966 II**, 264—265.
325. VALLOTTON, M. B., FORBES, A. P.: Autoimmunity in gonadal dysgenesis and Klinefelter's syndrome. Lancet **1967 I**, 648—651.
326. VOISIN, G. A., DELAUNAY, A., BARBER, M.: Sur des lésions testiculaires provoquées chez le cobaye par iso- et autosensibilisation. Ann. Inst. Pasteur **81**, 48—63 (1951).
327. VOISIN, G. A., TOULLET, F.: Étude sur l'orchite aspermatogénétique autoimmune et les autoantigènes de spermatozoides chez le cobaye. Ann. Inst. Pasteur **114**, 727—755 (1968).
328. VOISIN, G. A., TOULLET, F.: Relation between hypersensitivity responses to autoantigens and tissue damage in the male reproductive tract. In: Immunology and Reproduction (EDWARDS, R. G., Ed.), p. 93—105. London: International Parenthood Federation 1969.

329. VOLKOVA, L. S., MAYSKY, I. N.: Immunological interaction between mother and embryo. In: Immunology and Reproduction (EDWARDS, R. G., Ed.), p. 211—230. London: International Planned Parenthood Federation 1969.

330. VULCHANOV, V. H.: Personal communication (1967).

331. VULCHANOV, V. H.: Testicular damage and autoantibody formation in guinea-pigs immunized with homologous seminal vesicular fluid. In: Immunology and Reproduction (EDWARDS, R. G., Ed.), p. 136—147. London: International Planned Parenthood Federation 1969.

332. WAKSMAN, B. H.: Experimental allergic encephalomyelitis and the 'autoallergic' diseases. Intern. Arch. Allergy Appl. Immunol. (Suppl.) **14**, 25—32 (1959).

333. WAKSMAN, B. H.: A histologic study of the autoallergic testis lesion in the guinea pig. J. Exp. Med. **109**, 311—324 (1959).

334. WALSH, L. S. N.: Natural auto and homoio spermotoxins in guinea-pig serum. J. Immunol. **10**, 803—809 (1925).

335. WEIL, A. J.: Immunological differentiation of epididymal and seminal spermatozoa of the rabbit. Science **131**, 1040—1041 (1960).

336. WEIL, A. J.: Antigens of the adnexal glands of the male genital tract. Fertility Sterility **12**, 538—543 (1961).

337. WEIL, A. J., FINKLER, A. E.: Antigens of rabbit semen. Proc. Soc. Exp. Biol. Med. **98**, 794—797 (1958).

338. WEIL, A. J., FINKLER, A. E.: Isoantigenicity of rabbit semen. Proc. Soc. Exp. Biol. Med. **102**, 624—626 (1959).

339. WEIL, A. J., HERMAN, J. R., GOLDBERG, A. S., RODENBURG, J. M.: Immunological and chemical studies of spermatocele fluid. J. Urol. **85**, 665—667 (1961).

340. WEIL, A. J., KOTSEVALOV, O., WILSON, L.: Antigens of human seminal plasma. Proc. Soc. Exp. Biol. Med. **92**, 606—610 (1956).

341. WEIL, A. J., RODENBURG, J. M.: Immunological differentiation of human testicular (spermatocele) and seminal spermatozoa. Proc. Soc. Exp. Biol. Med. **105**, 43—45 (1960).

342. WEIL, A. J., RODENBURG, J. M.: The seminal vesicle as the source of the spermatozoa-coating antigen of seminal plasma. Proc. Soc. Exp. Biol. Med. **109**, 567—570 (1962).

343. WEIL, A. J., STEFANOVIC, D.: Spermatozoa-coating antigen (SCA): Its persistence in the genital tract of female rabbits. Fertility Sterility **20**, 689—692 (1969).

344. WILLIAMS, W. L., POLAKOSKI, K. L., ZANEVELD, L. J. D.: Purification of a proteolytic enzyme from rabbit acrosomes. Biol. Reprod. **6**, 23—29 (1972).

345. WILLIAMS, W. L., ZANEVELD, L. J. D., POLAKOSKI, K. L.: Properties of a proteolytic enzyme from rabbit sperm acrosomes. Biol. Reprod. **6**, 30—39 (1972).

346. WILSON, L.: Sperm agglutinins in human semen and blood. Proc. Soc. Exp. Biol. Med. **85**, 652—655 (1954).

347. YANTORNO, C., DEBANNE, M. T., VOTTERO-CIMA, E.: Autoimmune orchitis induced by autoimmunization with seminal plasma in the rabbit. J. Reprod. Fertility **27**, 311—320 (1971).

348. YANTORNO, C., SHULMAN, S., GONDER, M. J., SOANES, W. A.: Studies in cryo-immunology. I. The production of antibodies to urogenital tissue in consequence of freezing treatment. Immunology **12**, 395—410 (1967).

349. YANTORNO, C., SHULMAN, S., GONDER, M. J., SOANES, W. A., WITEBSKY, E.: Studies on organ specificity. XVIII. Immunological and biophysical characterization of canine prostatic fluid. J. Immunol. **96**, 1035—1045 (1966).

350. ZAMBONI, L., HONGSANAND, C., MASTROIANNI, L., JR.: Influence of tubal secretions on rabbit tubal ova. Fertility Sterility **16**, 177—184 (1965).

351. ZAPPI, E., AHMED, U., DAVIS, J., SHULMAN, S.: Immunologic consequences of vasectomy. Federation Proc. **29**, 374 (1970).

352. ZAPPI, E., SHULMAN, S.: Sperm sedimentation patterns. A semi-micro method for evaluation of antibodies against spermatozoa. Intern. J. Fertility **16**, 75—86 (1971).

353. ZAPPI, E., SMITH, D. J., SHULMAN, S.: Preparative separation of rabbit seminal plasma and immunochemical study of the resulting fractions. Intern. J. Fertility **17**, 145—152 (1972).

354. ZIMMERMANN, H., KIPPING, D.: Erfahrungen mit der Immunoelektrophorese des Spermatoplasmas bei der Fertilitätsdiagnostik des Mannes. Dermatol. Wochschr. **153**, 945—949 (1967).

Chapter 6. The Eye

1. ALLANSMITH, M., HUTCHISON, D.: Immunoglobulins in the conjunctiva. Immunology **12**, 225—229 (1967).
2. ALLANSMITH, M., NEWMAN, L., WHITNEY, C.: The distribution of immunoglobulin in the rabbit eye. Arch. Ophthalmol. **86**, 60—64 (1971).
3. ALLANSMITH, M., NEWMAN, L., HUTCHISON, D.: Immunoglobulin G in the rabbit cornea. Arch. Ophthalmol. **82**, 229—231 (1969).

3a. ALLANSMITH, M. R., O'CONNOR, G. R.: Immunoglobulins: Structure, function and relation to the eye. Survey Ophthalmol. **14**, 367—402 (1970).

3b. ALLANSMITH, M. R., WHITNEY, C. R., MCCLELLAN, B. H., NEWMAN, L. P.: Immunoglobulins in the human eye. Arch. Ophthalmol. **89**, 36—45 (1973).

4. ARONSON, S. B.: The homoimmune uveitises in the guinea pig. Ann. N.Y. Acad. Sci. **124**, 365—376 (1965).
5. ARONSON, S. B.: Experimental allergic uveitis. Uveitis following immunization to homologous and heterologous uveal and retino-vitreous preparations. Arch. Ophthalmol. **80**, 235—242 (1968).
6. ARONSON, S. B.: Patterns in experimental uveitis. Arch. Ophthalmol. **79**, 490—501 (1968).
7. ARONSON, S. B.: Personal communication.
8. ARONSON, S. B., HOGAN, M. J., ZWEIGART, P.: Homoimmune uveitis in guinea pig. I. General concepts of auto- and homoimmunity, methods, and manifestations. Arch. Ophthalmol. **69**, 105—109 (1963).
9. ARONSON, S. B., HOGAN, M. J., ZWEIGART, P.: Homoimmune uveitis in guinea pig. II. Clinical manifestations. Arch. Ophthalmol. **69**, 203—207 (1963).
10. ARONSON, S. B., HOGAN, M. J., ZWEIGART, P.: Homoimmune uveitis in guinea pig. III. Histopathologic manifestations of disease. Arch. Ophthalmol. **69**, 208—219 (1963).
11. ARONSON, S. B., SCHNELLMANN, D. C., YAMAMOTO, E. A.: Uveal autoantibody in ocular disease. J. Am. Med. Assoc. **196**, 225—228 (1966).
12. ARONSON, S. B., YAMAMOTO, E., GOODNER, E. K., O'CONNOR, G. R.: The occurrence of an autoantiuveal antibody in human uveitis. Arch. Ophthalmol. **72**, 621—625 (1964).
13. ARONSON, S. B., ZWEIGART, P., PROCTOR, F. I.: Immunologic testing in homoimmune uveitis in the guinea pig. Am. J. Ophthalmol. **51**, 329—300 (1961).
14. AUGUSTEYN, R. C., SPECTOR, A.: α-Crystallin. Fractionation of subunits and sequence studies on an isolated polypeptide. Biochem. J. **124**, 345—355 (1971).
15. BASH, J. A., MILGROM, F., WITEBSKY, E.: Autoantibodies to vitreous body in sheep. Vox Sanguinis **18**, 190—192 (1970).

15a. BOURS, J., VAN DOORENMAALEN, W. J.: The presence of lens antigens in the intra-ocular tissues of the chick eye. Exp. Eye Res. **13**, 236—247 (1972).

16. BUCKLEY III, C. E., GILLS, J. P., JR.: Cyclophosphamide therapy of Behcet's disease. J. Allergy **43**, 273—283 (1969).
17. BURKE, V., SULLIVAN, N., PETERSEN, H., WEED, R.: Ontogenetic change in antigenic specificity of the organs of the chick. J. Infect. Diseases **74**, 223—233 (1944).
18. CLARK, R., ZIGMAN, S., LERMAN, S.: Studies on the structural proteins of the human lens. Exp. Eye Res. **8**, 172—182 (1969).
19. CLAYTON, R. M.: Localization of embryonic antigens by antisera labelled with fluorescent dyes. Nature **174**, 1059 (1954).
20. CLAYTON, R. M., CAMPBELL, J. C., TRUMAN, D. E. S.: A re-examination of the organ specificity of lens antigens. Exp. Eye Res. **7**, 11—29 (1968).
21. CLAYTON, R. M.: Properties of the crystallins of the chick in terms of their subunit composition. Exp. Eye Res. **8**, 326—339 (1969).

21a. COLLINS, R. C.: Experimental studies on sympathetic ophthalmia. Am. J. Ophthalmol. **32**, 1687—1699 (1949).

22. COOPER, W. C., HALBERT, S. P., MANSKI, W. J.: Immunochemical analysis of vitreous and subretinal fluid. Invest. Ophthalmol. **2**, 369—377 (1963).
23. CORRAN, P. H., WALEY, S. G.: Amino acid sequences around the cysteine residue of calf lens α-crystallin. Biochem. J. **124**, 61—68 (1971).
24. DENDUCHIS, B., KEFALIDES, N. A.: Immunochemistry of sheep anterior lens capsule. Biochim. Biophys. Acta **218**, 357—359 (1970).

25. duPree, A. L., Little, J., Langman, J.: Human lens proteins examined by immunochemical and ultracentrifugal techniques. Arch. Ophthalmol. **72**, 660—666 (1964).
26. Ehrlich, G., Halbert, S. P.: Cytotoxicity of anti-tissue antibodies. III. The embryological development of cell antigens involved in immune cytotoxicity (lens, cornea and heart). Intern. Arch. Allergy Appl. Immunol. **29**, 510—516 (1966).
27. Ehrlich, G., Halbert, S. P.: Cytotoxicity of anti-tissue antibodies. IV. Immunofluorescence studies. Intern. Arch. Allergy Appl. Immunol. **34**, 428—436 (1968).
28. Ehrlich, G., Halbert, S. P., Manski, W.: Cytotoxicity of anti-tissue antibodies. II. Effects of anti-lens sera in tissue culture. J. Immunol. **89**, 391—399 (1962).
29. Ehrlich, G., Halbert, S. P., Manski, W.: Immunological and biological comparison of anti-rabbit lens sera obtained by homologous and heterologous immunization. Federation Proc. **21**, 44 (1962).
30. Elschnig, A.: Studien zur sympathischen Ophthalmie. 2. Die antigene Wirkung des Augenpigmentes. Albrecht von Graefe's Arch. Ophthalmol. **76**, 509—546 (1910).
31. Elschnig, A., Salus, R.: Studien zur sympathischen Ophthalmie. IV. Die antigene Wirkung der Augenpigmente. Albrecht von Graefe's Arch. Ophthalmol. **79**, 428—441 (1911).
32. Epstein, W. V., Tan, M., Easterbrook, M.: Serum antibody to RNA and DNA in patients with uveitis. New Engl. J. Med. **285**, 1502—1506 (1971).
33. Flickinger, R. A., Stone, G.: Localization of lens antigens in developing frog embryos. Exp. Cell Res. **21**, 541—547 (1960).
34. François, J., Rabaey, M.: Agar microelectrophoresis at high tension of soluble lens proteins. Arch. Ophthalmol. **61**, 351—360 (1959).
35. François, J., Rabaey, M., Boyen-Rikkers, I.: Distribution of protein molecular groups in the normal and cataractous lens. Exp. Eye Res. **8**, 157—160 (1969).
36. François, J., Rabaey, M., Wieme, R. J.: New method for fractionation of lens proteins. Arch. Ophthalmol. **53**, 481—486 (1955).
37. Fukushi, S., Spiro, R. G.: The lens capsule. Sugar and amino acid composition. J. Biol. Chem. **244**, 2041—2048 (1969).
38. Gills, J. P., Buckley, III, C. E.: Oral cyclophosphamide in the treatment of uveitis. Trans. Am. Acad. Ophthalmol. Otolaryngol. **74**, 505—508 (1970).
39. Halbert, S. P., Ehrlich, G.: Some aspects of the immunologic factors on corneal grafts. Invest. Ophthalmol. **1**, 233—243 (1962).
40. Halbert, S. P., Fitzgerald, P. L.: Studies on the immunologic organ specificity of ocular lens. Am. J. Ophthalmol. **46**, 187—195 (1958).
41. Halbert, S. P., Locatcher-Khorazo, D., Swick, L., Witmer, R., Seegal, B., Fitzgerald, P.: Homologous immunological studies of ocular lens. I. In vitro observations. J. Exp. Med. **105**, 439—452 (1957).
42. Halbert, S. P., Locatcher-Khorazo, D., Swick, L., Witmer, R., Seegal, B., Fitzgerald, P.: Homologous immunological studies of ocular lens. II. Biological aspects. J. Exp. Med. **105**, 453—462 (1957).
43. Halbert, S. P., Manski, W.: Organ specificity with special reference to the lens. Progr. Allergy **7**, 107—186 (1963).
44. Hall, J. M., O'Connor, G. R.: Correlation between ocular inflammation and antibody production. I. Serum antibody response following intravitreal immunization with protein antigens. J. Immunol. **104**, 432—439 (1970).
45. Hall, J. M., O'Connor, G. R.: Correlation between ocular inflammation and antibody production. II. Hemolytic plaque formation by cells of the uveal tract. J. Immunol. **104**, 440—447 (1970).
46. Hallett, J. W., Wolkowicz, M. I., Leopold, I. H., Canamucio, C., Wijenski, E.: Autoimmune complement fixation test in endogenous uveitis. Arch. Ophthalmol. **68**, 168—171 (1962).
47. Hektoen, L., Schulhof, K.: Further observations on lens precipitins. Antigenic properties of alpha and beta crystallins. J. Infect. Diseases **34**, 433—439 (1924).
48. Kawerau, E., Ott, H.: The soluble proteins of the cornea. Paper and immunoelectrophoretic studies. Exp. Eye Res. **1**, 137—144 (1961).
49. Khodadoust, A. A., Silverstein, A. M.: Studies on the nature of the privilege enjoyed by corneal allografts. Invest. Ophthalmol. **11**, 137—148 (1972).

50. KIDD, J. G., FRIEDEWALD, W. F.: A natural antibody that reacts in vitro with a sedimentable constituent of normal tissue cells. I. Demonstration of the phenomenon. J. Exp. Med. **76**, 543—556 (1942).
51. KIDD, J. G., FRIEDEWALD, W. F.: A natural antibody that reacts in vitro with a sedimentable constituent of normal tissue cells. II. Specificity of the phenomenon: General discussion. J. Exp. Med. **76**, 557—578 (1942).
52. KODAMA, R.: Anaphylaxis produced by eye tissues. J. Infect. Diseases **30**, 418—432 (1922).
53. KRAUSE, A. C.: Chemistry of the lens. II. Composition of beta crystallin, albumin (gamma crystallin) and capsule. Arch. Ophthalmol. **9**, 617—624 (1933).
54. KRAUSE, U., RAUNIO, V.: The proteins of the pathologic human aqueous humour. An *in vivo* investigation. Brit. J. Ophthalmol. **160**, 280—287 (1970).
55. LANGMAN, J., MAISEL, H.: Formation and distribution of chick lens proteins. Invest. Ophthalmol. **1**, 86—94 (1962).
56. LANGMAN, J., PRESCOTT, B. D.: An immunological approach to the problem of lens regeneration. J. Embryol. Exp. Morphol. **7**, 549—555 (1959).
57. LERNER, II, E. M., STONE, S. H., MYERS, R. E., VON SALLMANN, L.: Autoimmune chorioretinitis in rhesus monkeys. Science **162**, 561—562 (1968).
58. LESSELL, S., BEHAN, P., LAMARCHE, F., KIES, M.: Sensitivity to encephalitogenic protein in optic neuritis. Brit. J. Ophthalmol. **54**, 731—735 (1970).
59. LUNTZ, M. H.: Immune reaction to autologous lens proteins induced in guinea pigs (summary of a lecture delivered in Capetown, South Africa). J. Am. Med. Assoc. **186**, 33 (1963).
60. LUNTZ, M. H.: Anti-uveal and anti-lens antibodies in uveitis and their significance. Exp. Eye Res. **7**, 561—569 (1968).
61. MAISEL, H.: Lens antigens in ocular tissues. An immunoelectrophoretic study. Arch. Ophthalmol. **68**, 254—260 (1962).
62. MAISEL, H.: The immunologic specificity of lens antigens. Am. J. Ophthalmol. **55**, 1208—1216 (1963).
63. MAISEL, H.: The serological specificity of lens alpha-crystallin. Arch. Ophthalmol. **72**, 829—831 (1964).
64. MAISEL, H., GOODMAN, M.: Analysis of mammalian lens proteins by electrophoresis. Arch. Ophthalmol. **71**, 671—675 (1964).
65. MAISEL, H., GOODMAN, M.: The ontogeny and specificity of human lens proteins. Invest. Ophthalmol. **4**, 129—137 (1965).
66. MAISEL, H., GOODMAN, M.: Comparative electrophoretic study of vertebrate lens proteins. Am. J. Ophthalmol. **59**, 697—704 (1965).
67. MAISEL, H., LANGMAN, J.: An immuno-embryological study on the chick lens. J. Embryol. Exp. Morphol. **9**, 191—201 (1961).
68. MAISEL, H., LANGMAN, J.: Lens proteins in various tissues of the chick eye and in the lens of animals throughout the vertebrate series. Anat. Record. **140**, 183—194 (1961).
69. MANSKI, W., AUERBACH, M., HALBERT, S. P.: The evolutionary significance of lens organ specificity. Am. J. Ophthalmol. **50**, 985—990 (1960).
70. MANSKI, W., HALBERT, S. P.: Immunochemical investigation on the phylogeny of lens proteins. In: Protides of the Biological Fluids, Bruges 1964 (PEETERS, H., Ed.), p. 117—134. Amsterdam: Elsevier Publishing 1965.
71. MANSKI, W. J., HALBERT, S. P., AUERBACH, T. P.: Immunochemical analyses of lens protein separations. Arch. Biochem. Biophys. **92**, 512—524 (1961).
72. MANSKI, W., HALBERT, S. P., AUERBACH-PASCAL, T., JAVIER, P.: On the use of antigenic relationships among species for the study of molecular evolution. I. The lens proteins of the agnatha and chondrichthyes. Intern. Arch. Allergy Appl. Immunol. **31**, 38—56 (1967).
73. MANSKI, W., HALBERT, S. P., JAVIER, P.: On the use of antigenic relationships among species for the study of molecular evolution. II. The lens proteins of the choanichthyes and early actinopterygii. Intern. Arch. Allergy Appl. Immunol. **31**, 475—489 (1967).
74. MANSKI, W., HALBERT, S. P., JAVIER, P., AUERBACH-PASCAL, T.: On the use of antigenic relationships among species for the study of molecular evolution. III. The lens proteins of the late actinopterygii. Intern. Arch. Allergy Appl. Immunol. **31**, 529—545 (1967).
74a. MANSKI, W., SPECTOR, A.: I. Immunochemical studies on alpha crystallin subunits. Exp. Eye Res. **13**, 194—204 (1972).

75. Maumenee, A. E.: The immune reaction to corneal homografts. In: The Transparency of the Cornea (Duke-Elder, W. S., Ed.), p. 193—207. Oxford: Blackwell Scientific Publications 1960.
76. Maumenee, A. E.: The contributions of immunology to clinical ophthalmology. Am. J. Ophthalmol. **58**, 230—238 (1964).
77. Maurice, D. M.: The structure and transparency of the cornea. J. Physiol. (London) **136**, 236—286 (1957).
78. Maurice, D. M., Watson, P. G.: The distribution and movement of serum albumin in the cornea. Exp. Eye Res. **4**, 355—363 (1965).
79. Mehta, P. D., Cooper, S. N., Rao, S. S.: Identification of species-specific and organ-specific antigens in lens proteins. Exp. Eye Res. **3**, 192—197 (1964).
80. Mehta, P. D., Maisel, H.: Subunit structure of bovine α-crystallin and albuminoid. Exp. Eye Res. **7**, 265—268 (1968).
81. Nelken, D., Nelken, E.: The serological specificity of the cornea. Immunology **5**, 595—602 (1962).
82. Nelken, E., Michaelson, I. C., Nelken, D., Gurevitch, J.: Studies on antigens in the human cornea and their relationship to corneal grafting in man. J. Lab. Clin. Med. **49**, 745—752 (1957).
82. Nelken, E., Michaelson, I. C., Nelken, D., Gurevitch, J.: Studies on antigens in the human cornea and their relationship to corneal grafting in man. J. Lab. Clin. Med. **49**, 745—752 (1957).
83. Nelken, E., Nelken, D., Michaelson, I. C., Gurevitch, J.: Late clouding of experimental corneal grafts. Arch. Ophthalmol. **65**, 584—591 (1961).
84. Nozaki, M., Foster, L., Sery, T. W.: Eye and kidney tissue reactions to heterologous anti-uveal antibodies. Am. J. Ophthalmol. **58**, 447—453 (1964).
85. Perkins, E. S., Wood, R. M.: Auto-immunity in uveitis. Brit. J. Ophthalmol. **48**, 61—69 (1964).
86. Rana, M. W., Maisel, H.: Subunit composition of chick lens α-crystallin. Exp. Eye Res. **8**, 216—219 (1969).
87. Rao, S. S., Kulkarni, M. E., Cooper, S. N., Radhakrishnan, M. R.: Analysis of proteins of bovine lens, vitreous, and aqueous by electrophoresis and by Oudin's gel diffusion technique. Brit. J. Ophthalmol. **39**, 163—169 (1955).
88. Rathbun, W. B., Johnson, J. A., Fusaro, R. M.: Antigenic relationships between lens, epidermis and other bovine tissues. Exp. Eye Res. **12**, 298—303 (1971).
89. Sery, T. W., Nagy, R. M., Barber, G.: Corneal hypersensitivity. I. Escape kinetics of antigen from sensitized corneas. J. Immunol. **106**, 217—225 (1971).
90. Sery, T. W., Nagy, R. M.: Corneal hypersensitivity. II. Specific binding of antigen in sensitized corneas. J. Immunol. **106**, 226—232 (1971).
91. Shapiro, A. L.: Subunit composition of rabbit lens beta crystallins. Invest. Ophthalmol. **7**, 544—550 (1968).
92. Silverstein, A. M., Weller, S., Zimmerman, L. E.: A progressive immunization reaction in the actively sensitized rabbit eye. J. Immunol. **86**, 312—323 (1961).
93. Silverstein, A. M., Zimmerman, L. E.: Immunologic endophthalmitis produced in the guinea pig by different pathogenetic mechanisms. Am. J. Ophthalmol. **48**, 435—447 (1959).
94. Spector, A., Katz, E.: The deaggregation of bovine lens α-crystallin. J. Biol. Chem. **240**, 1979—1985 (1965).
95. Spector, A., Zorn, M., Li, L.: Architecture of calf lens α-crystallin. Exp. Eye Res. **7**, 154—163 (1968).
96. Spiro, R. G., Fukushi, S.: The lens capsule. Studies on the carbohydrate units. J. Biol. Chem. **244**, 2049—2058 (1969).
97. Šterzl, J., Silverstein, A. M.: Developmental aspects of immunity. In: Advances in Immunology, Vol. 6 (Dixon, F. J., Humphrey, J. H., Eds.), p. 337—459. New York: Academic Press 1967.
98. Truman, D. E. S., Brown, A. G., Rao, K. V.: Estimation of the molecular weights of chick β- and δ-crystallins and their subunits by gel filtration. Exp. Eye Res. **12**, 304—310 (1971).
99. Uhlenhuth, P. T.: Zur Lehre von der Unterscheidung verschiedener Eiweißarten mit Hilfe spezifischer Sera. In: Festschrift zum Sechzigsten Geburtstag von Robert Koch, p. 49—74. Jena: Gustav Fischer 1903.
100. Vulchanov, V. H., Nikolou, L. S., Kehayov, I. R.: On the significance of the phacoautoantibodies demonstrated in the sera of patients with senile cataract. Immunology **12**, 321—325 (1967).

101. WACKER, W. B., BARBEE, J. Y., MACDONALD, R., JR.: Experimental allergic uveitis. III. Manifestations produced in the guinea pig by immunization with homologous retina. Invest. Ophthalmol. **8**, 381—392 (1969).
102. WACKER, W. B., DODD, M. C.: The immunologic response of rabbits to homologous and heterologous corneal and uveal tissue. J. Immunol. **86**, 690—703 (1961).
103. WACKER, W. B., LIPTON, M. M.: Experimental allergic uveitis: Homologous retina as uveitogenic antigen. Nature **206**, 253—254 (1965).
104. WACKER, W. B., LIPTON, M. N.: Experimental allergic uveitis. I. Production in the guinea pig and rabbit by immunization with retina in adjuvant. J. Immunol. **101**, 151—156 (1968).
105. WACKER, W. B., LIPTON, M. M.: Experimental allergic uveitis. II. Serologic and hypersensitivity responses of the guinea pig following immunization with homologous retina. J. Immunol. **101**, 157—165 (1968).
105a. WACKER, W. B., LIPTON, M. M.: The role of two retina antigens in production of experimental allergic uveitis and its suppression by mycobacteria. Intern. Arch. Allergy Appl. Immunol. **41**, 370—380 (1971).
106. WACKER, W. B., LIPTON, M. M., ONGCHUA, F. E.: Antibody production in the guinea pig to homologous uvea. Proc. Soc. Exp. Biol. Med. **117**, 150—154 (1964).
107. WALTMAN, S. R., BURDE, R. M., FAULKNER, H. W.: The ocular immune response. II. Immune rejection of penetrating corneal homografts. Early versus late treatment with antilymphocyte serum. Transplantation **8**, 147—151 (1969).
108. WALTMAN, S. R., FAULKNER, H. W., BURDE, R. M.: Modification of the ocular immune response. I. Use of antilymphocytic serum to prevent immune rejection of penetrating corneal homografts. Invest. Ophthalmol. **8**, 196—200 (1969).
109. WITMER, R. H.: Antibody formation in rabbit eye studied with fluorescein-labeled antibody. Arch. Ophthalmol. **53**, 811—816 (1955).
110. WOOD, D. C., MASSI, L., SOLOMON, E. L.: The isolation, crystallization, and properties of proteins from rabbit eye lens. J. Biol. Chem. **234**, 329—334 (1959).
111. WOODS, A. C.: Ocular anaphylaxis. III. The role of uveal pigment. Arch. Ophthalmol. **46**, 283—297 (1917).
112. WOODS, A. C.: Ocular anaphylaxis. IV. The antigenic properties of uveal tissue as shown by complement fixation. Arch. Ophthalmol. **46**, 503—517 (1917).
113. WOODS, A. C.: Sympathetic ophthalmia. Use of uveal pigment in diagnosis and treatment. Trans. Ophthalmol. Soc. U. K. **45**, 208—251 (1925).
114. YORK, A. T., MARTINEZ, C., MANSKI, W.: Immunochemical studies on crystallines and albuminoids in human senile cataracts. Ophthalmol. Res. **3**, 183—191 (1972).
115. ZOUZIAS, D., MANSKI, W.: II. Immunochemical studies on alpha crystallin subunits. Exp. Eye Res. **13**, 205—218 (1972).

Chapter 7. The Kidney

1. ANDRES, G. A., ACCINNI, L., HSU, K. C., ZABRISKIE, J. B., SEEGAL, B. C.: Electron microscopic studies of human glomerulonephritis with ferritin-conjugated antibody. J. Exp. Med. **123**, 399—412 (1966).
2. ANDRES, G. A., MORGAN, C., HSU, K. C., RIFKIND, R. A., SEEGAL, B. C.: Electron microscopic studies of experimental nephritis with ferritin-conjugated antibody. The basement membranes and cisternae of visceral epithelial cells in nephritic rat glomeruli. J. Exp. Med. **115**, 929—935 (1962).
3. BAO-LINH, D., HERMANN, G., GRABAR, P.: Étude immunochimique des protéines rénales de la souris. Identification des antigènes organo-spécifiques. Ann. Inst. Pasteur **106**, 670—678 (1964).
4. BECKER, C. G., MURPHY, G. E.: The experimental induction of glomerulonephritis like that in man by infection with group A streptococci. J. Exp. Med. **127**, 1—23 (1968).
5. BEISSWENGER, P. J., SPIRO, R. G.: Human glomerular basement membrane: Chemical alteration in diabetes mellitus. Science **168**, 596—598 (1970).

6. Benacerraf, B., Potter, J. L., McCluskey, R. T., Miller, F.: The pathologic effects of intravenously administered soluble antigen-antibody complexes. II. Acute glomerulonephritis in rats. J. Exp. Med. **111**, 195—200 (1960).
7. Berns, A. W., Owens, C. T., Hirata, Y., Blumenthal, H. T.: The pathogenesis of diabetic glomerulosclerosis. II. A demonstration of insulin-binding capacity of the various histopathological components of the disease by fluorescence microscopy. Diabetes **11**, 308—317 (1962).
8. Bisno, A. L., Svartman, M., Stollerman, G. H.: Cross-reacting and monotypic T antigens of nephritogenic pyoderma streptococci: The type 56 system. J. Immunol. **106**, 1493—1498 (1971).
9. Blau, M., Day, E. D., Planinsek, J., Pressman, D.: Specificity and cross-localization of anti-kidney antibodies. J. Immunol. **79**, 334—336 (1957).
10. Blau, M., Day, E. D., Pressman, D.: The rate of localization of anti-rat kidney antibodies. J. Immunol. **79**, 330—333 (1957).
11. Boss, J. H., Silber, E., Nelken, D.: Antibodies to species homologous tissue in the rat. II. Circulating antibodies during the development of autoimmune renal disease. Clin. Exp. Immunol. **2**, 455—465 (1967).
12. Boyns, A. R., Hardwicke, J.: The relationship between circulating soluble antigen-antibody complexes and the production of chronic glomerulonephritis in the rabbit. Immunology **14**, 367—378 (1968).
13. Braun, D. G., Holm, S. E.: Streptococcal anti-group A precipitins in sera from patients with rheumatic arthritis and acute glomerulonephritis. Intern. Arch. Allergy Appl. Immunol. **37**, 216—224 (1970).
14. Carpenter, D. F., Steinberg, A. D., Schur, P. H., Talal, N.: The pathogenesis of autoimmunity in New Zealand mice. II. Acceleration of glomerulonephritis by polyinosinic polycytidylic acid. Lab. Invest. **23**, 628—634 (1970).
15. Cavelti, P. A.: Pathogenesis of glomerulonephritis and rheumatic fever; in vivo activation of tissue antigens as result of streptococcic infection and consecutive formation of autoantibodies. Arch. Pathol. **44**, 119—125 (1947).
16. Cavelti, P. A.: The technic of collodion particle agglutination. J. Immunol. **57**, 141—154 (1947).
17. Cavelti, P. A., Cavelti, E. S.: Studies on the pathogenesis of glomerulonephritis. I. Production of autoantibodies to kidney in experimental animals. Arch. Pathol. **39**, 148—152 (1945).
18. Cavelti, P. A., Cavelti, E. S.: Studies on the pathogenesis of glomerulonephritis. II. Production of glomerulonephritis in rats by means of autoantibodies to kidney. Arch. Pathol. **40**, 158—162 (1945).
19. Cavelti, P. A., Cavelti, E. S.: Studies on the pathogenesis of glomerulonephritis. III. Clinical and pathologic aspects of experimental glomerulonephritis produced in rats by means of autoantibodies to kidney. Arch. Pathol. **40**, 163—172 (1945).
20. Centeno, E., Shulman, S.: Physicochemical characterization and isolation of rabbit kidney-specific autoantigens. Immunology **24**, 911—924 (1973).
21. Centeno, E. R., Shulman, S., Milgrom, F.: Studies on the isolation and identification of a rabbit kidney-specific autoantigen. In: Abstracts of the Sixth International Congress of Biochemistry, p. 145. New York 1964.
22. Centeno, E., Shulman, S., Milgrom, F., Witebsky, E.: Studies on adrenal glands. VI. The multiple nature of the rabbit adrenal autoantigens. Immunology **8**, 160—169 (1965).
23. Centeno, E., Shulman, S., Milgrom, F., Witebsky, E., Skelton, F.: Studies on organ specificity. XVII. Autoantigens of rabbit kidney. J. Immunol. **96**, 530—536 (1966).
24. Cochrane, C. G.: Mediation of immunologic glomerular injury. Transplantation Proc. **1**, 949—958 (1969).
25. Cochrane, C. G., Unanue, E. R., Dixon, F. J.: A role of polymorphonuclear leukocytes and complement in nephrotoxic nephritis. J. Exp. Med. **122**, 99—116 (1965).
26. Cole, L. R., Cromartie, W. J., Watson, D. W.: A specific soluble substance involved in nephrotoxic nephritis. Proc. Soc. Exp. Biol. Med. **77**, 498—501 (1951).
27. Cook, W. F., Pickering, G. W.: A rapid method for separating glomeruli from the rabbit kidney. Nature **182**, 1103—1104 (1958).
28. Cruickshank, B.: Localization of nephrotoxic antigens. Lancet **1959 I**, 50—51.
29. Cruickshank, B., Hill, A. G. S.: The histo-chemical identification of a connective-tissue antigen in the rat. J. Pathol. Bacteriol. **66**, 283—289 (1953).

30. Dinh, B. L., Brassard, A.: Induction of experimental glomerulonephritis in the rat by homologous major urinary protein. Clin. Exp. Immunol. **2**, 633—644 (1967).
31. Dixon, F. J.: The role of antigen-antibody complexes in disease. Harvey Lectures **58**, 21—52 (1963).
32. Dixon, F. J., Feldman, J. D., Vazquez, J. J.: Experimental glomerulonephritis: The pathogenesis of a laboratory model resembling the spectrum of human glomerulonephritis. J. Exp. Med. **113**, 899—920 (1961).
33. Dixon, F. J., Unanue, E. R., Watson, J. I.: Immunopathology of the kidney. In: Immunopathology, IVth International Symposium (Grabar, P., Miescher, P. A., Eds.), p. 363—373. Basel: Benno Schwabe 1965.
34. Edgington, T. S., Glassock, R. J., Dixon, F. J.: Autologous immune complex pathogenesis of experimental allergic glomerulonephritis. Science **155**, 1432—1434 (1967).
35. Edgington, T. S., Glassock, R. J., Dixon, F. J.: Autologous immune complex nephritis induced with renal tubular antigen. I. Identification and isolation of the pathogenetic antigen. J. Exp. Med. **127**, 555—572 (1968).
36. Edgington, T. S., Glassock, R. J., Watson, J. I., Dixon, F. J.: Characterization and isolation of specific renal tubular epithelial antigens. J. Immunol. **99**, 1199—1210 (1967).
37. Edgington, T. S., Lee, S., Dixon, F. J.: Persistence of the autoimmune pathogenetic process in experimental autologous immune complex nephritis. J. Immunol. **100**, 528—536 (1969).
38. Eisen, H. N., Pressman, D.: The zone of localization of antibodies. VIII. Some properties of the antigen responsible for the renal localization of anti-kidney serum. J. Immunol. **64**, 487—498 (1950).
39. Farquhar, M. G., Wissig, S. L., Palade, G. E.: Glomerular permeability. I. Ferritin transfer across the normal glomerular capillary wall. J. Exp. Med. **113**, 47—66 (1961).
40. Feldman, J. D.: Pathogenesis of ultrastructural glomerular changes induced by immunologic means. In: Immunopathology, IIIrd International Symposium (Grabar, P., Miescher, P. A., Eds.), p. 263—281. Basel: Benno Schwabe 1963.
41. Feldman, J. D., Hammer, D., Dixon, F. J.: Experimental glomerulonephritis. III. Pathogenesis of glomerular ultrastructural lesions in nephrotoxic serum nephritis. Lab. Invest. **12**, 748—763 (1963).
42. Fischel, E. E.: Immune reactions in human glomerulonephritis. J. Chronic Diseases **5**, 34—44 (1957).
43. Fiuke, M. T.: Immunoenzymological studies on kidney rhodanese in relation to the problem of cellular differentiation. Embryologia (Nagoya) **10**, 11—31 (1967).
44. Fiuke, M. T., Okada, T. S.: Changes in rhodanese content during primary spreading culture of embryonic kidney cells revealed by immunoenzymological method. Embryologia (Nagoya) **10**, 32—41 (1967).
45. Fogel, M., Sachs, L.: Studies on the antigenic composition of hamster tumors induced by polyoma virus, and of normal hamster tissues in vivo and in vitro. J. Nat. Cancer Inst. **29**, 239—252 (1962).
46. Freedman, P., Markowitz, A. S.: Immunological studies in nephritis. Lancet **1959 II**, 45—46.
47. Freedman, P., Markowitz, A. S.: Gamma globulin and complement in the diseased kidney, J. Clin. Invest. **41**, 328—334 (1962).
48. Furth, J., Kabat, E. A.: Immunological specificity of material sedimentable at high speed present in normal and tumor tissues. J. Exp. Med. **74**, 247—256 (1941).
49. Gajdusek, D. C.: An 'autoimmune' reaction against human tissue antigen in certain acute and chronic diseases. I. Serological investigations. Arch. Internal Med. **101**, 9—29 (1958).
50. Gery, I., Yagi, Y., Pressman, D.: Reactions of localizing antikidney antibodies with tissues of various species. J. Immunol. **94**, 950—958 (1965).
51. Glassock, R. J., Edgington, T. S., Watson, J. I., Dixon, F. J.: Autologous immune complex nephritis induced with renal tubular antigen. II. The pathogenetic mechanism. J. Exp. Med. **127**, 573—588 (1968).
52. Glassock, R. J., Watson, J. I., Edgington, T. S., Dixon, F. J.: Autologous immune complex glomerulonephritis. II. Studies on cellular and parabiotic transfer. J. Immunol. **102**, 194—205 (1969).
53. Glynn, L. E., Holborow, E. J.: Conversion of tissue polysaccharides to auto-antigens by Group-A beta-haemolytic streptococci. Lancet **1952 II**, 449—451.

54. GOODMAN, H. C., BAXTER, J. H.: Nephrotoxic serum nephritis in rats. II. Preparation and characterization of a soluble protective factor produced by trypsin digestion of rat tissue homogenates. J. Exp. Med. **104**, 487—499 (1956).

55. GOODMAN, M., GREENSPON, S. W., KRAKOWER, C. A.: The antigenic composition of the various anatomic structures of the canine kidney. J. Immunol. **75**, 96—104 (1955).

56. GREENSPON, S. W., BOLLINGER, F. W., KRAKOWER, C. A.: Some chemical properties of nephrotoxic antigen. Federation Proc. **11**, 416—417 (1952).

57. GREENSPON, S. W., KRAKOWER, C. A.: Direct evidence for the antigenicity of the glomeruli in the production of nephrotoxic serums. Arch. Pathol. **49**, 291—297 (1950).

58. GRUPE, W. E., KAPLAN, M. H.: A proximal tubular antigen in the pathogenesis of autoimmune nephrosis. Federation Proc. **26**, 573 (1967).

59. HAMMER, D. K., DIXON, F. J.: Experimental glomerulonephritis. II. Immunologic events in the pathogenesis of nephrotoxic nephritis in the rat. J. Exp. Med. **117**, 1019—1034 (1963).

60. HENLE, W., CHAMBER, L. A., GRUPÉ, V.: The serological specificity of particulate components derived from various normal mammalian organs. J. Exp. Med. **74**, 495—510 (1941).

61. HESS, E. V., ASHWORTH, C. T., ZIFF, M.: Transfer of an autoimmune nephrosis in the rat by means of lymph node cells. J. Exp. Med. **115**, 421—438 (1962).

62. HESS, E. V., ASHWORTH, C. T., ZIFF, M.: Nephrosis in the rat induced by rat kidney extracts. Ann. N. Y. Acad. Sci. **124**, 323—328 (1965).

63. HEYMANN, W., HACKEL, D. B., HARWOOD, S., WILSON, S. G. F., HUNTER, J. L. P.: Production of nephrotic syndrome in rats by Freund's adjuvants and rat kidney suspensions. Proc. Soc. Exp. Biol. Med. **100**, 660—664 (1959).

64. HEYMANN, W., HUNTER, J. L. P., HACKEL, D. B.: Experimental autoimmune nephrosis in rats. III. J. Immunol. **88**, 135—141 (1962).

65. HEYMANN, W., Hunter, J. L. P., HACKEL, D. B., CUPPAGE, F.: Transfer of experimental autoimmune nephrosis in rats. Proc. Soc. Exp. Biol. Med. **111**, 568—573 (1962).

66. HEYMANN, W., KMETEC, E. P., WILSON, S. G. F., HUNTER, J. L. P., HACKEL, D. B., CUPPAGE, F.: Experimental autoimmune renal disease in rats. In: Immunopathology, IIIrd International Symposium (GRABAR, P., MIESCHER, P., Eds.), p. 240—251. Basel: Benno Schwabe 1963.

67. HEYMANN, W., KMETEC, E. P., WILSON, S. G. F., HUNTER, J. L. P., HACKEL, D. B., OKUDA, R., CUPPAGE, F.: Experimental autoimmune renal disease in rats. Ann. N. Y. Acad. Sci. **124**, 310—322 (1965).

68. HILL, A. G. S., CRUICKSHANK, B.: A study of antigenic components of kidney tissue. Brit. J. Exp. Pathol. **34**, 27—34 (1953).

69. HIRAMOTO, R., JURANDOWSKI, J., BERNECKY, J., PRESSMAN, D.: Precise zone of localization of anti-kidney antibody in various organs. Proc. Soc. Exp. Biol. Med. **101**, 583—586 (1959).

70. HOLM, G.: In vitro cytotoxic effects of lymphoid cells from rats with experimental autoimmune nephrosis. Clin. Exp. Immunol. **1**, 45—60 (1966).

71. HOLM, S. E., BRAUN, D., JÖNSSON, J.: Antigenic factors common to human kidney and nephritogenic and non-nephritogenic streptococcal strains. Intern. Arch. Allergy Appl. Immunol. **33**, 127—130 (1968).

72. HUNTER, J. L. P., HACKEL, D. B., HEYMANN, W.: Nephrotic syndrome in rats produced by sensitization to rat kidney proteins: Immunological studies. J. Immunol. **85**, 319—327 (1960).

73. INTORP, H. W., MILGROM, F.: Thermostable kidney antigen and its excretion into urine. J. Immunol. **100**, 1195—1203 (1968).

74. JOHNSON, G. D., ASHERSON, G. L., KAKLAMANIS, E., DUMONDE, D. C.: Demonstration by immunofluorescence of autoantibody in the serum of rabbits given injections of rat tissue. J. Pathol. Bacteriol. **86**, 521—525 (1963).

75. KASUKAWA, R., ABEYOUNIS, C. J., RAY, D. K., MILGROM, F.: Studies on the serology of renal diseases. I. Reactions of patients' sera with mammalian cell cultures. Intern. Arch. Allergy Appl. Immunol. **32**, 490—495 (1967).

76. KASUKAWA, R., ANTHONE, R., ABEYOUNIS, C. J., MILGROM, F.: Studies on the serology of renal diseases. II. Unusual antibodies in glomerulonephritis sera. Intern. Arch. Allergy Appl. Immunol. **32**, 563—573 (1967).

77. KATZ, D. H., UNANUE, E. R., DIXON, F. J.: Nephritogenic properties of cross-reacting kidney-fixing antibodies to heart, spleen and muscle. J. Immunol. **98**, 260—268 (1967).

78. KAY, C. F.: The mechanism by which experimental nephritis is produced in rabbits injected with nephrotoxic duck serum. J. Exp. Med. **72**, 559—572 (1940).
79. KAY, C. F.: The mechanism of a form of glomerulonephritis. Nephrotoxic nephritis in rabbits. Am. J. Med. Sci. **204**, 483—490 (1942).
80. KAY, C. F., LUCCHESI, P. F., RUTHERFORD, R. B.: An experimental investigation of an immunologic mechanism as the cause of glomerulonephritis. J. Immunol. **42**, 369—380 (1941).
81. KELLY, D. K., WINN, J. F.: Renal lesions produced by group A, type 12, streptococci. Science **127**, 1337 (1958).
82. KLEIN, P., BURKHOLDER, P.: Ein Verfahren zur fluoreszenzoptischen Darstellung der Komplementbindung und seine Anwendung zur histo-immunologischen Untersuchung der experimentellen Nierenanaphylaxie. Deut. Med. Wochschr. **84**, 2001—2004 (1959).
83. KRAKOWER, C. A., GREENSPON, S. W.: Localization of the nephrotoxic antigen within the isolated renal glomerulus. Arch. Pathol. **51**, 629—639 (1951).
84. KRAKOWER, C. A., GREENSPON, S. W.: Factors leading to variation in concentration of 'nephrotoxic' antigen(s) of glomerular basement membrane. Arch. Pathol. **58**, 401—432 (1954).
85. KRAKOWER, C. A., GREENSPON, S. W.: The localization of the 'nephrotoxic' antigen(s) in extraglomerular tissues. Arch. Pathol. **66**, 364—383 (1958).
86. KRAKOWER, C. A., GREENSPON, S. W., WARREN, H. M.: Electron microscopic observations on the cell-free nature of glomerular basement membrane after treatment of isolated renal glomeruli with trichloroacetic acid. Exp. Cell Res. **13**, 230—233 (1957).
87. KRAMER, N. C., WATT, M. F., HOWER, J. H., PARRISH, A. E.: Circulating antihuman kidney antibodies in human renal disease. Am. J. Med. **30**, 39 (1961).
88. KURTZ, S. M., FELDMAN, J. D.: Experimental studies on the formation of the glomerular basement membrane. J. Ultrastruct. Res. **6**, 19—27 (1962).
89. LAMBERT, P. H., DIXON, F. J.: Pathogenesis of the glomerulonephritis of NZB/W mice. J. Exp. Med. **127**, 507—521 (1968).
90. LANGE, C. F.: Chemistry of cross-reactive fragments of streptococcal cell membrane and human glomerular basement membrane. Transplantation Proc. **1**, 959—963 (1969).
91. LANGE, K., GOLD, M. M. A., WEINER, D., SIMON, V.: Autoantibodies in human glomerulonephritis. J. Clin. Invest. **28**, 50—55 (1949).
92. LANGE, K., CRAIG, F., OBERMAN, J., SLOBODY, L., OGUR, G., LOCASTO, F.: Changes in serum complement during the course and treatment of glomerulonephritis. Arch. Internal. Med. **88**, 433—445 (1951).
93. LANGE, K., SEMAR, M., TY, A., TRESER, G.: A specific antigen and antibody in acute poststreptococcal glomerulonephritis. Trans. Assoc. Am. Physicians **82**, 188—198 (1969).
94. LANGE, K., TRESER, G., SAGEL, I., TY, A., WASSERMAN, E.: Routine immunohistology in renal diseases. Ann. Internal Med. **64**, 25—40 (1966).
95. LANGE, K., WACHSTEIN, M., TRESER, G., MCPHERSON, S. E.: The possible role of autoantibodies in chronic human and experimental glomerulonephritis. Ann. N. Y. Acad. Sci. **124**, 329—331 (1965).
96. LANGE, K., WASSERMAN, E., SLOBODY, L. B.: The significance of serum complement levels for the diagnosis and prognosis of acute and subacute glomerulonephritis and lupus erythematosus disseminatus. Ann. Internal Med. **53**, 636—646 (1960).
97. LANGE, K., WENK, E. J., WACHSTEIN, M., NOBLE, J.: The mechanism of experimental glomerulonephritis produced in rabbits by avian antikidney sera. Am. J. Med. Sci. **236**, 767—778 (1958).
98. LAYTON, J. M.: The structure of the kidney from the gross to the molecular. J. Urol. **90**, 502—515 (1963).
99. LERNER, R. A., DIXON, F. J.: Spontaneous glomerulonephritis in sheep. Lab. Invest. **15**, 1279—1289 (1966).
100. LERNER, R. A., DIXON, F. J.: Transfer of ovine experimental allergic glomerulonephritis (EAG) with serum. J. Exp. Med. **124**, 431—442 (1966).
101. LERNER, R. A., DIXON, F. J.: The induction of acute glomerulonephritis in rabbits with soluble antigens isolated from normal homologous and autologous urine. J. Immunol. **100**, 1277—1287 (1968).
102. LERNER, R. A., GLASSOCK, R. J., DIXON, F. J.: The role of antiglomerular basement membrane antibody in the pathogenesis of human glomerulonephritis. J. Exp. Med. **126**, 989—1004 (1967).

103. LINDBERG, L. H., ROSENBERG, L. T.: Nephrotoxic serum nephritis in mice, with a genetic deficiency in complement. J. Immunol. **100**, 34—45 (1968).
104. LINDBERG, L. H., VOSTI, K. L., RAFFEL, S.: Experimental streptococcal glomerulonephritis in rats. J. Immunol. **98**, 1231—1240 (1967).
105. LIPPMAN, R. W., CAMERON, G., CAMPBELL, D. H.: The specificity of anti-kidney antibody determined by its effect upon tissue culture explants. Proc. Nat. Acad. Sci. **36**, 576—580 (1950).
106. LIU, C. T., MCCRORY, W. W.: Autoantibodies in human glomerulonephritis and nephrotic syndrome. J. Immunol. **81**, 492—498 (1958).
107. LIU, C. T., MCCRORY, W. W., FLICK, J. A.: Cytotoxic effect of nephrotoxic serum on rat tissue culture. Proc. Soc. Exp. Biol. Med. **95**, 331—335 (1957).
108. LOEWI, G.: Effect of antibody on heterologous and homologous cells in tissue culture. Immunology **6**, 569—580 (1953).
109. MARKOWITZ, A. S.: Interactions of anti-glomerular basement membrane antisera. Immunology **3**, 117—125 (1960).
110. MARKOWITZ, A. S., ARMSTRONG, S. H., jr., KUSHNER, D. S.: Immunological relationships between the rat glomerulus and nephritogenic streptococci. Nature **187**, 1095—1097 (1960).
111. MARKOWITZ, A. S., CLASEN, R., NIDUS, B. D., AINIS, H.: Streptococcal related glomerulonephritis. II. Glomerulonephritis in rhesus monkeys immunologically induced both actively and passively with a soluble fraction from human glomeruli. J. Immunol. **98**, 161—170 (1967).
112. MARKOWITZ, A. S., LANGE, C. F., jr.: Streptococcal related glomerulonephritis. I. Isolation, immunochemistry and comparative chemistry of soluble fractions from type 12 nephritogenic streptococci and human glomeruli. J. Immunol. **92**, 565—575 (1964).
113. MARKOWITZ, A. S., NIDUS, B., AINIS, H.: Active and passive glomerulonephritis induced in monkey with soluble fraction from human glomerulus. Federation Proc. **25**, 697 (1966).
114. MASUGI, M.: Über das Wesen der spezifischen Veränderungen der Niere und der Leber durch das Nephrotoxin bzw. Hepatotoxin: Zugleich ein Beitrag zur Pathogenese der Glomerulonephritis und der eklamptischen Lebererkrankung. Beitr. Path. Anat. Allgem. Pathol. **91**, 82—112 (1933).
115. MASUGI, M.: Über die experimentelle Glomerulonephritis durch das spezifische Antinierenserum. Ein Beitrag zur Pathogenese der diffusen Glomerulonephritis. Beitr. Path. Anat. Allgem. Pathol. **92**, 429—466 (1934).
116. MCCLUSKEY, R. T., BENACERRAF, B., POTTER, J. L., MILLER, F.: The pathologic effects of intravenously administered soluble antigen-antibody complexes. I. Passive serum sickness in mice. J. Exp. Med. **111**, 181—194 (1960).
117. MCCLUSKEY, R. T., VASSALLI, P., GALLO, G., BALDWIN, D. S.: An immunofluorescent study of pathogenic mechanisms in glomerular diseases. New Engl. J. Med. **274**, 695—701 (1966).
118. MCPHAUL, J. J., jr., DIXON, F. J.: The presence of antiglomerular basement membrane antibodies in peripheral blood. J. Immunol. **103**, 1168—1175 (1969).
119. MCPHAUL, J. J., jr., DIXON, F. J.: Immunoreactive basement membrane antigens in normal human urine and serum. J. Exp. Med. **130**, 1395—1409 (1969).
120. MCPHAUL, J. J., jr., DIXON, F. J.: Basement membrane antigens in serum and urine. Transplantation Proc. **1**, 964—967 (1969).
121. MCPHAUL, J. J., jr., DIXON, F. J.: Characterization of human anti-glomerular basement membrane antibodies eluted from glomerulonephritic kidneys. J. Clin. Invest. **49**, 308—317 (1970).
122. MELLORS, R. C.: Autoimmune disease in NZB/BL mice. I. Pathology and pathogenesis of a model system of spontaneous glomerulonephritis. J. Exp. Med. **122**, 25—40 (1965).
123. MELLORS, R. C., ORTEGA, L. G.: Analytical pathology. III. New observations on the pathogenesis of glomerulonephritis, lipid nephrosis, periarteritis nodosa, and secondary amyloidosis in man. Am. J. Pathol. **32**, 455—500 (1956).
124. MICHAEL, A. F., jr., DRUMMOND, K. N., GOOD, R. A., VERNIER, R. L.: Acute poststreptococcal glomerulonephritis: Immune deposit disease. J. Clin. Invest. **45**, 237—248 (1966).
125. MILGROM, F., CENTENO, E., SHULMAN, S., WITEBSKY, E.: Autoantibodies resulting from immunization with kidney. Proc. Soc. Exp. Biol. Med. **116**, 1009—1013 (1964).
126. MILAZZO, S. C.: A study of the immunological properties of reticulin. J. Pathol. Bacteriol. **73**, 527—537 (1957).
127. MUKERJEE, H., SRI RAM, J., PIERCE, G. B., jr.: Basement membrane. V. Chemical composition of neoplastic basement membrane mucoprotein. Am. J. Pathol. **46**, 49—57 (1965).

128. MÜLLER-RUCHHOLTZ, W., FEDERLIN, K., SCHNEIDER, A., SCHMITT, G., RAHLWES, G., OSTNER, K. H., PFEIFFER, E. F.: Übertragungsversuche zur Lokalisation eines nephritisauslösenden Faktors bei Ratten. Verhandl. Deut. Ges. Inn. Med. **68**, 553—557 (1962).
129. MYERS, J., FREI, J. V., COHEN, J. J., ROSE, B., RICHTER, M.: Basement membrane specific antisera produced to solubilized tissue fractions. Immunology **11**, 155—162 (1966).
130. NAGASAWA, T., SHIBATA, S.: Immunofluorescence on the anatomic distribution of the soluble antigen responsible for the production of nephrotoxic serum nephritis. J. Immunol. **103**, 736—740 (1969).
131. NAIRN, R. C., GHOSE, T., FOTHERGILL, J. E., MCENTEGART, M. G.: Kidney specific antigen and its species distribution. Nature **196**, 385—387 (1962).
132. NAIRN, R. G., RICHMOND, H. G., MCENTEGART, M. G., FOTHERGILL, J. E.: Immunological differences between normal and malignant cells. Brit. Med. J. **1960 II**, 1335—1340.
133. OKADA, T. S.: Tissue-specificity in the soluble antigens in kidney microsomes. Nature **194**, 306—307 (1962).
134. OKADA, T. S.: Cellular distribution of some microsomal antigens in embryonic chicken kidneys. Exp. Cell Res. **33**, 584—587 (1964).
135. OKADA, T. S.: Changes in antigenic constitutions of embryonic chicken kidney cells during in vitro speading culture. Exp. Cell Res. **39**, 591—603 (1965).
136. OKADA, T. S.: Development of kidney specific antigens: An immunohistological study. J. Embryol. Exp. Morphol. **13**, 285—297 (1965).
137. OKADA, T. S.: Immunohistological studies on the reconstitution of nephric tubules from dissociated cells, J. Embryol. Exp. Morphol. **13**, 299—307 (1965).
138. OKADA, T. S., SATO, A. G.: Production of a highly tissue-specific antiserum against a particular sub-fraction separated from kidney microsomes. Nature **197**, 1216—1217 (1963).
139. OKADA, T. S., SATO, A. G.: Soluble antigens in microsomes of adult and embryonic kidneys. Exp. Cell Res. **31**, 251—265 (1963).
140. OKUDA, R., KAPLAN, M. H., CUPPAGE, F. E., HEYMANN, W.: Deposition of autologous gamma globulin in kidneys of rats with nephrotic renal disease of various etiologies. J. Lab. Clin. Med. **66**, 204—215 (1965).
141. ORTEGA, L. G., MELLORS, R. C.: Analytical pathology. IV. The role of localized antibody in the pathogenesis of nephrotoxic nephritis in the rat. J. Exp. Med. **104**, 151—170 (1956).
142. PARKS, A. E., SHANKS, G.: Studies on experimental lesions in the kidneys of rabbits. J. Lab. Clin. Med. **26**, 950—956 (1941).
143. PFEIFFER, E. F.: Nachweis, Natur und klinische Bedeutung eines nephritisauslösenden Faktors bei Nierenerkrankungen. Verhandl. Deut. Ges. Inn. Med. **68**, 413—433 (1962).
144. PFEIFFER, E. F.: Demonstration of and evidence for the lymphocyte bound nature of a secondary nephritis producing factor in nephrotoxic glomerulonephritis in rats. In: Immunopathology, IIIrd International Symposium (GRABAR, P., MIESCHER, P., Eds.), p. 220—239. Basel: Benno Schwabe 1963.
145. PFEIFFER, E. F., BRUCH, M. E.: Über den Nachweis von Autoantikörpern gegen menschliches Nierengewebe bei Nieren- und Hochdruckkranken mit der Kollodium-Partikel-Reaktion. Deut. Arch. Klin. Med. **199**, 613—632 (1952).
146. PFEIFFER, E. F., MERRILL, J. P.: Die Autoaggression in der Pathogenese der diffusen glomerulonephritis. Deut. Med. Wochschr. **87**, 934—944 (1962).
147. PINCUS, T., Haberkern, R., CHRISTIAN, C. L.: Experimental chronic glomerulitis. J. Exp. Med. **127**, 819—831 (1968).
148. PORTER, K. A., ANDRES, G. A., CALDER, M. W., DOSSETOR, J. B., HSU, K. C., RENDALL, J. M., SEEGAL, B. C., STARZL, T. E.: Human renal transplants. II. Immunofluorescent and immunoferritin studies. Lab. Invest. **18**, 159—171 (1968).
149. PRESSMAN, D., KORNGOLD, L., HEYMANN, W.: Localizing properties of anti-rat-kidney serum prepared in ducks. Arch. Pathol. **55**, 347—348 (1953).
150. RAMMELKAMP, C. H., jr.: The natural history of streptococcal infections. Bull. N. Y. Acad. Med. **31**, 103—112 (1955).
151. RAMMELKAMP, C. H., jr.: Microbiologic aspects of glomerulonephritis. J. Chronic Diseases **5**, 28—33 (1957).
152. RAMMELKAMP, C. H., jr., WEAVER, R. S.: Acute glomerulonephritis. The significance of the variations in the incidence of the disease. J. Clin. Invest. **32**, 345—358 (1953).

153. RHODIN, J. A. G.: Structure of the kidney. In: Diseases of the Kidney, 2nd ed. (STRAUSS, M. B., WELT, L. G., Eds.), p. 1—30. Boston: Little, Brown 1971.
154. ROTHBARD, S., WAISON, R. F.: Demonstration by immunofluorescence of the fixation of perfused antibody to human collagen in human kidney. J. Exp. Med. **125**, 595—606 (1967).
155. ROTHBARD, S., WATSON, R. F.: Comparison of reactions of antibodies to rat collagen and to rat kidney in the basement membranes of rat renal glomeruli. J. Exp. Med. **129**, 1145—1162 (1969).
156. ROTHER, K.: Kidney. In: Textbook of Immunopathology, Vol. II (MIESCHER, P. A., MÜLLER-EBERHARD, H. J., Eds.), p. 584—594. New York: Grune and Stratton 1969.
157. ROTHER, K., ROTHER, U., VASSALLI, P., MCCLUSKEY, R. T.: Nephrotoxic serum nephritis in C'6-deficient rabbits. I. Study of the second phase of the disease. J. Immunol. **98**, 965—971 (1967).
158. SCHWENTKER, F. F., COMPLOIER, F. C.: The production of kidney antibodies by injection of homologous kidney plus bacterial toxins. J. Exp. Med. **70**, 223—230 (1939).
159. SCOTT, D. G.: A study of the antigenicity of basement membrane and reticulin. Brit. J. Exp. Pathol. **38**, 178—185 (1957).
160. SEEGAL, B. C., ANDRES, G. A., HSU, K. C., ZABRISKIE, J. B.: Studies on the pathogenesis of acute and progressive glomerulonephritis in man by immunofluorescein and immunoferritin techniques. Federation Proc. **24**, 100—108 (1965).
161. SEEGAL, B. C., HSU, K. C., ROTHENBURG, M. S., CHAPEAU, M. L.: Studies on the mechanism of experimental nephritis with fluorescein-labeled antibody. II. Localization and persistence of injected rabbit or duck anti-rat-kidney serum during the course of nephritis in rats. Am. J. Pathol. **41**, 183—203 (1962).
162. SEMAR, M., TRESER, G., LANGE, K.: Quantitative comparative immunohistology. Clin. Chem. **15**, 505—508 (1969).
163. SHARP, J. T., ANDERSON, M. S., LIDSKY, M. D.: Studies on bovine glomeruli. II. Localization of glomerular collagen. J. Immunol. **99**, 1254—1263 (1967).
164. SHIBATA, S., MIYAKAWA, Y., NARUSE, T., NAGASAWA, T., TAKUMA, T.: A glycoprotein that induces nephrotoxic antibody: its isolation and purification from rat glomerular basement membrane. J. Immunol. **102**, 593—601 (1969).
165. SHIBATA, S., NARUSE, T., MIYAKAWA, Y., NAGASAWA, T.: Further purification of the glycoprotein that induces nephrotoxic antibody: Isolation of the active polysaccharide fraction mainly composed of glucose. J. Immunol. **104**, 215—223 (1970).
166. SHIBATA, S., NARUSE, T., NAGASAWA, T., TAKUMA, T., MIYAKAWA, Y.: Purification by starch block electrophoresis of renal antigen that induces nephrotoxic antibody. J. Immunol. **99**, 454—464 (1967).
167. SHULMAN, S., CENTENO, E.: Isolation and characterization of a rabbit non-tissue-specific auto-antigen which is shared by kidney, heart, adrenal, and liver. Immunology **24**, 925—937 (1973).
168. SHULMAN, S., WYPYCH, J.: Kidney antigens active in isoimmunization. I. The antigenic diversity. Immunology **17**, 641—652 (1969).
169. SKOGLUND, R. W., jr.: Preparation of a pure glomerular fraction. A modification. Invest. Urol. **8**, 284—285 (1970).
170. SNELLMAN, O.: A glycoprotein from reticulin tissue. Acta. Chem. Scand. **17**, 1049—1056 (1963).
171. SOLOMON, D. H., GARDELLA, J. W., FANGER, H., DETHIER, F. M., FERREBEE, J. W.: Nephrotoxic nephritis in rats. Evidence for the glomerular origin of the kidney antigen. J. Exp. Med. **90**, 267—272 (1949).
172. SPIRO, R. G., SPIRO, M. J.: Studies on the biosynthesis of the hydroxylysine-linked disaccharide unit of basement membranes and collagens. I. Kidney glucosyltransferase. J. Biol. Chem. **246**, 4899—4909 (1971).
173. SPIRO, M. J., SPIRO, R. G.: Studies on the biosynthesis of the hydroxylysine-linked disaccharide unit of basement membranes and collagens. II. Kidney galactosyltransferase. J. Biol. Chem. **246**, 4910—4918 (1971).
174. SPIRO, R. G., SPIRO, M. J.: Studies on the biosynthesis of the hydroxylysine-linked disaccharide unit of basement membranes and collagens. III. Tissue and subcellular distribution of glycosyltransferases and the effect of various conditions on the enzyme levels. J. Biol. Chem. **246**, 4919—4925 (1971).
175. STAVITSKY, A. B., HACKEL, D. B., HEYMANN, W.: Reduction of serum complement following in vivo tissue antigen-antibody reactions. Proc. Soc. Exp. Biol. Med. **85**, 593—597 (1954).

176. STEBLAY, R. W.: Glomerulonephritis induced in sheep by injections of heterologous glomerular basement membrane and Freund's complete adjuvant. J. Exp. Med. **116**, 253—272 (1962).

177. STEBLAY, R. W.: Glomerulonephritis induced in monkeys by injections of heterologous glomerular basement membrane and Freund's adjuvant. Nature **197**, 1173—1176 (1963).

178. STEBLAY, R. W.: Glomerulonephritis induced in sheep and monkeys by injections of heterologous glomerular basement membrane and Freund's adjuvant. In: Immunopathology, IIIrd International Symposium (GRABAR, P., MIESCHER, P., Eds.), p. 252—262. Basel: Benno Schwabe 1963.

179. STEBLAY, R. W.: Studies on autoimmune nephritis in sheep and rats. IV. The relative efficacy of heterologous, homologous and autologous glomerular basement membrane (GBM) in inducing nephritis. Federation Proc. **26**, 531 (1967).

180. STEBLAY, R. W., LEPPER, M. H.: The nephrotoxic properties of rabbit antiserum prepared by immunizing rabbits with purified human glomerular basement membrane or dog glomerular basement membrane. J. Lab. Clin. Med. **46**, 956—957 (1955).

181. TEAGUE, P. O., YUNIS, E. J., RODEY, G., FISH, A. J., STUTMAN, O., GOOD, R. A.: Autoimmune phenomena and renal disease in mice. Role of thymectomy, aging, and involution of immunologic capacity. Lab. Invest. **22**, 121—130 (1970).

182. TRESER, G., EHRENREICH, T., ORES, R., SAGEL, I., WASSERMAN, E., LANGE, K.: Natural history of 'apparently healed' acute poststreptococcal glomerulonephritis in children. Pediatrics **43**, 1005—1017 (1969).

183. TRESER, G., SEMAR, M., MCVICAR, M., FRANKLIN, M., TY, A., SAGEL, L., LANGE, K.: Antigenic streptococcal components in acute glomerulonephritis. Science **163**, 676—677 (1969).

184. TRESER, G., SEMAR, M., TY, A., SAGEL, I., FRANKLIN, M. A., LANGE, K.: Partial characterization of antigenic streptococcal plasma membrane components in acute glomerulonephritis. J. Clin. Invest. **49**, 762—768 (1970).

185. UNANUE, E. R.: Immunopathology of rabbits immunized to kidney fractions. Federation Proc. **25**, 659 (1966).

186. UNANUE, E., DIXON, F. J.: Experimental glomerulonephritis. IV. Participation of complement in nephrotoxic nephritis. J. Exp. Med. **119**, 965—982 (1964).

187. UNANUE, E. R., DIXON, F. J.: Experimental glomerulonephritis. V. Studies on the interaction of nephrotoxic antibodies with tissues of the rat. J. Exp. Med. **121**, 697—714 (1965).

188. UNANUE, E. R., DIXON, F. J.: Experimental allergic glomerulonephritis induced in the rabbit with heterologous renal antigens. J. Exp. Med. **125**, 149—162 (1967).

189. UNANUE, E. R., DIXON, F. J.: Experimental glomerulonephritis: Immunological events and pathogenetic mechanisms. Adv. Immunol. **6**, 1—90 (1967).

190. UNANUE, E. R., DIXON, F. J., FELDMAN, J. D.: Experimental allergic glomerulonephritis induced in the rabbit with homologous renal antigens. J. Exp. Med. **125**, 163—176 (1967).

191. UNANUE, E. R., DIXON, F. J., FELDMAN, J. D.: Experimental immunologic diseases of the kidney. In: Textbook of Immunopathology, Vol. I (MIESCHER, P. A., MÜLLER-EBERHARD, H. J., Eds.), p. 164—178. New York: Grune and Stratton 1968.

192. UNANUE, E. R., DIXON, F. J., LEE, S.: Experimental glomerulonephritis. VIII. The in vivo fixation of heterologous nephrotoxic antibodies to, and their exchange among, tissues of the rat. Intern. Arch. Allergy Appl. Immunol. **29**, 140—150 (1966).

193. UNANUE, E. R., MARDINEY, M. R., jr., DIXON, F. J.: Nephrotoxic serum nephritis in complement intact and deficient mice. J. Immunol. **98**, 609—617 (1967).

194. VOGT, A., BOCKHORN, H., KOZIMA, K., SASAKI, M.: Electron microscopic localization of the nephrotoxic antibody in the glomeruli of the rat after intravenous application of purified nephritogenic antibody ferritin conjugates. J. Exp. Med. **127**, 867—878 (1968).

195. WAGNER, V., ZAVÁZAL, V., KASALOVÁ, D., MALÝ, V., MECL, A., PROKOP, J.: Immunology of toxemias of pregnancy. I. Findings of organ-specific antibodies. Experientia **15**, 24—25 (1959).

196. WARD, P. A., COCHRANE, C. G., MÜLLER-EBERHARD, H.: The role of serum complement in chemotaxis of leukocytes in vitro. J. Exp. Med. **122**, 327—346 (1965).

197. WEILER, E.: Antigenic differences between normal hamster kidney and stilbestrol induced kidney carcinoma; complement fixation reactions with cytoplasmic particles. Brit. J. Cancer **10**, 553—559 (1956).

198. WEILER, E.: A cellular change in hamster kidney cultures: Loss of tissue-specific antigens. Exp. Cell Res. Suppl. **7**, 244—262 (1959).

199. Williams, R., Steblay, R. W.: Glomerulonephritis induced in goats by injections of human glomerular basement membrane (HGBM) and Freund's adjuvant (FA). Federation Proc. **24**, 243 (1965).
200. Wypych, J., Shulman, S.: Kidney antigens active in isoimmunization. II. Fractionation of saline extracts. In preparation.
201. Yagi, Y., Korngold, L., Pressman, D.: Purification of kidney components capable of neutralizing kidney localizing anti-rat-kidney antibodies. J. Immunol. **77**, 287—293 (1956).
202. Zabriskie, J. B., Lewshenia, R., Moller, G., Wehle, B., Falk, R. E.: Lymphocytic responses to streptococcal antigens in glomerulonephritic patients. Science **168**, 1105—1108 (1970).

Chapter 8. Mechanisms of Immunopathology

1. Doebbler, T., Rose, N. R.: The role of adjuvants in experimental autoimmune thyroiditis. Federation Proc. **20**, 39 (1961).
2. Felix-Davies, D., Waksman, B. H.: Passive transfer of experimental immune thyroiditis in the guinea pig. Arthritis Rheumat. **4**, 416—417 (1961).
3. Flax, M. H.: Experimental allergic thyroditis in the guinea pig. II. Morphologic studies of development of disease. Lab. Invest. **2**, 199—213 (1963).
4. Flax, M. H., Billote, J. B.: Experimental allergic thyroiditis in the guinea pig. III. Correlation of morphologic and functional changes in early lesions. Ann. N. Y. Acad. Sci. **124**, 234—246 (1965).
5. Flax, M. H., Jankovic, B. D., Sell, S.: Experimental allergic thyroiditis in the guinea pig. I. Relationship of delayed hypersensitivity and circulating antibody to the development of thyroiditis. Lab. Invest. **12**, 119—129 (1963).
6. Friedman, R. M., Buckler, C. E., Baron, S.: The effect of aminomethylpterylglutamic acid on the development of skin hypersensitivity and on antibody formation in guinea pigs. J. Exp. Med. **114**, 173—183 (1961).
7. Genghof, D. S., Battisto, J. R.: Antibody production in guinea pigs receiving 6-mercaptopurine. Proc. Soc. Exp. Biol. Med. **107**, 933—936 (1961).
8. Hoyer, J., Condie, R. M.: Suppression of delayed hypersensitivity in guinea pigs and rabbits with 6-mercaptopurine. Federation Proc. **21**, 277 (1962).
9. McMaster, P. R. B., Lerner, R. M.: The transfer of allergic thyroiditis in histocompatible guinea pigs by lymph node cells. J. Immunol. **99**, 208—213 (1967).
10. McMaster, P. R. B., Lerner, E. M., Exum, E. D.: The relationship of delayed hypersensitivity and circulating antibody to experimental allergic thyroiditis in inbred guinea pigs. J. Exp. Med. **113**, 611—623 (1961).
11. McMaster, P. R. B., Lerner, E. M., II, Kyriakos, M., Mueller, P. S.: The influence of the dose of thyroid extract and mycobacteria upon experimental autoimmune thyroiditis in inbred histocompatible and random-bred guinea pigs. J. Immunol. **99**, 201—207 (1967).
12. Miescher, P., Gorstein, F., Benacerraf, B., Gell, P. G.: Studies on the pathogenesis of experimental immune thyroiditis. Proc. Soc. Exp. Biol. Med. **107**, 12—16 (1961).
13. Nakamura, R. M., Weigle, W. O.: Transfer of experimental autoimmune thyroiditis by serum from thyroidectomized donors. J. Exp. Med. **130**, 263—285 (1969).
14. Packalén, T., Wasserman, J.: Inhibition of migration of normal guinea pig blood leukocytes by homologous immune γ_2-globulin in the presence of specific antigen. Intern. Arch. Allergy Appl. Immunol. **41**, 790—796 (1971).
15. Roitt, I. M., Jones, H. E. H., Doniach, D.: Mechanisms of tissue damage in human experimental autoimmune thyroiditis. In: Mechanism of Cell and Tissue Damage Produced by Immune Reactions, Second International Symposium on Immunopathology (Grabar, P., Miescher, P., Eds.), p. 174—183. Basel: Benno Schwabe 1962.
16. Rose, N. R., Kite, J. H., jr., Doebbler, T. K.: Experimental autoimmune thyroiditis. In: Mechanism of Cell and Tissue Damage Produced by Immune Reactions, Second International Symposium on Immunopathology (Grabar, P., Miescher, P., Eds.), p. 161—173. Basel: Benno Schwabe 1962.

17. RUDDLE, N. H., WAKSMAN, B. H.: Cytotoxicity mediated by soluble antigen and lymphocytes in delayed hypersensitivity. I. Characterization of the phenomenon. J. Exp. Med. **128**, 1237—1252 (1968).
18. RUDDLE, N. H., WAKSMAN, B. H.: Cytotoxicity mediated by soluble antigen and lymphocytes in delayed hypersensitivity. II. Correlation of the in vitro response with skin reactivity. J. Exp. Med. **128**, 1255—1265 (1968).
19. RUDDLE, N. H., WAKSMAN, B. H.: Cytotoxicity mediated by soluble antigen and lymphocytes in delayed hypersensitivity. III. Analysis of mechanism. J. Exp. Med. **128**, 1267—1279 (1968).
20. SHULMAN, S., GHAYASUDDIN, M., WITEBSKY, E.: Studies on organ specificity. XX. Molecular forms in the antibody response to isoimmunization with thyroid protein. J. Immunol. **101**, 1059—1067 (1968).
21. SPIEGELBERG, H. L., MIESCHER, P. A.: The effect of 6-mercaptopurine and aminopterin on experimental immune thyroiditis in guinea pigs. J. Exp. Med. **118**, 869—890 (1963).
22. TERPLAN, K. L., WITEBSKY, E., ROSE, N. R., PAINE, J. R., EGAN, R. W.: Experimental thyroiditis in rabbits, guinea pigs and dogs, following immunization with thyroid extracts of their own and of heterologous species. Am. J. Pathol. **36**, 213—239 (1960).
23. WAKSMAN, B. H.: Auto-immunization and the lesions of autoimmunity. Medicine **41**, 93—141 (1962).
24. WASSERMAN, J., PACKALÉN, T.: Immune responses to thyroglobulin in experimental allergic thyroiditis. Immunology **9**, 1—10 (1965).
25. WEIGLE, W. O., High, G. J., NAKAMURA, R. M.: The role of mycobacteria and the effect of proteolytic degradation of thyroglobulin on the production of autoimmune thyroiditis. J. Exp. Med. **130**, 243—262 (1969).

Appendix

A number of general reference works that can provide additional information are listed here for the convenience of the reader. There are very few books or review articles on the subject of tissue specificity. Only one of the available reviews can be recommended. This is:

DUMONDE, D. C.: Tissue-Specific Antigens. Advan. Immunol. **5**, 245—412 (1966). The coverage is extensive, rather than detailed.

However, there are many books and reviews on the closely related subjects, of autoimmunity, autoimmune disease, or immunopathology. A few of the most useful and recent are:

1. GLYNN, L. E., HOLBOROW, J.: Autoimmunity and Disease. Philadelphia: F. A. Davis 1965.
2. SAMTER, M. (Ed.): Immunological Diseases, 2nd ed. Boston: Little, Brown 1971.
3. DAMESHEK, W., WITEBSKY, E., MILGROM, F. (Eds.): Autoimmunity-Experimental and Clinical Aspects. Ann. N. Y. Acad. Sci. **124**, 1965.
4. MIESCHER, P. A., MÜLLER-EBERHARD, H. J. (Eds.): Textbook of Immunopathology. New York: Grune and Stratton; Vol. I, 1968; Vol. II, 1969.

Many reviews in this field are contained in several Monograph series:

1. Advances in Immunology. New York: Academic Press; Vols. 1—17 (1961—73).
2. Progress in Allergy. Basel: S. Karger; Vols. 1—17 (1939—73).
3. International Symposium on Immunopathology. Basel: Benno Schwabe; New York: Grune and Stratton; Vols. 1—5 (1959—68).

The 20 papers of the series on organ specificity by Witebsky and his colleagues constitute a useful compendium:

1. WITEBSKY, E., ROSE, N. R., SHULMAN, S.: Studies on organ specificity. I. The serological specificity of thyroid extracts. J. Immunol. **75**, 269—281 (1955).
2. ROSE, N. R., WITEBSKY, E.: Studies on organ specificity. II. Serological interrelationships among thyroid extracts of various species. J. Immunol. **75**, 282—290 (1955).
3. SHULMAN, S., ROSE, N. R., WITEBSKY, E.: Studies on organ specificity. III. Ultracentrifugal and electrophoretic examinations of thyroid extracts. J. Immunol. **75**, 291—300 (1955).
4. WITEBSKY, E., ROSE, N. R.: Studies on organ specificity. IV. Production of rabbit thyroid antibodies in the rabbit. J. Immunol. **76**, 408—416 (1956).

5. ROSE, N. R., WITEBSKY, E.: Studies on organ specificity. V. Changes in the thyroid glands of rabbits following active immunization with rabbit thyroid extracts. J. Immunol. **76**, 417—427 (1956).

6. ROSE, N. R., WITEBSKY, E.: Studies on organ specificity. VI. Cross-reactions of thyroid autoantibodies with thyroids of other species. J. Immunol. **83**, 34—40 (1959).

7. WITEBSKY, E., ROSE, N. R.: Studies on organ specificity. VII. Production of antibodies to rabbit thyroid by injection of foreign thyroid extracts. J. Immunol. **83**, 41—48 (1959).

8. ROSE, N. R., METZGAR, R. S., ISAACS, E.: Studies on organ specificity. VIII. Serologic interrelationships among thyroid extracts of various species revealed by gel-diffusion precipitation techniques. J. Immunol. **84**, 649—658 (1960).

9. SHULMAN, S., WITEBSKY, E.: Studies on organ specificity. IX. Biophysical and immunochemical studies on human thyroid autoantibody. J. Immunol. **85**, 559—567 (1960).

10. WITEBSKY, E., ROSE, N. R., NADEL, H.: Studies on organ specificity. X. The serological specificity of pancreas extracts. J. Immunol. **85**, 568—574 (1960).

11. ROSE, N. R., METZGAR, R. S., WITEBSKY, E.: Studies on organ specificity. XI. Isoantigens of rabbit pancreas. J. Immunol. **85**, 575—587 (1960).

12. SHULMAN, S., WITEBSKY, E.: Studies on organ specificity. XII. Fractionation of hog thyroid, preparation of thyroglobulin and thyralbumin. J. Immunol. **88**, 221—228 (1962).

13. ROSE, N. R., SHULMAN, S., WITEBSKY, E.: Studies on organ specificity. XIII. Immunological analysis of thyroglobulin and thyralbumin. J. Immunol. **88**, 229—239 (1962).

14. BEUTNER, E. H., WITEBSKY, E.: Studies on organ specificity. XIV. Immunofluorescent studies of thyroid reactive autoantibodies in human sera. J. Immunol. **88**, 462—475 (1962).

15. BEUTNER, E. H., WITEBSKY, E.: Studies on organ specificity. XV. Immunohistologic evaluation of reactions produced by thyroid autoantibodies. J. Immunol. **91**, 204—209 (1963).

16. SHULMAN, S., YANTORNO, C., SOANES, W. A., GONDER, M. J., WITEBSKY, E.: Studies on organ specificity. XVI. Urogenital tissues and autoantibodies. Immunology **10**, 99—113 (1966).

17. CENTENO, E., SHULMAN, S., MILGROM, F., WITEBSKY, E., SKELTON, F.: Studies on organ specificity. XVII. Autoantigens of rabbit kidney. J. Immunol. **96**, 530—536 (1966).

18. YANTORNO, C., SHULMAN, S., GONDER, M. J., SOANES, W. A., WITEBSKY, E.: Studies on organ specificity. XVIII. Immunological and biophysical characterization of canine prostatic fluid. J. Immunol. **96**, 1035—1045 (1966).

19. SHULMAN, S., RIERA, C., YANTORNO, C.: Studies on organ specificity. XIX. Antigenic specificity of seminal plasma and the formation of autoantibodies. J. Immunol. **100**, 682—688 (1968).

20. SHULMAN, S., GHAYASUDDIN, M., WITEBSKY, E.: Studies on organ specificity. XX. Molecular forms in the antibody response to isoimmunization with thyroid protein. J. Immunol. **101**, 1059—1067 (1968).

A complete listing of all the papers of WITEBSKY and his coworkers is contained as part of the dedication in:

ROSE, N. R., MILGROM, F. (Eds.): International Convocation on Immunology, Buffalo, N. Y. 1968. Basel: S. Karger 1969.

Subject Index

MIX
Papier aus verantwortungsvollen Quellen
Paper from responsible sources
FSC® C105338

If you have any concerns about our products,
you can contact us on
ProductSafety@springernature.com

In case Publisher is established outside the EU,
the EU authorized representative is:
Springer Nature Customer Service Center GmbH
Europaplatz 3, 69115 Heidelberg, Germany

Printed by Libri Plureos GmbH
in Hamburg, Germany